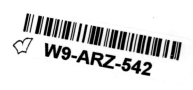

W9-ARZ-542

This book is dedicated to Norm, Marie, Fred, and our children, *who have lent their support for the long hours spent on this book. Without their patience, we could not have completed this task.*

Table of Contents

Foreword xi

Acknowledgments xiii

Introduction xv

Contributors xix

PART I—   PROGRAM DEVELOPMENT AND DELIVERY .   1

Chapter 1—   Designing Health Education Programs   3
Victoria J. Marsick, PhD

Steps in Program Design   7
Choosing a Model   10
Guidelines for Developing a Design Strategy   12
Belief Systems   13
Educational Paradigms   15
Organizational Delivery Systems   21
Abandoning the Linear Approach   22
Some Obstacles   26
Empowerment   27
Summary   28

Chapter 2—   Financing Patient Education Programs   31
Edward E. Bartlett, DrPH

Essential Knowledge   32
Improving the Financing of Patient Education   38

Implications for the Future of Patient Education
Financing 46

Chapter 3—   **Assessing Health Education Needs: A
Multidimensional-Multimethod Approach** 49
Charles E. Basch, PhD

Ambiguity about Needs and Needs Assessment 50
Values and Needs Assessment 52
Three Distinctions of Needs 53
Dimensions of Needs 55
Data Collection Methods for Assessing Health
Education Needs 60
Integrating Perceptions of Needs and Data in an
Organizational Context 65
Planning a Needs Assessment 66

Chapter 4—   **Marketing for Health Educators** 75
Elizabeth F. Dunn, PhD

Why Marketing? 75
Marketing Fundamentals 77
Your Strategy for Success 82
A Closing Word 86

Chapter 5—   **Ethics and Health Education: Issues in Theory and
Practice** 87
Marc D. Hiller, DrPH

Can We Move Forward? 88
Ethics, Values, and Morals 90
Ethical Principles in Health Education 94
Levels of Ethical Analysis 99
Using Ethics in Health Education 101
"Doing Ethics" in Health Education: Six Steps 102
Summary 104
Organizations to Contact for Further Information 105

PART II—   **PROGRAM TOOLS** 109

Chapter 6—   **Humor As a Health Education Tool** 111
*William Carlyon, PhD, and Pauline Carlyon, MS,
MPH*

The Cousins Connection 112
The Nature of Humor 112

Humor in Patient Care 116
Health Promotion 117
Summary 119
Suggested Resources 119

Chapter 7—   The Use of Computers in Health Education 123
Laurel Burch-Minakan, MPH

Hardware 123
How To Choose the Right Software 124
Software for Health 125
Interactive Microcomputer-Based Health Risk
    Appraisal Software 125
Software on Health Topics 126
Health and Fitness Software 127
Nutrition Software 128
Combined Exercise and Nutrition Program 128
Psychological Software 130
Integrated Software 130
Future Implications of Interactive Computer Software
    Programs and Health Education 131
Appendix 7-A 135
Appendix 7-B 137

Chapter 8—   Incentive Systems for Changing Health Behaviors . 145
Larry S. Chapman, MPH

What Are Incentives? 146
Why Utilize Incentives? 147
Advantages and Disadvantages of Incentives 147
What Kinds of Incentive Pay Values Are There? 149
How Should Incentives Be Designed? 149
Opportunities for the Use of Incentives 153
Strength of Incentives 153
Summary 158
Appendix 8-A 161

Chapter 9—   Creating the Healing Connection 167
John L. Coulehan, MD, FACP, and Marian R. Block,
MD

Patient-Centered Health Care 168
The Process of Creating Patient Involvement 172
Interactive Decision Making: Negotiation 178

Personal Change 182
Summary 185

PART III— STRATEGIES FOR PARTICIPATION **187**

Chapter 10— Self-Care Education **189**
Barbara Caporael-Katz, RN, MSN, and
Lowell S. Levin, EdD, MPH

Some Definitions 189
The Emergence of Self-Care 190
What Is a Self-Care Program? 191
The Outcomes of Self-Care 192
Self-Care vs. Traditional Health Education 193
Self-Care Education—A Case Study 194
Tailoring Programs to Client Needs 195
Organizational Integration and Self-Care 197
Reinforcing Clients' Self-Care Knowledge 197
Access to Health Information 198
Participative Learning in Self-Care Education 199
Client Involvement in Program Maintenance 200
Evaluation of Self-Care Learning 201
The People Puzzle in Self-Care 202
Problems and Obstacles in Self-Care 203
Self-Care and the Future 204

**Chapter 11— Evaluation of Medical Information: The Role of
Health Educators** **209**
Arthur Aaron Levin, MPH

Objectives 210
Informed Consent 211
Empowerment 211
Information Overload 212
Lack of Agreement 213
Subjective Decisions 214
Informed Consent As Therapy 215
The Risks of Progress 216
Medications—Helpful and Harmful 216
Surgery—The Double Edged Scalpel 217
Risks of Health Promotion and Disease Prevention ... 219
Skills for Assessing Medical Information 220
Randomized Controlled Trials 220
Validity 221

Conclusion 224
Appendix 11-A 228

PART IV—   **STRATEGIES FOR SPECIFIC POPULATIONS** ..   **229**

Chapter 12—   **A Healthy Old Age: Health Education with Older
People** **231**
Stephanie FallCreek, DSW

Addressing Elder Needs in Health Education/Health
Promotion   232
Obstacles and Opportunities for Health Education   234
Programs for Older Adults   236
Future Implications   241
Demographic Trends   244
Where Are We Now?   247
Appendix 12-A   254

Chapter 13—   **Community Health Advocacy** **261**
Sally Kohn, MPH

Health Advocacy Programs: Two Case Studies   262
Factors That Promote Advocacy   266
The Role of Health Professionals in Advocating for a
Community Group   271
Summary   276
Appendix 13-A   279

Chapter 14—   **Workplace Health Promotion** **281**
Michael P. Eriksen, ScD

Why Wellness in the Workplace   282
The Status of U.S. Wellness Programs   283
Current Level of Practice: Overview   285
Smoking Control   287
Nutrition Education Programs   291
Fitness Programs   295
Weight Control   298
High Blood Pressure Control   300
Stress Management   302
Cancer Screening and Early Detection Programs   304
Critical Issues and Future Trends   305
Appendix 14-A   319

Index **321**

Foreword

The theme of *The Handbook of Health Education, Second Edition,* is particularly important for several reasons. We are constantly increasing our understanding of the importance of lifestyle and health behaviors on rates of morbidity and mortality. In addition, we are beginning to generate some clear and defensible evidence that health promotion and education can have positive impacts on lifestyle and behavior. Second, we are beginning to realize the potential breadth of opportunity of health education at all ages of the life cycle, and in all settings. Third, we have begun to identify our health education needs more precisely, and more than that—gaps in service. This has allowed us to identify barriers to successful implementation of health education programs in many settings. The aggregation of three points allows us to plan for the future in order to carefully examine what works and what does not, and to generate new questions that demand attention. These points are:

1. recognition of needs
2. evidence of effectiveness
3. identification of gaps in service and barriers

After speaking with the editors of this book, I realized that the potential readers are not a homogeneous group. Hospital based personnel, community agency people, school based health educators, university based health educators, and a variety of others are all likely readers. While this mixture creates a special challenge of trying to satisfy the needs of different groups within one handbook, it also provides the opportunity to address a realistic community of professionals together. All too often we exist in our separate worlds, compete for the same limited resources, and fail to understand how we must work together. All other things aside, there appears to be a consensus building on one aspect of health policy that is of special significance to health education: the relative importance of prevention and health promotion, and the consequent crucial role of each individual, each family, and each community to shape our health futures.

The editors have undertaken a difficult task—and I think have provided a remarkably broad based response to that task. Though the chapters in this handbook are diverse, and in many cases nontraditional, it should serve our community well.

Robert S. Gold, PhD, DrPh
Director of Graduate Studies
Division of Human and Community Resources
College of Physical Education, Recreation, and Health
University of Maryland
January 1987

Acknowledgments

We would like to thank our editor, Barbara Tansil, who has encouraged and assisted us over the last two years to help put together this comprehensive book. We would also like to acknowledge Dr. Stephen Brookfield from Teachers College, Columbia University, for the contribution of his ideas. A special thanks to Melissa Harrington, who helped us get our manuscripts into final form.

Introduction

Today, new pressures and paradoxes challenge practitioners responsible for designing and delivering health education programs. Since the publication of the first edition of *The Handbook of Health Education,*[1] the field has changed. New trends in morbidity and mortality, different demographic patterns, changing lifestyles, expansion of alternative health care settings and products, and redefined practitioner-client relationships warrant new approaches.

This edition of *The Handbook of Health Education* provides practitioners and program managers with practical concepts and strategies for designing and implementing health education programs in the context of today's health care environment. The present cost-containment climate is strongly influencing decision making in medical practice, reimbursement schemes, consumer choices in health services, and the growth of alternative ambulatory care settings. The emergence of Diagnostic Related Groups (DRGs) is placing new restrictions on service availability. These changes are demanding new approaches in local communities and within service systems.

Health education activities have an important role in responding to these problems and opportunities. For example, health education programs, established to involve patients in their treatment plan and increase their ability to alter their health habits, have resulted in decreased length of hospital stays while retaining quality medical care and reducing the need for unnecessary surgery. In workplaces, health education programs have helped employees stay fit and recognize behaviors harmful to their health while at the same time reducing employers' medical and health care costs.

Though administrators may regard health education as an important component of comprehensive health services or cost-containment strategies, such programs may also be regarded as superfluous, especially when setting budget priorities. Thus in the face of economic and organizational uncertainty, it is vitally important for practitioners to strengthen their skills in designing, financing, marketing, and evaluating programs for which they are responsible.

As the health care education field has become more sophisticated, interpretations of what constitutes health education have also broadened. Several labels are ascribed to activities, materials, and programs that purport to be health education. In this handbook, the editors acknowledge that terms like "health promotion," "patient education," "wellness," "community health," and "health counseling" are used interchangeably despite differences in definitions. Labeling has often added to confusion over what is and who "does" health education.

Green's definition of health education can serve as a common reference: ". . . any combination of learning methods, designed to facilitate voluntary adaptation of behavior conducive to health."[2] Green also distinguishes between health education and health promotion in aim and scope, noting that "health promotion can be defined as any combination of health education related to organizational, economic, and environmental supports for behavior conducive to health."[3]

Health education draws upon a diversity of theories, data bases, and experiences from other disciplines. People with different professional affiliations, job titles, or preparation have generated a wide range of health education programs. This diversity has both challenged and enriched the field. For this reason contributing authors have been selected from fields that have contributed theory and practical experience. They represent backgrounds in health education, social work, adult education, organizational and staff development, medicine, nursing, marketing, and health care administration.

This second edition of *The Handbook of Health Education* is intended to serve as a resource for program ideas and models and as a guide for tools and information relevant for health education programs. The organization of the chapters allows the reader to proceed, systematically, from fundamentals of program development to program approaches for specific populations.

The chapters are organized into four parts. Part I presents principles and strategies applicable for establishing and sustaining comprehensive programs. Clearly, no single approach exists to identifying needs, selecting participative program models, and financing or marketing a program. However, these are all important components for any strategy. Ethical issues that can complicate the delivery of a program must also be considered. In Part II, three creative tools for strengthening programs are presented. Chapters include discussions of the use of humor, incentives, and computer software. All of these tools can add new dimensions to program design and outcomes. Part III presents specific approaches to increase the participation and involvement of patients and consumers in their health and medical care. Chapters cover strategies for establishing self-care programs and the importance, usefulness, and methods for creating access to medical information for consumers. Methods to strengthen the relationship and opportunities for learning between practitioners and patients are also presented. Part IV addresses anticipated needs for the next decade by focusing on examples of programs for older adults, urban communities, and worksites. The importance of appropriate programming and service strategies for creating advocacy is also stressed.

The perspectives and positions regarding health care expressed through these chapters by no means represent a consensus. The editors' and authors' points of view have been shaped by their work in a variety of practice and academic settings. Nevertheless, the importance of engaging individuals and communities in an active process of inquiry, self-responsibility, and behavior change is shared by all who contributed to this book. The result of such efforts should be the creation of greater consumer empowerment, as well as an increased role for consumers in their health care and health care decisions. The ultimate goal, of course, is a more healthy public.

Today, responsibility is shifting to a more mutual relationship between both clients and practitioners. For health care practitioners it has become essential to facilitate this process. This second edition of *The Handbook of Health Education* aims at furthering these goals in a manner tailored to today's health care environment and consumer needs.

NOTES

1. Lazes, Peter M., *Handbook of Health Education* (Rockville, Md.: Aspen Publishers, 1979).

2. Green, L. et al., *Health Education Planning: A Diagnostic Approach* (Palo Alto, Calif.: Mayfield, 1980).

3. Matarazzo, Joseph, and Associates, eds. *Behavioral Health—A Handbook of Health Enhancement and Disease Prevention* (New York: John Wiley, 1984).

SUGGESTED READINGS

American Hospital Association. *Planning Hospital Health Promotion Services for Businesses and Industry.* Chicago: American Hospital Association. 1982.

Cleary, Helen. *Advancing Health Through Education: A Case Study Approach.* Palo Alto, Calif.: Mayfield, 1985.

DHHS. *Healthy People.* The Surgeon General's Report on Health Promotion and Disease Prevention. Washington, D.C. 1979.

DHHS. *Promoting Health/Preventing Disease. Objectives for the Nation.* Washington, D.C.: Government Printing Office. 1980.

Lange, M.E., and A. Wolf. *Promoting Community Health Through Innovative Hospital-Based Programs.* Chicago: American Health Association. 1984.

Mullen, P.D., and J. Zapka, eds. *Guidelines for Health Promotion and Education Services in HMO's.* Washington, D.C.: Government Printing Office. 1982.

Mullen, Kathleen, D. et al. *Connections for Health.* Dubuque: Iowa: William C. Brown, 1986.

Contributors

Edward E. Bartlett, DrPH
Associate Adjunct Professor
Department of Community and Family
    Medicine
Georgetown University
Washington, D.C.
    and
Edward Bartlett, Associates
President
Rockville, Maryland

Charles E. Basch, PhD
Assistant Professor
Department of Health Education
Teachers College
Columbia University
New York, New York

Marian R. Block, MD
Assistant Professor
Chief, Division of Family Medicine
Department of Community Medicine
University of Pittsburgh School of Medicine
Pittsburgh, Pennsylvania

Laurel Burch-Minakan, MPH
Manager
South New England Telephone Company
Reach Out for Health
New Haven, Connecticut

**Barbara Caporael-Katz, RN,
    MSN**
Health Education Coordinator
Community Health Care Plan
New Haven, Connecticut

Pauline Carlyon, MS, MPH
Regional Coordinator for U.S. Corporate
    Health Management
Chicago, Illinois

William Carlyon, PhD
Director of Health Education Projects
American Medical Association
Chicago, Illinois

Larry S. Chapman, MPH
President
Corporate Health Designs
Seattle, Washington

John L. Coulehan, MD, FACP
Associate Professor
Department of Community Medicine
University of Pittsburgh School of Medicine
Pittsburgh, Pennsylvania

Elizabeth F. Dunn, PhD
Vice President, Marketing and Planning
West Jersey Health System
Camden, New Jersey

Michael P. Eriksen, ScD
Director of Behavior Research
Department of Cancer Prevention
M.D. Anderson Hospital
University of Texas
Houston, Texas

Stephanie FallCreek, DSW
Director
The Institute for Gerontological Research
    Education
Las Cruces, New Mexico

Karen A. Gordon, MPH
Director of Health Education
University Health Services
Princeton University
Princeton, New Jersey

Marc D. Hiller, DrPH
Associate Professor
Department of Health Administration and
    Planning
School of Health Studies
University of New Hampshire
Durham, New Hampshire

**Laura Hollander Kaplan, MPH,
    OTR**
Coordinator of Special Projects
Reach Out for Health
South New England Telephone Company
New Haven, Connecticut

Sally Kohn, MPH
Director of Planning and Program
    Development
Planned Parenthood of New York City, Inc.
New York, New York

Peter M. Lazes, PhD
Director and Visiting Associate Professor
Programs for Employment and Workplace
    Systems
New York State School of Industrial and
    Labor Relations
Division of Extension and Public Service
Cornell University
Ithaca, New York

Arthur Aaron Levin, MPH
Director
Center for Medical Consumers and Health
    Care Information
New York, New York

Lowell S. Levin, EdD, MPH
Professor of Public Health
Department of Epidemiology and Public
    Health
Yale School of Medicine
Yale University
New Haven, Connecticut

Victoria J. Marsick, PhD
Assistant Professor
AEGIS/Department of Higher and Adult
    Education
Teachers College
Columbia University
New York, New York

Part I

Program Development and Delivery

Chapter 1

Designing Health Education Programs

Victoria J. Marsick, PhD

You may be directly in charge of designing health education programs, either of a complex nature for thousands of people or of a simple nature for one small community. Or you may be only indirectly involved in program design by virtue of your role as part of a team of people who interpret and implement plans developed by others. In either case, this chapter will assist you to develop better programs by reviewing different models of program design and identifying ways in which the designer can maximize a program's resources and results through fuller participation of clients and staff in the process.

This chapter is written from the point of view of an adult educator with experience in international primary health care, staff development, and training in a variety of health, community, and business settings. The author's experience has been that, while the "objective" quality of program design is important, it is equally important that the people involved in implementing and receiving services participate in its design. This is particularly important when programs address complex issues of social change. Participation, while not a panacea, provides a vehicle for more accurately assessing which problems people want to address, for creating better solutions, and for adjusting the program when planned conditions change.

Research and practice in educational professions outside health support this focus on participation. Innovative businesses, for example, have been experimenting with worker participation through quality of work life/ employee involvement activities as a mechanism for designing changes in work habits.[1] Active participation in identifying and solving problems has also been a central focus of community development programs.[2]

Program development is defined as the process by which a series of activities are selected and planned to meet goals that are expected to solve problems considered important to clients.[3] In health education, program design usually includes both learning activities as well as service or other

3

noneducational activities that influence and reinforce changes in health behavior. "Program design" is used interchangeably with "program development," even though "design" refers to learning strategies for delivering the program, while "program development" encompasses everything needed to plan, implement, and evaluate the program. The designer is the person who catalyzes, coordinates, and is responsible for leading the process.

While design models generally follow similar steps, these steps are interpreted and sequenced differently depending on who, when, and how people are involved. This chapter will discuss such variation. It will also examine several educational belief systems that influence both participation and the resultant program design.

The following three scenarios illustrate these three belief systems. Suppose you are a health educator assigned to a cluster of public health clinics in a large, multiethnic, multiracial city. You are new to the program and are collecting information from staff in order to decide on alternative approaches to health education even though the program in place is considered reasonably well run. In reality, staff are always plagued by insufficient time and resources in reaching a large number of clients and find themselves doing little more than "putting out fires."

One staff member sees the job primarily in terms of making sure that clients have the right information and treatment. Health education for him means well-designed materials on common diseases that can be discussed with the client. A second staff member wants to do more than give the facts. He wants to talk with people about the way they live, what they mean by health, how their lifestyles may contribute to disease, and what plans they can make to solve problems they identify. He does this through home visits and as a public speaker in the community.

A third staff member has been involved in a Women's Health Alliance in her spare time and wants to try out this approach in the clinic's work. This would mean holding workshops for community members in which persons affected by specific health problems would facilitate their own discussion of the problem, drawing on resource persons as needed and on reading materials distributed in advance. People would be supported in their roles as health care providers for themselves, not in place of physicians, but as active partners with them. Implementing this approach, however, would require a shift in policy since the staff member could not concurrently continue other responsibilities.

The above scenarios describe a set of different perspectives on health education. To the first person, health education means providing the client with information and perhaps skills to solve a problem identified by the program. The client and his or her environment in this model are seen as recipients of program action. The problem with this approach is that knowing what to do and how to do it does not always result in behavior change, as, for example, in telling people why they should stop smoking.

The second example starts with the client's definition of a health problem. Clients are helped through education to recognize their behavior as a problem and to use the program to modify unhealthy habits. The environment is taken into account as an influence on behavior, but there is no probing below the surface for underlying forces that influence action. While people might change their behavior, this approach often requires external motivation and reinforcement that the program cannot give. For example, smokers can learn to identify times when they are more likely to smoke and to substitute other activities, but the program cannot monitor and reinforce every such occurrence.

The third example takes the interaction between program and client to another level. Health education here focuses on helping people see themselves differently vis-à-vis the program by probing below surface behavior to the culture, assumptions, and beliefs that mold their health decisions. To influence change, health education helps people analyze the way in which these larger forces have encouraged them to resist change and to see themselves as capable of taking action despite these forces. In the case of smoking, individuals would be helped to see what influenced their decision to smoke and to view themselves as nonsmokers. Change might well involve steps similar to those of the second example, but in this example, the process would go one step further to ground action in internal motivation and self-reliance.

Figure 1-1 illustrates the three approaches to program development in the above scenarios. In each of the spheres, "P" represents the program system and "C" the client system. These systems are influenced by, and impact on, the larger social, cultural, organizational, political, and economic forces within the environment ("E") in which programs operate. Unfortunately, these forces are not always taken into account in designing programs.

Thus, program development can be carried out as in the top two spheres, where the primary consideration is either the impact of the program on the clients or their reciprocal impact on one another, but without much consideration of how they are grounded in or influenced by these larger environmental forces. The lower left sphere illustrates how programs must consider the way the client's actions impact on his or her immediate environment. The lower right sphere illustrates a three-dimensional interaction of program and client systems that takes into account the ways environmental forces fundamentally influence programs and clients.

Kilmann's use of a three-dimensional model to explain organizational change parallels the rationale for such an approach. Kilmann pointed out

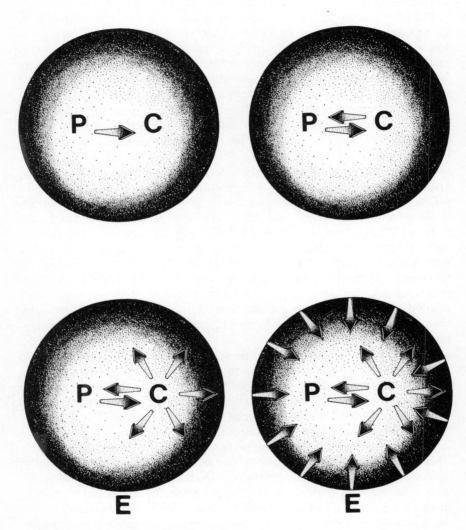

Figure 1–1 Program Development Approaches

In the top two spheres, program development takes place in a one- or two-dimensional plane of interaction between program (P) and client (C) systems.. In the lower two spheres, a third dimension—the environment—is considered. Concept by V. Marsick. Illustrations by George Williams.

that an organization is often looked at either one-dimensionally, as a simple machine with parts that can be replaced if they break down, or two-dimensionally, as an interactive open system in which change in one component impacts on other parts of the system. A three-dimensional model, on the other hand, shows how the open system is grounded in underlying assumptions, cultural factors, and psyches that operate below the surface to influence action and interaction.[4]

The top left sphere in Figure 1-1 illustrates a one-dimensional view of program development such as was found above in the first scenario. A program of correct information is provided, but little attention is paid to whether or how it is received or affected by either clients or the environment. Program development is viewed two-dimensionally in the top right sphere as in the second scenario. This scenario also allows for some interaction with the environment, as in the lower left sphere, but primarily as a nonchangeable set of conditions.

The third scenario resembles the lower right sphere or open system in which larger environmental forces shape decisions and are mirrored in the way the clients understand their health behavior. The norms set by these systems are internalized by the clients and must be critically examined for long-term change to take place.

This chapter begins by discussing the steps commonly advocated in program design. Three program approaches are examined, each of which reflects aspects of the one- , two- , and three-dimensional programming models illustrated in Figure 1-1. The chapter then places each model within the context of an educational belief system and further discusses considerations for strengthening program design drawn from the literature and practice. Following a discussion of obstacles that may arise in implementation, the chapter concludes with a discussion of the concept of health education as empowerment.

STEPS IN PROGRAM DESIGN

While it is not possible to recommend one simple formula for program design, models minimally include the following steps. First, someone identifies a problem in a specific target group. The problem is then analyzed in order to confirm its dimensions through a needs assessment. Choices are then made as to which priorities should be addressed. Priorities are then translated into objectives and activities designed within the boundaries of assessed resources. A plan is developed, staff oriented to the plan, and a strategy designed for monitoring progress and evaluating outcomes.

In order to compare differences in the way these steps are interpreted, this section illustrates three different approaches to program design. The first is the PRECEDE framework developed by Green, Kreuter, Deeds, and Partridge, selected because this "diagnostic" approach is commonly advocated in health education.[5] Two other models from adult education, also used in health settings, provide contrast because they call for a different kind of participation of clients and health staff in program design: Knowles' concept of adragogy[6] and Freire's use of culture circles.[7]

PRECEDE

PRECEDE is an acronym for predisposing, reinforcing, and enabling causes in educational diagnosis and evaluation. Predisposing factors provide the motivation for behavior; enabling factors allow the motivation to be realized; and reinforcing factors provide the incentives, rewards, or punishments that maintain or stop continuation of the behavior. PRECEDE provides a framework for making choices about which behaviors can best be addressed through educational strategies. PRECEDE also reminds the designer that the outcomes, although at times difficult to assess, are more important than specific activities, even though activities completed are easier to examine. The PRECEDE framework begins with epidemiological and social diagnoses of health and nonhealth factors affecting quality of life, and it works backward through behavioral, educational, and administrative diagnoses to identify the desired content and delivery of a program.[8]

PRECEDE has been applied successfully to planning comprehensive programs in many different settings. An important component to the success of the model is the ways designers have drawn health staff and clients into the process of diagnosing health problems and developing educational solutions. For example, in one instance involving the design of a project to educate the community about services available through the local health department, staff and community steering committees were formed and involved in the project throughout phases of data collection and analysis. Another example is an industrial health program where the diagnosis was based on data gained by participation in informal discussions with workers and co-analysis of data by specialists and workers.[9]

Knowles' Andragogy

A second model is that of andragogy, developed by Malcolm Knowles to address the learning needs of adults as distinct from children. The term *andragogy* is derived from the Greek *agogus* (meaning "leading"), whereas the root word of pedagogy is *paid* (meaning "child"). Andragogy takes into account the fact that adults need to be independent and self-directed, that they are interested in learning from their experience, that they learn best when education is based on practical life problems, and that they want to apply new knowledge and skills immediately to these problems.[10] Based on these assumptions, Knowles suggests the following approach to program development:

1. The establishment of a climate conducive to adult learning;
2. The creation of an organizational structure for participative planning;
3. The diagnosis of needs for learning;
4. The formulation of directions for learning (objectives);
5. The operation of the activities;
6. The rediagnosis of needs for learning (evaluation).[11]

Knowles' approach has been applied successfully to staff development programs for health care professionals.[12] One of the distinguishing characteristics of this model is its emphasis on collaboration with the learner in all phases of design. Sweetwood, for example, developed an andragogical model for training reentry nurses built around a system for ongoing dialogue between nurses and instructors as to what should be learned and how individuals could customize a learning plan for themselves.[13] Walsh points out that continuing education in the health professions is seldom based on such needs assessment even though it is recommended.[14] An andragogical framework corrects for this by building in a feedback loop.

Freire's Approach

A third model of program design is based on Paolo Freire's work with illiterates directed at empowering people to recognize and act on their ability to change themselves and their environments. Freire never set out to develop general program guidelines, yet the approach he developed for literacy education has been applied to health and other adult learning settings.[15] The essence of Freire's approach is problem posing. The facilitator helps learners probe for what is problematic about objects or activities in their daily life, seeing the taken-for-granted from different viewpoints in order to question roles, definitions, and meanings usually uncritically learned through socialization.

For example, nurses might examine the roles they have accepted vis-à-vis doctors and begin to negotiate for different responsibilities. Freire's approach is liberating in that it helps people break out of the roles they have passively accepted. However, to do this people usually have to work together to influence larger social, political, economic, or cultural forces.

To continue with the above example, nurses might have to join together to press for new guidelines and changed job descriptions.

Minkler and associates in California have linked Freire's ideas with social support theory in the design of health education programs for elderly residents of the Tenderloin area of San Francisco. They held a series of health fairs in different hotels where the unreached elderly lived to provide screening for certain common ailments as well as a forum for interaction among people who are often isolated. This was followed up by the formation of support groups to discuss and resolve social and health problems. Themes for discussion were generated with a small group of residents.[16]

Apps analyzed the way Freire's approach can be applied generically to program development. The heart of the process is thematic research to identify concerns important to people. Once themes have been developed, people work with a facilitator in groups called culture circles to critically analyze the themes. The facilitator uses photos, drawings, or other visual aids to provide a starting point for decoding the meaning they carry for participants. Apps points out that while Freire provides guidelines for his approach to program design, a lack of specific steps makes the approach difficult for many designers to follow.[17]

CHOOSING A MODEL

Table 1-1 illustrates some selected differences in emphasis among these three models. Distinctions are drawn more sharply than one would perhaps find in an actual situation. The table enables a designer to identify more clearly which models are now operative in his or her context and which ones might be drawn upon in the future.

The view that the designer holds about his or her role and that of clients in identifying problems and planning solutions is central to making a choice among models. In the PRECEDE framework, the specialist retains more control over identifying the problem, even though clients can participate as well. The Freire approach puts most control over the process in the hands of the clients, with the facilitator acting as a catalyst for critical reflection and analysis. The andragogical model falls somewhere in between.

Another related difference is the degree to which the designer expects the clients to accept the program's interpretation of desired health behavior and practice within the existing social, political, economic, and cultural system. The PRECEDE and andragogical models are built more on acceptance of social norms as to desirable health practice and delivery of service. The PRECEDE formula does suggest caution in determining who is responsible for a problem, the client or the system in which he or she lives. Drawing on

Table 1-1 Different Program Design Emphases

	PRECEDE	Andragogy	Freire
Criterion of success	Accurate assessment of nature of health problem and how it impacts on quality of life leading to most effective technical solutions	Establishment of climate and structure for mutual planning, negotiation, and adjustment of program to meet learner needs	Critical analysis of problems from different perspectives leading to deeper awareness and self-reliant action planning
Role of clients in program design	Consumer who at times is asked to help flesh out dimensions of identified problem, select or validate priorities within an established framework, and evaluate options offered by program	Co-designer who is asked to identify "felt" needs, decide on the best way to learn material and take responsibility for directing and assessing progress toward goals	Co-director who is asked to probe "felt" needs in order to name and frame the problem, set own priorities, and decide on/take individual and social action to change conditions or resolve problem
Role of educator in program design	Planner, technical resource, coordinator of inputs, adviser, diagnostician	Facilitator who creates a "warm" climate conducive to personal development, resource in designing learning and reaching goals	Critical facilitator who probes situations, helps learners pose and analyze problems, brings values and assumptions to surface for examination, links individual experience with internalized group norms
Emphasis in needs assessment and objective setting	Systematic identification of gap between current and desired behaviors expressed in specific statement of behavioral objectives that form the basis of program design	Dialogue around "felt" needs throughout program in order to reassess and modify learner's objectives, which are developed by learner in consultation with facilitator and expressed in behavioral terms	Analysis of the way individual-perceived needs are shaped by social norms, with emphasis on process objectives leading to empowerment rather than predefined behavioral outcomes
Emphasis in learning design	Instructional technology approach in which methods are selected to best master information and skills to reach objectives	Creative design approach in which facilitator works with learner to draw out experience as framework for solving problems and applying new concepts and skills	Culture circles in which learners analyze materials based on thematic research of their lives by probing relationships, reasons, causes, values, assumptions in dialogue

Ryan, the authors point out that unqualified acceptance of the views of some health care providers may lead to "blaming the victim" instead of identifying the real cause of a problem.[18] The Freire model, on the other hand, assumes that a critical analysis of situations will probably lead to questioning and changing the status quo.

Whatever the model, Boyle points out that program design also differs with the purpose served. He differentiates among three types: developmental, institutional, and informational. Developmental programs address complex programs of social change involving a number of different client groups, each of whom takes a different view of the problem, as, for example, a drug problem among youth in a community. Institutional programs are developed to help individuals master new knowledge and skills that an institution can provide. Staff development is often guided by institutional purposes, as are health agencies, since they are usually funded and founded to meet specific health needs of different clientele. Boyle, for example, suggests that a developmental community drug program might include institutional programs for various groups who need to cooperate in solving this problem. Informational programs, by contrast, aim primarily at providing knowledge when a problem has already been acknowledged by a group motivated to do something about it. A mass media program is a typical example of an informational program.[19]

Health education programs must frequently address developmental problems, although institutional and informational programs are far easier to design. Developmental program design calls for participation from many groups of people since success depends on the clients' acknowledgment of the problem and the action they take to resolve it.

GUIDELINES FOR DEVELOPING A DESIGN STRATEGY

Program development does not take place in a vacuum. Theories and models provide an idealized version of reality based on principles abstracted from experience that took place in a specific context. The program designer must step back and analyze both the problem and the context in which the program is being developed to decide on a strategy.

Program success does not depend solely on the brilliance, creativity, or comprehensiveness of a solution. Success also depends on the support of people who have a stake in the program. Design should be built on the best analysis of available data about the problem and the clientele, but it must also take into account these more elusive factors of human interaction. The following summarizes guidelines for such a strategy, each of which is then elaborated.

First, program design is based on the designer's interpretation of beliefs of stakeholders, filtered through the organization's mission statement. The designer should identify these beliefs and negotiate "buying in" to the problem and to approaches in program design.

Second, beliefs reflect different educational paradigms. Designers should become aware of how paradigms affect their choices in program design. One key choice is problem setting as opposed to problem solving, a step not often given sufficient attention in design models.

Third, programs are designed for clients, but are delivered through organizations. The designer can use a strategic planning framework to better understand the climate and politics of change within an organizational delivery system.

Fourth, program design must be based on accurate needs assessment. Ideally, such analysis is done comprehensively before goals and strategies are finalized. The designer should abandon the linear model of design in which the stated program goals and objectives are based only on an initial needs assessment. Instead, an interactional model should be employed. Here, a preliminary analysis and synthesis is refined through several stages of consultation with key actors as the program is designed and implemented.

Fifth, program design should include a plan for monitoring and evaluation. However, indicators of success should include process objectives as well as behavioral performance objectives. Monitoring and evaluation should incorporate sensitivity to departures from program design that clearly represent participant refinement of goals, procedures, and desired outcomes.

BELIEF SYSTEMS

Program design begins with the beliefs held by the designer and other stakeholders, such as staff within the organization, policymakers, funding agencies, advisory groups, influential community leaders, and members of other organizations whose cooperation is desired. The designer must consider both individual beliefs as well as group values reflected in statements about an organization's or community's mission, goals, and clientele.

In order to select a program development model, the designer needs to identify and compare competing belief systems with respect to the situation at hand. For example, a designer of a family planning education program in a small town might be concerned about extending services to minority groups of lower socioeconomic income levels. The Executive Director might prefer that the Advisory Board set directions on clientele even though representatives currently prefer a policy of reaching middle-class women in the neighborhood. The funding agency might be most concerned with expanding coverage quickly to maximize its resources, irrespective of the target group. Several minority community groups might resist the exploratory efforts of the agency, claiming that the program attempts to interfere with their rights to a large family. Staff in the organization might be less concerned with whom they serve than with power balances within the organization or the Advisory Board.

Belief systems such as these are seldom clearly labeled, but must be inferred by examining the choices people make about factors such as priorities, goals, where time and money are spent, who is consulted in the decision-making process, or criteria of success.

Negotiating agreement among belief systems is not an easy process. Organization development theory suggests that consensus decisions are desirable when people must work together as a team to implement a goal.[20] Likewise, the more that program success depends on the cooperation of a

---

Exhibit 1-1 Steps in Force Field Analysis

1. Identify and assemble together a group of informed respondents who represent key actors in the program.
2. Clarify the goals of the program you are designing.
3. Brainstorm a list of all positive and negative forces that might affect program success. In brainstorming, participants should be encouraged to generate the widest possible range of responses without first screening them for reasons they might not work.
4. Review the list and reach consensus on the most important forces likely to affect program success. Consensus decisions are based ideally on full agreement of the group after weighing the arguments, not on a simple majority vote or on the basis of the strongest voices raised.
5. Assign each force a value from 1 to 10 based on the degree to which the group believes each force will affect outcomes. Make criteria by which values are assigned explicit.
6. Map these forces on a graph against a horizontal line that represents the present equilibrium being held in place by these positive and negative forces. Use bars or lines to graph the positive forces above the line and the negative forces below the line against a grid of values from 1 to 10 in both directions.
7. Look at the composite picture of forces and brainstorm a list of people who have some control over these forces. If you wish, you might also develop a list of strategies to strengthen positive forces and overcome negative forces.
8. Contact key people to discuss their views about the proposed program, assess their beliefs, and determine how and when they might be involved in later stages of program design.

wide range of people, the more pressing it is that the designer seek consensus about program goals, policy guidelines, and the criteria by which a program will be judged successful.

In many cases, there is little time to conduct such a thorough consultation prior to initiating a program. An alternative is to begin the program with as much agreement as possible and then build flexibility into the design to accommodate subsequent changes. The designer must then choose a course of action based on an assessment of which belief systems are most important, which are most powerful, or which are most likely to achieve a modicum of success.

Force field analysis can be used to identify stakeholders and their belief systems. This tool was developed by social psychologist Kurt Lewin to identify the positive and negative forces that can influence successful goal achievement.[21] Exhibit 1-1, and Figure 1-2 outline how to do a force field analysis and use it as a starting point in negotiating agreement among people with different belief systems.

Negotiating agreement requires skills in influencing others over whom the health educator has no direct authority. A spinoff of this negotiation is getting stakeholders to "buy in" to the problem and the approach to its solution. People are more likely to take responsibility for solutions if they feel they "own" the program.

EDUCATIONAL PARADIGMS

Belief systems affect not only choices made about educational methods and materials, but also more fundamental concerns such as what is considered a problem and how that problem is defined. Belief systems represent different paradigms or frameworks for explaining a phenomenon. The scenarios at the beginning of this chapter, for example, illustrates three different paradigms of health education.

Carr and Kemmis examine three educational paradigms that explain the above scenarios and reflect characteristics of the three program design models discussed.[22] They are the technical paradigm that resembles some dimensions of PRECEDE, the practical paradigm that resembles andragogy and other dimensions of PRECEDE, and the strategic paradigm that resembles the Freire model. Table 1-2 compares the essential characteristics of each of these paradigms.

Most educators are accustomed to the technical paradigm because it has been most commonly used in teaching. The technical paradigm is particularly inappropriate when the client does not see something as a problem or

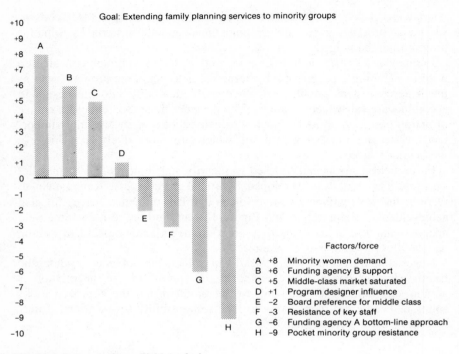

Figure 1–2 Sample Force Field Analysis

know enough about it to ask questions to clarify understanding. The first staff member illustrates this approach in his search for providing the best technical advice to clients. Another example might be a primarily informational program on sexually transmitted diseases based on the assumption that clients understand their dangers even though they may not, as, for example, with immigrants from countries where public awareness of these diseases is low.

Carr and Kemmis point out that the technical paradigm does not sufficiently consider the context in which people make decisions. Both clients and program staff are influenced by differences in ethnic or racial backgrounds, socioeconomic levels, and lifestyles. Both interact in a specific organization and community where encounters are filtered through individual fears, stereotypes, needs, and anxieties. Organizational factors also come into play, such as time pressures or lack of privacy to establish rapport.

Carr and Kemmis consider a second way of understanding the work of educators that takes this context into consideration: the practical paradigm. This paradigm goes beyond the technical paradigm by helping learners understand better why they act the way they do and how their behavior is shaped by other people and events around them. It is illustrated by the second health educator, who was concerned with helping the client understand how behavior and lifestyle shape health.

The practical paradigm helps people identify ways in which behavior contributes to poor health and how it is reinforced by conditions in the environment. The emphasis, however, is primarily on individual change within these parameters. A health educator using the practical paradigm to educate people about smoking would not just tell people about its dangers and consequences, but would help the learner examine how smoking is part of a lifestyle that he or she needs to change.

Table 1–2 Three Educational Paradigms

| | Types of Paradigms | | |
Characteristics	Technical	Practical	Strategic
Philosophical basis	Logical positivism	Interpretive social sciences	Critical social science
Type of learning emphasized	Instrumental, i.e., identifying and applying principles of cause and effect	Practical, i.e., better understanding of why and how people act in situation	Emancipatory, i.e., psychoanalytic method of self-reflection
Learning design principle	Selection of best alternative technology to reach given ends	Process approach with experienced educator choosing means to guide learner	Problem-posing approach to investigating and analyzing situations
Role of educator	Craftsmen who scientifically mold interaction into desired shape	Professional guided by inspiration to act responsibly to develop learner	Strategist and tactician who uses every situation for critical reflection
Emphasis	Systematization and institutionalization of education for efficiency and effectiveness	Individualization of experience through ethical intervention and social interaction	Location within history and integral connection of individual and social action

Carr and Kemmis discuss a third paradigm that goes one step further than the practical paradigm in empowering people to make changes in their lives: the strategic paradigm. This framework pushes people to examine how they have internalized and accepted limiting ways of looking at themselves and to confront these internalized values and norms in both themselves and society when making changes. Individual change is often linked with group action to change limiting conditions in the environment.

The health educator who was involved with the Women's Health Alliance was working within this paradigm, questioning the way people often give over power to a physician for their own health care. A health educator dealing with smoking under this paradigm might help a person see how the expectations of others and personalities in the media influence smoking habits, how to envision oneself as a nonsmoker, and how to take group action to change environmental conditions such as the banning of smoking in public places.

Paradigms are strongly influenced by the culture, so to speak, of a profession. Health education, while a marriage of several disciplines, has been molded by the medical sciences. Medicine's emphasis on objectivity, scientific method, diagnosis, and cure carries over into program design that focuses on the soundest research and most accurate analysis of disease and its prevention or cure.

Schön discusses the limits to what he calls "technical rationality," his term for this heavy emphasis on scientific objectivity. Technical rationality calls for application of existing theory to problems found in practice, but, as Schön points out, problems are seldom packaged as found in the literature. Practitioners spend a good deal of time in first interpreting the problem before they can even begin to solve it. However, theories and models seldom pay enough attention to this art of problem setting.[23]

Schön's investigation of how practitioners identify and solve problems is relevant because this process is at the heart of program design. Many design models start with assumptions about a problem, but do not make these assumptions explicit or build into the process attention to this critical first phase of problem setting: naming the problem and framing it within the larger context. This first stage is often quite complex in health programs because the problem is posed differently by different people.

Taking the above family planning illustration, for example, the Executive Director might assume that acceptability to the most influential leaders in the community is the supreme criterion of success. She will define the problem in terms of reaching a socially acceptable target group with socially acceptable contraceptives and information. By contrast, her program designer might consider such a program ineffective because she frames the problem in terms of reaching minority groups even if this means potentially controversial efforts such as counseling women on abortions and lobbying for sex education in the schools.

Schön discusses the way practitioners can develop their skills in naming and framing the problem. Problem framing is a reflective conversation with the situation, in which the professional constructs "virtual worlds," a representation of the real world, and then tries out different viewpoints evolved from past experience. He or she projects the consequences of each viewpoint, looking for the unexpected and focusing on the best fit between reality and possible theories of action.[24]

This reflective conversation can be carried out by the specialist alone or through dialogue with others. The PRECEDE, andragogical, and Freire models illustrate different approaches to this often-neglected phase of program design as illustrated below. It should be noted that no design model is purely representative of one paradigm. However, the thrust of each model will be exaggerated in the following section to illustrate distinctly different paradigms and draw out contrasts in alternative programming choices.

Programming under Different Paradigms

Consider the problem of designing a family planning education program for a mixed-minority population. Perhaps some husbands associate begetting children with virility, and while their wives may wish for fewer children, women may not be economically independent or culturally able to oppose their husbands' point of view. Having a child may be considered a status symbol among some young girls, whether or not they are married. Children may be important for helping to raise and support other members of the family. Religious beliefs may militate against birth control.

For purposes of this example, the PRECEDE model will be interpreted from a viewpoint of technical rationality even though it does not have to be so construed. Interpreted narrowly, PRECEDE would emphasize an accurate technical diagnosis of the problem. The designer might consult with clients and community leaders in problem setting, but the primary purpose would be to discuss the problem in order to develop the best professional solution. The belief system behind setting priorities, deciding on objectives, and selecting educational strategies would be that given an accurate diagnosis of the problem, the right message and media can be selected to change attitudes and catalyze adoption of new birth control practices.

Specialists might decide that a key factor for program success is changing male attitudes toward family planning even though the target group might not define this as the problem. The program might use radio and billboard advertising to legitimize smaller family size by utilizing well-known minority male sports or movie heroes. Educational materials would be developed to provide information and persuade the clients to adopt new practices. Programming might thus be more institutional and informational than developmental.

If one were to use an andragogical model, programming would be a more mutual developmental process. The designer would involve clients and community members as well as other key actors in both defining the problem and selecting a strategy for solving it. The designer might form one or more advisory groups to collect information on needs and interpret this from the point of view of the clients' perceived needs. These groups could be called upon at various stages of program design and might even be involved in some way in launching the program or in monitoring its progress. Perceived client needs might stand in contrast with the specialists' analysis of their needs, but would be used as the point of departure for educational strategies.

For example, an andragogical model might not attempt to change male attitudes toward family size even though this might be acknowledged by the designer as important. Instead, the program might begin with problems that the client group sees as important, such as the health and welfare of the children parents already have. Educational materials and strategies would be designed to elicit experience and problems these parents face and would then work gradually toward an examination of how having fewer children could improve the quality of life for the parents and their families. While mass media might be used in this kind of program, it might focus less on information about new norms than on helping clients see their experience in typical life situations as related to the quality of their lives.

If one were to design a program using Freire's approach, the starting point would be identification of concerns the client group members have around family size. Themes selected might go far beyond the diagnosis of immediate influences on the practice of birth control or even the welfare of living children. For example, instead of trying to change male attitudes toward family size, education would provide a forum for analyzing why these attitudes exist. Themes to explore might include the welfare system, which enables women to raise children, family and community support systems, or unemployment.

Designers might utilize an advisory board for identifying themes, but these themes would be posed as problems to the clients themselves for diagnosis, drawing on the help of facilitators trained more in the process of critical reflection and analysis than in the content of family planning. Program design might be phased to allow for a beginning stage of client analysis of problems followed by client selection of priorities and their decisions about what action they are willing to take and what resources they need to implement their decisions.

ORGANIZATIONAL DELIVERY SYSTEMS

Program design models are primarily concerned with impact on clientele. However, there are also "hidden clients" who should be involved in planning, that is, staff and other agencies within the organizational delivery system that also have an interest in outcomes.

Too often, staff are viewed primarily in terms of a resource analysis or an inventory of supplies, material, people, and money needed to carry out the program. Other agency resources might not even be considered. One cannot assume, however, that people will automatically carry out plans. Low levels of enthusiasm or commitment can ruin the best-laid plans, unless they are compensated for by other motivating factors such as financial incentives or the disincentive of being fired or not promoted. Even then, subtle forms of sabotage can be utilized. For example, reports can be filled out with fictitious data; potential clients can be "unavailable" when field staff want to reduce their workload; or supplies can be "on order" for a long time.

One tool for involving staff constructively in this process is strategic planning, a tool that can improve short-term operations planning for many reasons, including the fact that a search for alternatives to goals draws staff into a creative look at maximizing resources. Dorfman summarized the steps of strategic planning as follows:

1. Identify problems, needs, and long-range goals.
2. Conduct a strategic audit of current programs, resources and services to accurately assess one's present position.
3. Using the best possible data, forecast future conditions within three to five years with the highest possible degree of confidence.
4. Design alternative paths to achieving long-range goals in light of this forecast, weighing costs and benefits of each alternative.
5. Develop your strategic plan, using clearly identified priorities to select among alternative paths.
6. Translate long-term plans into operational plans.
7. Monitor progress, using knowledge of conditions and alternatives to adjust your plans for unanticipated or new developments.[25]

Strategic planning requires input from a wide range of staff. It also broadens thinking about available resources because it forces a look at the larger organizational delivery system. Take, for example, the above illustration of a family planning education program in a small town. Suppose that staff decided to increase contraceptive, fertility, and maternal/child health services to both middle-class and minority groups, particularly for women aged 16 through 25, by 15 percent within three years.

Consideration of alternative paths to reaching this goal might reveal that this program competes for clients with public health community clinics and that several youth clubs also educate teenagers even though they do not provide services. The implications for health educators might include forging new lines of communication with these agencies to discuss issues such as complementarity of messages, appeal to different sectors of the market, duplication or gaps in providing services, and experience with learning design. Without this longer-range perspective, health educators might operate within different agencies in isolation from one another. Interagency rivalries could easily set limits on linkages as agencies battle for turf and compete with one another for the same population sector.

Strategic planning might also highlight the need to look beyond the agency to both community groups and higher-level policymakers of the town. For example, a proposal that the agency notify parents when their children use services could split the public opinion of town leaders, including key members of the agency's Advisory Board. Health education may have to include a strategy for advocacy through personal communication and contact with radio, newspapers, and other media. Advocacy efforts may extend to state or federal legislators.

Strategic planning includes the need to look at the organization itself—particularly at its culture, the climate for change, and the internal politics of the situation. Much of this analysis usually takes place informally because of its sensitive nature. It may turn out that although one solution is objectively preferable to another, an alternative path is pursued, professional judgment to the contrary.

ABANDONING THE LINEAR APPROACH

Traditional models of program development suggest a sequential, linear planning process. A three-dimensional interactional model is presented instead in which the program designer works simultaneously at several levels within and outside the organization to achieve consensus about a problem and how it should be solved.

Figure 1-3 illustrates schematically this interactional model of programming. Each level of programming represents steps needed to arrive at a vision of the program's design, which becomes successively refined as one moves higher up the spiral. The process does not stop with the initiation of the program. It continues throughout implementation in the form of formative (ongoing) evaluation with program refinement and concludes with a

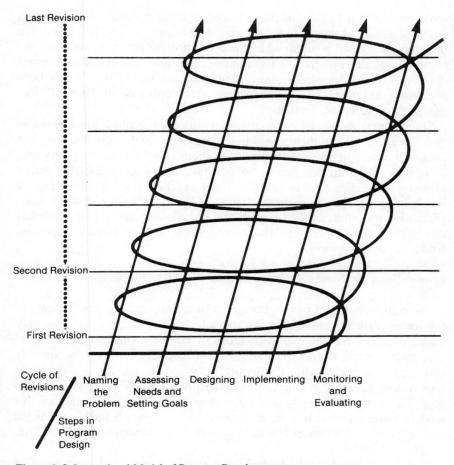

Last Revision

Second Revision

First Revision

Cycle of
Revisions

Naming
the
Problem

Assessing
Needs and
Setting Goals

Designing

Implementing

Monitoring
and
Evaluating

Steps in
Program
Design

Figure 1–3 Interactional Model of Program Development

summative (final) evaluation that ideally feeds back into the beginning of another cycle of design.

Each level could represent the entire process of problem naming, needs assessment, goal setting, design, implementation, and evaluation; or it could represent exploration and elaboration of one or another component. The diagram could include additional vertical axes representing other components or subcomponents and would look more like undulating blades of grass than straight poles since the timing of each step at successive plateaus might vary.

This interactional model of program development is based on maximizing the involvement of people in the program and client systems. In a sense, the program developer is more like the conductor of an orchestra than the composer of the symphony. By contrast, in linear models, the program developer invites people to play a new piece of music after it has been composed. In effect, staff and clients are often "enlisted" or "enticed" into providing or accepting services.

The interactional model of programming turns this around. Designers can build consultation into their planning through individual discussion with key opinion leaders, or they can utilize workshops, conferences, and networks to provide a forum for people to generate and select ideas for action planning. Sometimes, this can involve local media or other means of highlighting the event, such as drama, a booth at a local "street fair," graduation speeches, or the opening of a community center. Staff meetings and agency newspapers can be utilized for a similar education process within the health agency.

Implications for Needs Assessment and Objective Setting

For active co-design of programs, the linear approach is insufficient. In the linear planning approach, any mutual effort is often a one-time-only stage, which is fraught with difficulties in knowing which instruments to use, which people to involve, and how to collect and analyze data quickly enough to use the results. Consequently, while lip service is paid to its importance, needs assessment often either does not take place or results in data that are not sufficiently utilized in program design. In the interactional model, while an extensive needs assessment may be planned and carried out, less complex forms can be used at later stages to supplement, build on, or refine results.

Needs assessment can be looked upon as educational, and as an ongoing process, it can be a useful way of getting clients to "buy in" to a problem, to discover over time what their needs are, and to design or modify solutions. Agency reports and discussions with a few knowledgeable persons can serve to map out the territory and provide a basis for decisions about critical numbers to be reached. A variety of techniques can then be used to involve persons in interpreting and redefining their own needs as they are reached by the program.

For example, the designer of a smoking cessation program might rely on existing research data on the needs of people who wish to stop smoking and find that all that is necessary to launch a program is demographic data on participants. However, the program would be greatly strengthened, and very possibly modified, if people develop their own goals and periodically reasses them in order to customize treatment plans. Designers might also begin their programs with a discussion of data on the entire group, mutual negotiation of the way in which the program will be conducted, and consciousness raising as to why people buy into Madison Avenue's wishes for them in the first place.

The linear model advocates the development of observable, quantifiable, measurable outcomes around which programs are designed and evaluated. The interactional model does not discourage the designer from being as specific as possible about the program's statement of desired outcomes. However, objectives are seen as descriptive starting points for discussion and negotiation as clients reflect on their own needs and move toward a process of defining the directions they are willing to take to make lifestyle changes.

The interactional model thus assumes that people seldom know what they need until they have gathered sufficient information and related this to other concerns in their lives within some meaningful framework. Program design takes advantage of this by offering a definition clients can either accept or modify, by using a similar process but starting with definitions of the problem, or by opening a more discovery-oriented Freire-type dialogue about conditions in client lives that lead to analysis and probing until a problem is named and acted upon.

Implications for Monitoring and Evaluation

Monitoring may be defined as a system for noting whether or not events take place as planned and adjusting the program design accordingly. Evaluation, on the other hand, involves collection and analysis of data about progress in order to make judgments about success or failure so that programs can be improved. Scriven distinguishes between formative evaluation, which takes place while the program is being implemented in order to refine its operations, and summative evaluation, which takes place after the program is completed in order to determine actual effects.[26]

In the interactional model, monitoring and evaluation are focused on decisions about continuous refinement of program design as the designer moves from one plateau to the next. The emphasis is therefore on a process of transformation of objectives more than on evaluation against a final set of behavioral outcomes. Thus, designers have to build into their design sensitivity to evaluating against both process and outcome indicators of progress as well as against both proposed and revised objectives.

Indicators of this kind of progress must be considered along a continuum of change in a desired direction. In addition, at times, program directions are modified to meet new perceptions of need. So, for example, an evaluation of a family planning program might find that the program reached only 50 percent of its target of new acceptors. However, further investigation might also reveal that the health educator spent her time creating a teen discussion group, which was now ready to set up forums for dialogue with parents so teens could more easily accept services.

Process evaluation often requires the use of qualitative methods such as observation and interview since these tools allow for probing of relationships and are open to unanticipated outcomes that might otherwise be missed. Kinsey argues for the involvement of participants in internal evaluations for these and other reasons, even though he also identifies conditions under which this kind of evaluation is not warranted. Participatory evaluation often promotes learning on the part of both clients and staff, can improve awareness about programs, and increase commitment and support.[27]

SOME OBSTACLES

The obstacles to effective program design are many. There is seldom enough time to do a thorough analysis of a problem or need, the people who are enmeshed in it, the reasons why it should or should not be addressed, and all possible causes and consequences. Estimates often serve as the basis for setting targets, determining indicators of success, and sometimes for the baseline data itself. Extensive planning may thus be sacrificed because of time pressure to get the program implemented rapidly. Planning models might be used systematically to think through what one wants to accomplish and to get funding, but once implementation begins, real-life factors change the actual program into something vastly different.

Practitioners thus find themselves programming "by the seat of their pants," sometimes because of practical constraints and sometimes because of conceptual limitations of existing models. Practitioners often find that playing their hunches brings better results than following the rules since intuition includes human aspects not always factored into models.

In this chapter the author has been advocating an interactional model of program development built on a philosophy and practice of involvement to turn some of these weaknesses into strengths. The author has argued that practitioners can and should become reflective practitioners who build their own theories of practice, drawing on existing theory as appropriate but not simply applying it before naming and framing the problem. However, there are obstacles to this approach as well. While arguing persuasively for participatory management, Kanter identifies 23 dilemmas of managing this process at various stages of project design and implementation.[28] Participation can become abdication of leadership, risk taking, and responsibility. While participation can enhance the quality of programs, it increases the time needed for planning and unless properly managed, it can result in duplication of effort and in inefficiency.

Strategic planning is also a time-consuming process involving many people. Health educators are not always placed high enough in the hierarchy to change the organization's policy on planning. Moreover, strategic planning has been most successful in business environments that take a proactive stance toward achieving bottom-line results ultimately measured in terms of profits. Health organizations, by contrast, often work toward outcomes that are less easily measured or controlled. Health agencies are also more vulnerable to rapid changes in funding sources and are often accountable to the public.

Building a program along either the Knowles or Freire models requires skilled staff who are willing and able to assist learners in redefining their needs. People accustomed to a passive role with respect to both examining their needs and directing change in their lives may not be willing to modify these habits. Moreover, changing health habits still requires more than heightened awareness of the problem.

Finally, most programs are set up to serve certain purposes and are seldom flexible enough to respond to other identified needs. Organizational climates in bureaucracies are not generally innovative, adaptable, risk-taking, or conducive to cooperation among units or across other organizational boundary lines—all qualities facilitative of a bottom-up approach to programming.

EMPOWERMENT

Recognizing that health change is complex, health educators are broadening their understanding of strategies for healthy living. In the United States, this movement is spelled out in *Healthy People*[29] and *Objectives for the Nation*.[30] Green points out how health education has moved toward support of a combination of preventive health services, health protection and health promotion. He shows that behavior influences health not only directly (through individual self-care and lifestyle), but also through the environment by social action and environmental risks. Health promotion is a comprehensive strategy that takes this into consideration.

Ideally, health promotion enables people to define their own health problems, see how something in their lives causes them, and decide how they can be changed. It may require groups of people working together toward change in the social, cultural, or physical environment so that they can live healthy lives, as for example, with no-smoking laws or pressure on employers for exercise facilities and wellness-in-the-workplace programs. In short, it requires a concerted effort toward full *empowerment* of people in deciding what health means to them and how they want to preserve and practice it.

SUMMARY

To return to Figure 1-1, health promotion thus operates most effectively when practitioners view the world three-dimensionally because of the way interactions of clients and the program are embedded in larger social, cultural, economic, historic, and political forces. This strategic model of programming facilitates health promotion because it also emphasizes empowerment.

Green highlights trends in health education that show the profession's awareness of a paradigm shift from the technical to strategic viewpoint: from health information to health promotion, from an emphasis on activities to outcomes, from diagnosis to prognosis, from a biomedical model to a biosocial model, from concern with acute conditions to concern with chronic conditions, from cure to prevention, from the reliance on the "expert" for health to self-reliance of consumers in managing their own health.[31]

However, changing passive habits of reliance on experts is not necessarily the first priority of the people who stand to benefit in the long run from empowerment. Health educators must not only be convinced that empowerment is worth working toward, they must also develop strategies for building it into program design that enable clients at all levels to see its advantages.

A strategic view of learning emphasizes the fact that educators are not passive instruments in delivering educational change any more than the clients are. Educators are active participants in the process, who make choices that affect outcomes and who themselves grapple with issues regarding empowerment that are similar to those of the client. The educator enters into a partnership in the change process, practicing for himself or herself the same principles that are advocated for the client and working toward a "peerness" with the client in which each shares his or her strengths.

NOTES

1. Rosabeth Moss Kanter, *The Changemasters* (New York: Simon & Schuster, 1983); and Thomas J. Peters and Robert H. Waterman, Jr., *In Search of Excellence* (New York: Warner Books, 1984).

2. David C. Korten and Felipe B. Alfonso, eds., *Bureaucracy and the Poor: Closing the Gap* (Manila, Philippines: McGraw-Hill for Asian Institute of Management, 1981); and David Deshler and Donald Sock, "Community Development Participation: A Concept Review of the International Literature" (Paper presented at the First Annual Conference of the International League for Social Commitment in Adult Education, Sweden, July 22–26, 1985).

3. Patrick G. Boyle, *Planning Better Programs* (New York: McGraw-Hill, 1981); and Malcolm Knowles, *The Modern Practice of Adult Education*, rev. ed. (New York: Cambridge Books, 1980).

4. Ralph H. Kilmann, "Managing All Barriers to Organizational Success," *Training and Development Journal* (September 1985): 64–72.

5. Lawrence W. Green et al., *Health Education Planning: A Diagnostic Approach* (Palo Alto, Calif.: Mayfield, 1980).

6. Knowles, *Modern Practice.*

7. Paolo Freire, *Pedagogy of the Oppressed* (New York: Seabury Press, 1973).

8. Green et al., *Health Education Planning,* 10–16, 68–70.

9. Ibid., 180–181, 221–224.

10. Knowles, *Modern Practice,* 40–45.

11. Ibid., 59.

12. Malcolm Knowles, *Andragogy in Action* (San Francisco: Jossey-Bass, 1984), 297–340.

13. Hannelore Sweetwood, "A Framework for Re-Entry into Nursing Practice" (Ed.D. diss., Teachers College, Columbia University, 1986).

14. Patrick Walsh, "Planning and Developing Programs Systematically," in *Continuing Education for the Health Professions,* ed. J. Green et al. (San Francisco: Jossey-Bass, 1984), 138–139.

15. Phyllis Noble, *Formation of Freirian Facilitators* (Chicago: The Latino Institute, 1983); and A. Hope, S. Timmel, and C. Hodzi, *Training for Transformation: A Handbook for Community Workers* (Gweru, Zimbabwe: Mambo Press, 1984).

16. Meredith Minkler and Kathleen Cox, "Creating Critical Consciousness in Health: Applications of Freire's Philosophy and Methods to the Health Care Setting," *International Journal of Health Services,* 10:2 (1980): 311–322; and Meredith Minkler, Sheryl Frantz, and Robin Wechsler, "Social Support and Social Action Organizing in a 'Grey Ghetto': The Tenderloin Experience," *International Quarterly of Community Health Education,* 3:1 (1982–83): 3–15.

17. Jerald Apps, "Problems with Planning Approaches," in *Problems in Continuing Education,* ed. Jerald Apps (New York: McGraw-Hill, 1979), 112–134.

18. Green et al., *Health Education Planning,* 77.

19. Boyle, *Planning Better Programs,* 6–12.

20. Rensis Likert, *New Patterns of Management* (New York: McGraw-Hill, 1961); and Chris Argyris, *Integrating the Individual and the Organization* (New York: John Wiley, 1964).

21. Duane Dale and Nancy Mitiguy, *Planning for a Change: A Citizens' Guide to Creative Planning and Program Development* (Amherst: University of Massachusetts, Citizen Involvement Training Project, 1978), 32–35.

22. Wilfred Carr and Stephen Kemmis, *Becoming Critical: Knowing through Action Research* (Victoria, Australia: Deakin University Printery, 1984).

23. Donald A. Schön, *The Reflective Practitioner* (New York: Basic Books, 1983), 128–133.

24. Ibid., 157–162.

25. Sharon Dorfman, "Thinking Like a Manager" (Taped presentation in Health Education Section Session, Sixty-third Annual Meeting of the American College Health Association, Washington, D.C., May 31, 1985).

26. Michael Scriven, "The Methodology of Evaluation," in *Evaluating Action Programs: Readings in Social Action and Education,* ed. Carol Weiss (Boston: Allyn & Bacon, 1972).

27. David C. Kinsey, "Participatory Evaluation in Adult and Nonformal Education," *Adult Education,* 31:3 (1981): 158–160.

28. Kanter, *Changemasters.*

29. *Healthy People: The Surgeon General's Report on Health Promotion and Disease Prevention* (Washington, D.C.: Office of the Assistant Secretary for Health, Public Health Service, U.S. Department of Health and Human Services, 1979).

30. *Objectives for the Nation* (Washington, D.C.: Office of the Assistant Secretary for Health, Public Health Service, U.S. Department of Health and Human Services, 1980).

31. Lawrence W. Green, "Emerging Federal Perspectives on Health Promotion," *Health Promotion Monographs,* ed. John P. Allegrante, 1 (July 1981): 20–21.

SUGGESTED READINGS

Santo Pietro, Daniel, ed. *Evaluation Sourcebook for Private and Voluntary Organizations.* New York: American Council of Voluntary Agencies for Foreign Service, 1983.

"Special Report: Adult Education and Primary Health Care." *Convergence* 15 (1982): 1–81.

Chapter 2

Financing Patient Education Programs

Edward E. Bartlett, DrPH

Imagine having to choose among three different restaurants with the intention of consuming a delectable vegetarian meal. At the first restaurant, the deal is "Salad Bar—$1.95 per bowl." At the second establishment, the sign reads "Salad Bar—All You Can Eat—$3.49." And the third possibility advertises "Salad Bar—12 cents per ounce." And consider your behavior at the first restaurant—you would pile everything possible into the bowl, being careful to select a minimum of lettuce because the leaves occupy too much space. In the second location, you might try to gorge yourself, knowing that your next meal will not be as tantalizing (or filling) as this one. At the third establishment, exceptionally conscious of the weights of different foods, you skimp on the salad dressing and load up on nuts and cauliflower.

What accounts for this seemingly irrational behavior? Can it be explained in terms of contradictory culinary impulses that strike your fancy? Probably not. A more reasonable explanation is that the financial arrangements are exerting a powerful effect on your gastronomic preferences. The same holds true in medical care. At first glance, the behavior of medical institutions may appear irrational and inexplicable. Such is the all-too-familiar case of hospitals dauntlessly constructing new wings in a community already burdened with excessive beds. However, when the existing financing arrangements are examined more closely (which we will do in this chapter), the behavior becomes completely understandable. If our own food preferences are radically altered by just a few pennies, we should not be surprised by

Note: This work was supported in part by a Cooperative Agreement between the UAB School of Public Health; the Centers for Disease Control, Center for Health Promotion and Education; and the Association of Schools of Public Health.

The author thanks the Diabetes Control Program, Michigan Department of Public Health, for sharing information regarding reimbursement activities for outpatient diabetes education.

31

the revenue-driven behavior of administrators when millions of dollars are at stake.

Health educators traditionally have paid scant attention to understanding financing mechanisms and how these mechanisms influence their programs. This attitude can be perilous, as demonstrated by the recurrent difficulty of health education programs attempting to acquire a stable funding base after their initial seed monies have terminated. This chapter explains important concepts in financing, the current status of financing patient education programs, and strategies that health educators can undertake to improve the financial stability of their own programs. The discussion is not a comprehensive examination of this complex topic, but it will equip the patient educator with the basic vocabulary, understanding, and "savvy" necessary to ensure adequate funding.

Emphasis will be on the ambulatory rather than the inpatient setting; however, because most reimbursement programs focus on hospital care, that arena must be considered, too. Some of the terminology and concepts of financing are somewhat technical, but understanding how the financing system works will greatly increase the chances of improving the funding and longevity of one's program.

Some of the confusion arises from the fact that medical care financing is currently undergoing a revolutionary metamorphosis from cost-based to prospective and capitation financing. Thus, patient educators must understand both systems in order to make their way in the current environment. Because this chapter stresses the outpatient setting, and because prospective pricing applies only to inpatient care at the present time, more attention is placed on cost-based reimbursement.

Two notes about terminology. The definition of patient education is fashioned by the Delphi Group on Patient Education Terminology: "a planned learning experience using a combination of methods such as teaching, counseling, and behavior modification techniques which influence patient's knowledge and health behavior . . . [and] involve an interactive process between patient and professional which assists patients to participate actively in their health care."[1] Also, because most insurance plans exclude coverage for preventive services, it is a misnomer to refer to them as "health insurance." Thus, the term "medical insurance" is used, although "illness care insurance" is more accurate.

ESSENTIAL KNOWLEDGE

This section presents the essential knowledge that is a prerequisite to effective advocacy efforts toward improving patient education financing.

Basic Financing Concepts

It is important to distinguish between the words "financing" and "reimbursement." Financing refers to *any* means of paying for a health care service, whether from the organization's operating funds, reimbursement from an insurance company, a bank loan, an external grant, or philanthropy. Reimbursement is a more specific term and indicates the payment of funds to the health care "provider" (a hospital, an HMO, or a physician) by a third-party carrier for a specified service or procedure. The third-party carrier could be Medicare, Medicaid, Blue Cross/Blue Shield, or a commercial insurance company.

The first medical insurance programs in the United States were established when the Depression threatened the ability of patients to pay their hospital and medical bills. The first Blue Cross plan for hospital insurance was established in 1929 in Dallas, and the forerunner to the first Blue Shield plan was initiated by the California Medical Association in 1939. As commercial insurance companies flourished in the subsequent decades by selling group policies to businesses and corporations, it became increasingly clear that the elderly and poor were being denied access to medical care because of inadequate insurance coverage. Hence, Medicare (a federal program for the elderly) and Medicaid (a state-run program for persons with low income) were passed as Titles XVIII and XIX of the Social Security Amendments of 1965.

With the growth of these third-party insurance programs came the perplexing problem of determining (1) the unit of payment and (2) the amount of payment. For the unit of payment, should clinics and hospitals be reimbursed on the basis of the number of procedures performed (e.g., x-rays, lab tests), the number of office visits or hospital days, or the total number of patients cared for during a specified time period? And once the unit of payment was set, how much should be paid?

Regarding the first question, insurance companies settled on a combination of paying for both procedures and visits (outpatients) or days (inpatients). And to determine the proper amount, they either employ a fee schedule that pays a fixed amount to providers regardless of the actual charge or use the "usual, customary, and reasonable" (UCR) method. UCR means that the provider is reimbursed according to whatever his or her charges may be, as long as two conditions are met:

1. All patients are charged the same amount, regardless of the insurance plan covering them.
2. The charge is in line with what other providers in the same community are charging.

In addition, Medicare established the magnanimous policy of reimbursing hospitals on a so-called "cost-plus" basis. This means that hospitals could bill to cover the charge of whatever procedures their physicians deemed were necessary, *plus* the interest payments for new construction or equipment.

These "cost-based" reimbursement policies were reinforced by the peculiar fact in medical care that physicians determine both the *demand* and the *supply* for medical services.[2] They influence the demand because they recommend to patients how frequently to make follow-up visits, whether diagnostic tests are indicated, whether surgery is necessary, and which hospital to use. And they determine the supply because they themselves are the providers of these services.

Given these factors, it is easy to see why national health expenditures have consistently risen faster than the Consumer Price Index over the past two decades, representing 6.0 percent of the Gross National Product in 1965 and 10.9 percent in 1983.[3] These policies, popularly referred to as "blank check" reimbursement, undergirded the rapid rise of medical care costs, which set the stage for the recent advent of prospective and capitation financing (discussed later in this chapter).

Medical Care Financing: Carriers, Services, and Populations

In order to comprehend the total picture, the patient educator must understand which are the most important carriers in the United States and the nature of their coverage:

1. *Private insurance.* Benefits offered by Blue Cross, Blue Shield, and commercial insurance companies range from coverage of basic hospital and physician expenses, to "Major Medical" policies, to catastrophic insurance. About 85 percent of the U.S. population has some type of private insurance coverage, often offered as an employee fringe benefit.

2. *Medicare.* Medicare covers persons 65 years and older plus end-stage renal disease (ESRD) patients. Part A covers hospital expenses, and Part B ("supplementary medical insurance") includes physician and outpatient fees. Medicare is available to about 10 percent of the population as an entitlement benefit. In 1983, Medicare began to phase in the prospective pricing system for financing its recipients' hospital care (described below). More recently, Medicare has begun to actively support "capitation" payments to HMOs for Medicare beneficiaries.

3. *Medicaid.* Medicaid serves low-income persons, representing less than 10 percent of the population. It is operated by the state governments but receives about 25 percent federal funding. Because it is state run, eligibility criteria and coverage are highly variable. Previously, Medicaid programs were the most comprehensive of all the medical insurance plans, providing

such services as Early Periodic Screening, Detection, and Treatment (EPSDT) for children. However, budget changes since 1980 have reduced the extent of medical coverage in most states.

4. *Health Maintenance Organizations.* HMOs represent a radical departure in health care financing for two principal reasons: the unit of payment is the *person* (not the procedure, office visit, or hospital day), and the provider and insurer are contractually merged. This system shares the financial risk of paying the medical expenses between the *providers* (physician and hospital) and the *insurer,* and thus imposes a financial incentive on both parties to reduce expenses. Although one might expect HMOs to be primary advocates of prevention and health education, this has not been necessarily true,[4] leading some to prefer the term "prepaid group practice" over "health maintenance organization." About 6 percent of the population currently are members of an HMO.

In general, these programs (with the exception of HMOs) favor inpatient and therapeutic services over outpatient and preventive programs. Additional information on the range of benefits covered by various sources of funds is shown in Table 2-1. This table indicates that in 1983, the health dollar was split among hospital care (42 cents), physicians' services (19 cents), nursing home care (8 cents), drugs (7 cents), government public health activities (2 cents), and other expenses (22 cents).

It also should be noted that about 10 percent of the American population has no medical insurance. These persons must pay their own medical expenses, request free care, or remain deprived of needed services.

Recent Developments in Financing

Two important developments in medical care financing in recent years portend the demise of the traditional cost-based reimbursement systems. The first, referred to above, is the steady growth of capitation financing (i.e., the unit of payment is the person), as represented by the increased prominence of Health Maintenance Organizations around the country. This development means that to the extent that health education and patient education services can be demonstrated to reduce medical costs and improve the quality of care, these programs should expand in the future.

The second development is the inception of the prospective pricing system (PPS) in 1983 to cover hospital charges for Medicare patients. Under prospective pricing, the unit of payment is the *patient admission* ("case"), not the number of procedures or hospital days. One of 467 diagnostic categories, referred to as Diagnosis Related Groups ("DRGs"), is assigned to each hospital patient, and each DRG is assigned a weight that determines how much the hospital will be reimbursed for that patient. Thus, a hypothetical hospital would be reimbursed $20,962 for DRG 106 ("Coronary

Table 2–1 National Health Care Expenditures, by Type of Expenditure and Source of Funds—1983

Type of Expenditure	Total	Private			Public	
		Consumer			Federal	State and Local
		Direct	Insurance	Other*		
	Aggregate Amount (000,000,000 Omitted)					
1983 (Estimated)						
Total	$362.3	$103.8	$95.2	$12.1	$104.2	$46.9
Health Services and Supplies	347.4	103.8	95.2	5.2	98.7	44.5
Personal Health Care	323.6	103.8	85.3	4.5	94.6	35.5
Hospital Care	154.7	19.3	51.3	2.3	62.0	19.8
Physicians' Services	69.8	27.1	23.1	—	15.4	4.1
Dentists' Services	21.6	15.2	5.6	—	0.5	0.4
Other Professional Services	7.9	4.5	1.5	0.1	1.5	0.4
Drugs and Medical Sundries	24.9	19.6	3.0	—	1.1	1.1
Eyeglasses and Appliances	6.0	4.7	0.4	—	0.8	0.1
Nursing Home Care	30.3	13.4	0.3	0.2	8.9	7.5
Other Health Services	8.5	—	—	2.0	4.4	2.1
Program Administration and Net Cost of Insurance	16.0	—	10.0	0.6	2.9	2.4
Government Public Health Activities	7.8	—	—	—	1.2	6.6
Research and Construction of Medical Facilities	14.9	—	—	7.0	5.5	2.4
Research	5.8	—	—	0.4	4.9	0.5
Construction	9.1	—	—	6.6	0.6	1.9

*Spending by philanthropic organizations, industrial in-plant services, and privately financed construction.
Note: Details may not add to totals due to rounding.

Source: U.S. Department of Health and Human Services, Health Care Financing Administration, Health Care Financing Review, March 1983 and Fall 1983.

bypass, with cardiac catheterization"), regardless of the patient's length of stay or consumption of other hospital services. In a number of states, prospective pricing now is being extended to cover Medicaid and private insurance patients.

The implications of prospective pricing are truly revolutionary. First, hospitals now have a powerful incentive to improve efficiency and reduce expenses. If they do not, hospitals are headed for imminent bankruptcy. Second, it is now much more practical for people (including prospective patients) to compare hospitals in terms of number of admissions, procedures, and complication rates on a disease-specific basis. Before, there were over 7,000 ICD (International Classification of Diseases) diagnoses; now there are only 467 classifications. Third, insurers now have an efficient means of controlling their hospital payments (and thus, their overall medical care payments) by adjusting their reimbursement rate for each DRG. Fourth, third-party payers, aided by local quality assurance groups (Peer Review Organizations—"PROs"), can determine which medical procedures are deemed unproven, unaffordable, or inappropriate for treatment in the hospital setting. For example, DRG 103, Heart Transplant, has a severity weighting of 0, meaning that it is not reimbursable under prospective pricing. The same approach is being used to shift care to the ambulatory care setting for such diagnoses as diabetes and cataract surgery. Clearly, they who pay the piper will be calling the tune more often, and putative assertions of "medical necessity" will carry less weight in the years ahead.

Under prospective pricing, patient education services for inpatients will be paid for from the lump sum provided to the hospital to cover a patient's hospital stay. How much of that sum will be allocated to patient education is a key question. For example, part of that amount will cover the salary expenses of unit nurses, pharmacists, and dietitians who are carrying much of the patient education responsibility.

How much money is budgeted to the patient education department is a decision that rests entirely with the hospital administrator. From 0.3 to 0.5 percent of the institution's total budget is recommended.[5] Patient education managers will be able to make a convincing case for increasing their budgets if they can successfully link patient education with the accomplishment of the institution's strategic planning objectives, such as providing high-quality medical care. Under prospective pricing, patient education has been enjoying greater administrative support (for reasons outlined in the next section), which seems likely to grow in the years ahead.

Can Patient Education Reduce Medical Costs?

With the advent of prospective pricing, the principal question is, How can we reduce expenses while at the same time maintaining high quality of care? Fortunately, a growing body of research now indicates that patient education can save on medical expenses for selected conditions.[6] This research indicates that the following patient education strategies (i.e., aggregations of educational approaches and techniques) will expand under prospective pricing:

1. *Preoperative education*—prepares and supports patients undergoing surgery or other invasive procedures.

2. *Discharge planning education*—prepares patients for their discharge from the hospital, by locating community resources and training them to perform necessary self-care activities.
3. *Early discharge programs*—allows patients to be discharged one or more days earlier from the hospital. The most common example is short-stay maternity programs.
4. *Home care education*—assists patients who require continued care at home, frequently for a severe illness.
5. *Medication self-administration programs*—trains patients to administer their own injections, intravenous medications, or home dialysis treatments.
6. *Cooperative care units*—actively involves patients and family members in providing their own routine care in the hospital setting.
7. *Outpatient education*—shifts education previously accomplished in the hospital to the ambulatory setting, accomplished either before or after the hospitalization.
8. *Family education*—educates family members to better support and care for the patient.
9. *Peer educators*—utilizes former or current patients who educate patients in practical means of coping with the illness.

Of particular interest is the fact that the research indicates that patient education can not only save medical costs, but also improve the quality of patient care. For example, studies indicate that preoperative education can reduce a broad range of postsurgical complications[7]; that parents of children with disabling conditions prefer to care for their children at home rather than keeping them in the hospital[8]; that family members prefer to play an active caregiving role in the hospital[9]; that patients requiring dialysis treatments experience less dependence and better rehabilitation when they perform the dialysis at home[10]; that patients administering their own medications commit no more drug errors than health professionals[11]; that peer educators can assist patients to better cope with their illness[12]; and that behaviorally oriented patient education can improve adherence and control of chronic conditions.[13] In short, a better quality of care can be provided at less cost. Less is more!

IMPROVING THE FINANCING OF PATIENT EDUCATION

This section provides information on how patient education is financed currently and strategies that have been used to improve patient education reimbursement.

How Much of the Health Care Dollar Is Allocated to Health Education?

Before discussing the ways to increase patient education financing, it would be helpful to gauge how well health education and patient education are financed. Unfortunately, the available data are not extensive or always up to date.

Recent epidemiological evidence indicates that *behavior* (smoking, diet, exercise, etc.) accounts for 55–75 percent of factors determining a person's health condition.[14] This remarkable finding contrasts strikingly with the level of funding for health education programs. According to the President's Committee on Health Education,[15] less than one-fourth of 1 percent of the 1973 budget of the United States Public Health Service was allocated specifically for programs in health education, and less than one half of the budgets of state health departments were devoted to this purpose. Similarly, Dever[16] concluded that only 1.2 percent of the federal health budget for 1974–1976 was allocated to lifestyle change programs.

Regarding patient education, the percentage figure is more difficult to ascertain, because patient education is accomplished by nurses, physicians, and other caregivers as part of their regular patient care activities. Observational studies of medical practice indicate that physicians devote from 19 to 41 percent of their direct patient care time in ambulatory settings to patient education and counseling.[17] Data on nurses are less extensive, but one observational study found that hospital nurses devote 25.8 percent of their total time to patient teaching, although much of this time was concurrently devoted to such clinical activities as taking vital signs, administering medications, and the like.[18] Although it is not possible to fix a precise percentage figure, it is nonetheless clear that a substantial portion of the $323.6 billion spent for personal health care in 1983 was devoted to the provision of patient education services.[19]

If one accepts the premise that 1 percent of the national health budget is a woefully inadequate sum for lifestyle programs, this analysis suggests that for community health education programs, the main problem is to *increase* funding levels. In contrast, for *patient* education, it is apparent that considerable amounts of time, and hence resources, currently are devoted to this activity. Thus the major challenge for patient education is not simply increasing funds but also improving its visibility and effecting a better consolidation of its resources.

How Do Third-Party Carriers Cover Patient Education under Cost-Based Reimbursement?

In order to discuss financing for patient education services under cost-based reimbursement policies, it is necessary to distinguish patient educa-

Exhibit 2-1 Patient Education Reimbursement Policy by Medicare and Medicaid

---

80 Patient Education Programs

80-1 Institutional and Home Care Patient Education Programs

While the law does not specifically identify patient education programs as covered services, reimbursement may be made under Medicare for such programs furnished by providers of services (i.e., hospitals, SNFs, HHAs, and OPT providers) to the extent that the programs are appropriate, integral parts in the rendition of covered services which are reasonable and necessary for the treatment of the individual's illness or injury. For example, educational activities carried out by nurses—teaching patients to give themselves injections, follow prescribed diets, administer colostomy care, administer medical gases, and carry out other inpatient care activities—may be reimbursable as a part of covered routine nursing care. Also, the teaching by an occupational therapist of compensatory techniques to improve a patient's level of independence in the activities of daily living may be reimbursable as a part of covered occupational therapy. Similarly, the instruction of a patient in the carrying out of a maintenance program designed for him by a physical therapist may be reimbursed as a part of covered physical therapy.

However, where the educational activities are not closely related to the care and treatment of the patient, such as programs directed toward instructing patients or the public generally in preventive health care activities, reimbursement cannot be made since the law limits Medicare payment to covered care which is reasonable and necessary for the treatment of an illness or injury. For example, programs designed to prevent illness by instructing the general public in the importance of good nutritional habits, exercise regimens, and good hygiene are not reimbursable under the program.

Source: Reprinted from *Medicare and Medicaid Guide,* Section 27201, p. 9023, Health Care Financing Administration, Baltimore, MD.

---

tion conducted as *incidental to care* (e.g., a physician's instructions about prescribed medications) versus education conducted as a *separate activity* (e.g., diabetes education classes, smoking cessation counseling, or cardiac rehabilitation classes). Although it could be argued that diabetes classes in fact should be "incidental to care," insurance companies nonetheless enforce the distinction between education conducted by the usual providers of treatment services, and education that is conducted by others. (Note that under prospective pricing, the difference between incidental and separate patient education is less important because the budget allocation decision is made by the hospital administrator.)

Under current third-party payer regulations, basic patient education activities that are incidental to care *and* therapeutically oriented are reimbursable by Medicare (Exhibit 2-1) and Blue Cross/Blue Shield. *Preventive* patient education is less often reimbursable than education that is therapeutic and incidental to care.

Table 2-2 indicates the general level of financing for therapeutically oriented patient education activities, broken down by setting, provider (MD, others), form of payment (DRG, non-DRG), and type of education (incidental to care, separate from care).[20] Table 2-2, which is based on the Blue Cross/Blue Shield survey and the author's own knowledge of reimbursement practices, indicates that financing inpatient education that is part of the usual diagnostic and treatment activities generally is not problematic. As a rule, educational services accomplished as incidental to care are

Table 2–2 Coverage of Therapeutically Oriented Patient Education by Third-Party Carriers

	Incidental to Care	*Separate Activity*
Inpatient		
1. DRG-based reimbursement	Yes	Varies, depending on support by administrator
2. Non-DRG-based reimbursement—by RN and other staff	Yes	Varies, depending on support by administrator and/or specific approval by third-party carrier
3. MDs	Yes	NA
Outpatient		
1. MDs	Yes	NA
2. Other staff in MD office or clinic	Yes	Varies, depending on support by physician and/or specific approval by third-party carrier
3. RN, RD, etc. in independent practice	No	No
4. Hospital-sponsored outpatient department	Yes	Varies, depending on support by administrator and/or specific approval by third-party carrier (can be financed either as part of DRG payment for inpatient care or as a separate reimbursable item)
HMO	Yes	Varies, depending on support by administrator and/or clinical staff

NA = Not Applicable

"buried" in the fee for the overall office visit (outpatient) or room charge (inpatient), whereas education conducted separate from care is more stable if it can be reimbursed as a separate charge. However, this latter approach can require prolonged negotiations with the third-party carrier, as the case study later in this chapter illustrates.

Considering that patient education is widely reimbursed as long as it is incidental to the care process, and that third-party carriers prefer to pay for patient education buried in the office visit or room charge, *why are patient educators attempting to secure separate reimbursement?* There are four important reasons:

1. Several conditions (such as asthma and diabetes) require a major educational component for their management, and this education cannot be achieved on an "incidental" basis.
2. Patient education often lacks visibility, and separate reimbursement greatly enhances visibility.
3. It is easier to ensure the quality of patient education when it is organized and paid for separately.
4. Separate reimbursement ensures greater financial stability.

Improving Reimbursement for Patient Education: A Case Study

In order to demonstrate how knowledge of these concepts will assist the patient education advocate to achieve better funding, a chronicle of the experiences of a group that worked in Michigan to obtain third-party reimbursement for ambulatory diabetes education programs is outlined in Exhibit 2-2.

Exhibit 2-2   A Case Study

1979—Michigan Department of Public Health created a Task Force on Third Party Reimbursement for Diabetes Patient Education and Ambulatory Care. The objective of the Task Force was to achieve reimbursement for diabetes ambulatory education by all insurers in Michigan.

1980—The Task Force collected data indicating that there were 350,000 diabetics in Michigan (38 percent eligible for Medicare) and 26,000 hospitalizations caused by diabetes occur annually, costing over $93.6 million per year. These data indicated that hospital care for diabetes patients consumed a considerable sum of money. Task Force decided to focus on initial efforts on reimbursement by Medicare.

January 1981—Task Force held initial discussions with Michigan Medicare Contractor (Blue Cross/Blue Shield of Michigan). Task Force was told that separate billing of

Exhibit 2-2 *Continued*

educational services could not be made unless services were part of a "documented therapeutic regimen," and that it was preferable that education be billed as incidental to routine nursing services. Task Force also became aware of the need to assure high quality diabetes patient education and began to develop standards.

May 1981—Medical staff of Medicare Contractor ruled that programs meeting diabetes education standards of Task Force were not covered under Medicare reimbursement.

June 1981—Task Force contacted Region V, Office of the Health Care Financing Administration (HCFA) in Chicago, to discuss patient education reimbursement policies and criteria development. Concurrently, the Michigan Diabetes Policy Advisory Committee approved Program Standards. These standards were subsequently used as a basis for awarding seed monies by the Michigan Department of Public Health for a new diabetes patient education program.

September 1981–February 1981—Discussions and letters between the Task Force and the HCFA Region V staff (Chicago) led to a request for clarification from the HCFA central office (Baltimore) regarding reimbursement for diabetes patient education. This resulted in an encouraging letter from region V HCFA to the Task Force outlining the specific circumstances under which Medicare would reimburse for such services.

April 1982—Task Force representatives met with Medicare Contractor to formulate eligibility criteria.

June 1982–March 1983—During the course of several communications, Contractor appeared to contradict earlier letter from HCFA by indicating that Program Standards were too complex, that diabetes patient education was of little proven value in reducing costs, and that the Contractor would not reimburse separately for such services.

April 1983—Task Force reassessed the strategy. Consistent with Medicare policies prohibiting payment for preventive services, Task Force decided to emphasize the fact that *diabetes patient information was integral to management of disease* and deemphasized patient education as a *means of preventing morbidity and saving costs*. The Task Force also decided to contact HCFA Region V staff to clarify the responsibility of the Contractor in implementing reimbursement that HCFA had authorized in February 1982. In addition, the Task Force contacted Michigan Congressional representatives, known to be supportive of health-related legislation.

June 1983—Administrator of HCFA Region V responded favorably to Task Force letter of April 1983, indicating "outpatient education programs for diabetics were the only such programs for which Medicare would make reimbursement as a separate service which need not be included as part of another service." Administrator also indicated the problem that "the specific coverage of these unique programs and the related reimbursement and cost accounting procedures were not addressed in the manual" and requested additional information to resolve these questions. Task Force responded to these concerns.

Exhibit 2-2 *Continued*

August 1983—HCFA Region V sent letter specifically instructing Michigan Contractor to initiate reimbursement for outpatient diabetes education.

September 1983—Task Force met with Contractor to review procedures to implement separate coverage of outpatient diabetes patient education.

October, 1983—Contractor distributed a bulletin to all Medicare-certified hospitals in Michigan regarding new coverage.

Subsequent efforts by the Task Force were directed toward securing reimbursement by Medicaid and by private insurance companies. There is not space to describe the steps followed by the Task Force in working with the other third-party carriers. Medicaid has agreed to the Task Force's request, and universal coverage for outpatient diabetes education in Michigan will be a major breakthrough.

Problems in Financing Patient Education

Patient education rests on weaker ground when it is accomplished as a separate activity. Given the fact that patient education *is* widely reimbursable when it is incidental to usual caregiving activities, what are the problems faced in trying to improve the financing for patient education services as a separate charge? As illustrated by the case in Michigan, the problems are both technical and political in nature. These are highlighted as follows:

1. *Defining the benefit design.* In order to reimburse for patient education, the insurer must know the *what, where,* and *who* of the service it is paying for. For example, how many sessions will an asthma outpatient education program consist of, over what period of time, using what educational methods? Will it be performed in physicians' offices, in hospital outpatient departments, by county health departments, in free-standing educational centers, or all of these? Who will do the educating—nurse, physician, health educator, nutritionist, pharmacist, or others?
2. *Maintaining quality.* How will the insurer be assured that the program will represent high standards of educational practice? By setting

standards and accrediting programs? By providing special training and certification to the educators? By accomplishing chart reviews to review documentation of educational activities? By allowing only certain providers (e.g., hospital outpatient departments) to be reimbursed?

3. *Establishing the benefit rating.* How much will the educational service add to subscribers' premiums, and will there be co-payments or deductibles?

4. *Setting up claims review procedures.* These procedures include designing the claim form, verifying the eligibility of persons who request patient education services (e.g., should education of spouses of patients be reimburseable?), and establishing administrative procedures for claims review and payment.

5. *Minimizing administrative costs.* Processing each claim costs money, and insurers prefer not to process small claims (say, less than $100) in order to restrain administrative costs.

6. *Addressing the procedural bias.* Insurance companies prefer to reimburse for services they can easily measure and count. Thus, procedural services (like an x-ray or surgery) fare better than so-called "cognitive" services such as education and counseling.

7. *Restricted coverage of outpatient services.* Limited reimbursement for outpatient services in general may preclude coverage of ambulatory patient education.

8. *Cost containment mind set.* One barrier that has arisen in the past few years is convincing insurers to add a new benefit with increased short-term costs, in an era emphasizing cost containment and cutbacks in services.

9. *Gaining increased visibility for patient education as a service.* Because patient education is widely considered as an incidental component of medical care, it lacks visibility. Thus, it probably receives less attention from administrators and third-party payers than it deserves.

10. *Addressing the double standard.* Medical insurance plans were established with the explicit purpose of supporting medical services rendered by physicians. Hence, new diagnostic or therapeutic procedures generally are expected only to demonstrate *"medical necessity."* In contrast, persons advocating the separate reimbursement of educational services find themselves being asked not only to demonstrate medical necessity but also *effectiveness* and *cost savings.* These stricter criteria make it more difficult to obtain third-party reimbursement for patient education.

IMPLICATIONS FOR THE FUTURE OF PATIENT EDUCATION FINANCING

What do these findings say to patient educators with interests broader than diabetes? First, to the extent that traditional cost-based mechanisms for third-party reimbursement continue, patient educators will need to work with insurers on a disease-by-disease basis. Likely candidates for future attention are hypertension, asthma, and cardiac rehabilitation.

At the same time, patient educators must be aware of the inexorable trend toward prospective and capitation financing. This means that budget allocation decisions will be made more by administrators of HMOs, clinics, and hospitals and less by third-party carriers. As this trend becomes firmly established, patient educators will need to direct more of their advocacy efforts *within* rather than *outside* their organizations. Above all, health educators need to keep in mind these key issues and strategies:

- Having adequate resources is essential to success of any program. Keep your mind on the bottom line.
- Scientific studies show that patient education can reduce medical costs and improve the quality of care. Master these studies, and incorporate them into your arsenal of advocacy strategies.
- Financing for health care services currently is undergoing revolutionary changes—changes that bode well for patient education. This shift is propelling patient education into the mainstream of health care, and will require novel approaches by patient educators.
- Improving the financing for patient education requires overcoming a variety of technical and political obstacles. Use your creativity, determination, and patience to become an effective advocate of improved patient education financing.

NOTES

1. E.E. Bartlett, "At Last, A Definition," *Patient Education and Counseling* 7 (1985): 323–324.

2. S.R. Eastaugh, *Medical Economics and Health Finance* (Boston: Auburn House, 1981).

3. *Sourcebook of Health Insurance Data* (Washington, D.C.: Health Insurance Association of America, 1984).

4. P.D. Mullen and J.G. Zapka, *Guidelines for Health Promotion and Education Services in HMOs* (Washington, D.C.: Office of Disease Prevention and Health Promotion, 1982).

5. E.E. Bartlett and B.A. Manzella, *Innovative Solutions to PPS: Focus on Patient Education* (Birmingham: University of Alabama, 1985).

6. E.E. Bartlett, *Assessing the Benefits of Patient Education Under Prospective Pricing* (Birmingham: University of Alabama, 1984); E.E. Bartlett, "Social Consumption or Social Investment?" *Patient Education and Counseling* 7 (1985): 223–224.

7. E. Mumford et al., "The Effects of Psychological Intervention on Recovery From Surgery and Heart Attacks: An Analysis of the Literature," *American Journal of Public Health* 72 (1982): 141–151.

8. Bartlett, *Assessing the Benefits.*

9. B. Berg, "A Touch of Home in Hospital Care," *New York Times Magazine,* 27 Nov. 1983, pp. 90–95.

10. P.G. Jenkins et al., "Self-Hemodialysis: The Optimal Mode of Dialytic Therapy," *Archives of Internal Medicine* 136 (1976): 357–361.

11. C.J. Roberts and W.A. Miller, "Clinical Pharmacy, Self-Administration, and Technician Drug Administration Services in a 72-Bed Hospital," *Drug Intelligence and Clinical Pharmacy* 6 (1972): 408–415.

12. L.W. Green et al., "Research and Demonstration Issues in Self-Care: Measuring the Decline of Mediocentrism," *Health Education Monographs* 5 (1977): 161–189.

13. S.A. Mazzuca, "Does Patient Education in Chronic Disease Have Therapeutic Value?", *Journal of Chronic Disease* 35 (1982): 521–529.

14. E.E. Bartlett, "Forging an Educational Model of Health Care," *Patient Education and Counseling* 7 (1985): 3–5.

15. President's Committee on Health Education, *Report of the President's Committee on Health Education* (New York, 1974), 24.

16. G.E.A. Dever, "An Epidemiological Model for Health Policy Analysis," *Social Indicators Research* 2 (1977): 453–466.

17. E.E. Bartlett, "The Contributions of Consumer Health Education for Primary Care Practice: A Review," *Medical Care* 18 (1980): 862–871.

18. L.A. Bukowski, "Patient Education and the Nursing Process: Nurses' Observed and Reported Activities" (Master's thesis, School of Nursing, University of Illinois, Chicago, 1983).

19. *Sourcebook of Health Insurance Data.*

20. P. Lebrun et al., *Financing for Health Education Services in the United States* (Chicago: Blue Cross and Blue Shield Association, 1980).

SUGGESTED READINGS

American Dietetic Association. *Nutrition Services Payment System.* Chicago, 1984 (430 N. Michigan Ave., Chicago, IL 60611).

American Nurses' Association. *Obtaining Third Party Reimbursement: A Nurse's Guide to Methods and Strategies.* Kansas City, MO , 1984 (2420 Pershing Rd., Kansas City, MO 64108).

Bartlett, E.E. *Assessing the Benefits of Patient Education Under Prospective Pricing.* Birmingham: University of Alabama, 1984 (720 S. 20th St., Birmingham, AL 35294).

Fielding, J. *Corporate Health Management.* Reading, MA: Addison-Wesley, 1984.

LeBrun, P., et al. *Blue Cross and Blue Shield Plan Support for Health Education Services: A Discussion of Issues.* Chicago: Blue Cross and Blue Shield Associations, 1982 (430 N. Michigan Ave., Chicago, IL 50611).

_____. *Financing for Health Education Services in the United States.* Chicago: Blue Cross and Blue Shield Associations, 1980 (Attn: Research and Development—Publications, 676 St. Clair St., 11th Floor, Chicago, IL 60611).

"Prospective Pricing: The Impact of DRGs on Patient Education." *Patient Education and Counseling* 6, no. 2(1984) (Elsevier Scientific Publishers, PO Box 85, Limerick, Ireland).

Reimbursement Committee, Public Health Education Section, American Public Health Association (1015 Fifteenth Street, NW, Washington, DC 20005).

Chapter 3

Assessing Health Education Needs: A Multidimensional-Multimethod Approach

Charles E. Basch, PhD

Although planning and program design are often carried out in a haphazard fashion, a health education practitioner should make every effort to be systematic. How does one respond to an opportunity such as: "We have $4,000 to spend on a health education program for this department. Which problems are the top priorities that we should address in the program"? The person responsible for health education programming must make some key decisions about the needs of the population served by the department and how the money can be used most effectively.

Needs assessment is one of the key elements in planning, developing, implementing, and evaluating a health education program. There are many possible approaches to and functions of needs assessment. The approach presented in this chapter focuses on ways of gathering information and defining needs in order to clarify community health problems that lend themselves to health education strategies and interventions.

The main ideas in the framework that will be described are:

1. Needs should be identified using three dimensions—importance, feasibility, and desirability
2. Multiple methods should be used when collecting data about these dimensions of needs.

A framework for conceptualizing needs assessment approaches can be used for prioritizing health problems that can be addressed through health education programs. The framework for needs assessment discussed in this chapter is oriented toward identifying and prioritizing problems, but it does not focus on determining specific educational methods or learning needs.

As a preamble to discussing the dimensions that underlie the proposed framework and the data collection methods used in needs assessment, three issues are considered: (1) ambiguity about the concepts of need and needs assessment, (2) the relationship between values and needs assessment, and (3) distinctions between different aspects of needs.

AMBIGUITY ABOUT NEEDS AND NEEDS ASSESSMENT

Need is not a universally defined and easily accepted concept. Rather its meaning differs depending on context and values.

> Thus we hear of the need for food, the need for a cigarette, the need for a telephone, the need for trained doctors, and the need for all pupils to study mathematics. It soon becomes obvious that there are subtle but important differences between these senses of the term as well as definite similarities.[1]

Definitions and distinctions related to the concept of need reveal that the way in which need is defined will have implications for selecting appropriate measurement methods and will influence the results of needs assessment.

Many additional definitions related to the concept of need have been discussed elsewhere.[2] In summary:

> Need is at best a relative concept and the definition of need depends primarily on those who undertake the identification and assessment effort . . . [needs] are based on values, culture, past history, and experiences of the individual and the community . . . needs are not singular, easily identifiable entities, but are diffuse and interrelated. Communities and their needs are dynamic and in a constant state of flux.[3]

Given the ambiguity surrounding the concept of need, it is not surprising that needs assessment has been defined in a variety of ways also.[4] Reviewing the many definitions of needs assessment found in the literature seems to result in greater confusion than clarification. A better sense for conceptualizing a needs assessment can be gained by considering the specific functions that needs assessment may serve. The function a needs assessment is

Exhibit 3-1 Examples of Purposes of Needs Assessment and Functions of Needs Assessment Data

---

Purposes

Assess appropriateness of goals, objectives, and activities
Plan new goals, objectives, and activities
Provide guidelines at the state level to help programs meet local needs
Provide accountability information about prevention activities and services
Identify duplication of services and unmet needs

Functions

Identify unmet needs
Identify new target or high-risk populations
Identify duplication of services
Provide baseline data for evaluation
Research the community's perception of the problem
Research the community's perception of the need for services
Identify barriers to the target population utilization of available services
Support request for funding
Support the development of a state plan
Validate current activities
Provide accountability data
Help make decisions about allocation of new funds
Help make decisions about reallocation of funds
Refine agency goals and objectives
Plan new programs
Identify existing services or produce a directory

Source: A Needs Assessment Workbook for Prevention Planning, Vol. II, by National Institute of Drug Abuse, DHHS Publication No. (ADM) 81-1061, Washington, D.C.: U.S. Government Printing Office, 1981.

---

intended to serve may vary considerably. The assessment may focus on identifying and prioritizing problems and be used as a guide in formulating goals and objectives for a new program or it may focus on determining the most appropriate intervention strategies and methods to address alternative needs. Needs assessment may occur at a single point in time to define a new program or it may occur on an ongoing basis to reassess priorities in light of changing needs and opportunities, which in turn can be used to revise goals of an existing program. The data collected in an initial needs assessment may serve as baseline measures in summative evaluation studies. Examples of purposes of needs assessment and functions of needs assessment data are shown in Exhibit 3-1.

VALUES AND NEEDS ASSESSMENT

Defining needs for health education programs will depend in part on the values of those who propose definitions. When health educators are conducting needs assessment or assisting community members in conducting needs assessment, reflection on how their values may be different from those of community members is essential for a successful participative approach. How these differences will be resolved should also be considered as part of planning a needs assessment.

The values of health educators may be in contrast with the target population they are intending to serve.[5] For example, some health educators may personally place a high value on safety and longevity while individuals in a population they are working with may value excitement derived from risk-taking behaviors such as excessive alcohol use or driving over the speed limit. Green and colleagues point out that determinants of personal health behavior are often conflicting. Consider the exchange between two people:

He: Did I hear you say that you are going to try skydiving?
She: Absolutely not!
He: Why not?
She: Because I value my life, that's why not!
He: Do you also value your health?
She: Of course I do.
He: Then why do you smoke cigarettes?
She: Because I enjoy smoking and it helps me relax.
He: If that's the case, can you honestly say that you really value life?
She: Sure I can. It is not that I don't value my life and health but that I value other things too, among them the pleasure of smoking. What's wrong with that?[6]

In a similar vein, data collected for an organization or population are likely to reflect conflicting perceptions of needs and health.

Values are a key issue in defining need and conducting needs assessment. Typically, there is a great deal of competition for resources to conduct health promotion and disease prevention programming and development. Professionals working in various agencies and settings must justify why their problem has the greatest need for resolution. Needs assessment may be biased as groups with vested interests search for data to justify their existing or proposed mission. Often in identifying priorities the best interests of community members are not served. Needs assessment studies are sometimes undertaken primarily as a means to provide program accountability and justify continued resources for a given program rather than identifying top priorities.

If needs assessment is intended to determine what a program's objectives should be, and thus decide how limited resources should be allocated, political, social, and economic values are a key issue. Guba and Lincoln describe six ways that values influence the way the needs assessment is conducted:

1. selecting target states (e.g., physical, psychological, social, etc.) that will be measured;
2. selecting target states that will be used as standards;
3. determining how target states and actual conditions will be measured;
4. determining criteria that will be utilized to judge the extent to which there are discrepancies between actual and target conditions;
5. determining benefit priorities; and
6. determining what constitutes an unsatisfactory condition.[7]

Some needs represent absolute necessities (e.g., food for survival) while other needs represent luxuries (e.g., ice cream). In some cases, however, what constitutes an unsatisfactory condition and absolute necessity in a community context is a value-laden decision.

THREE DISTINCTIONS OF NEEDS

Scriven and Roth identified three distinctions of needs:[8]

1. Motivational vs. functional
2. Performance vs. treatment
3. Basic vs. incremental

These distinctions are useful for both planning a needs assessment and interpreting the findings. Different aspects of needs are more or less relevant at different stages of the planning, implementation, and evaluation cycle. Familiarity with these distinctions should help practitioners to beware of some conceptual and pragmatic traps in conducting needs assessment.

Motivational vs. Functional

The motivational concept is derived from a drive and is equated with felt needs, desires, and cravings, while the functional concept is related to an organic state of deficiency or excess equated with real or genuine needs. Using an individual's felt needs exclusively can be inadequate even when the majority of people within a given community report having a common perception of need.[9] The main problem with relying on felt needs (also referred to as perceived needs or wants) is that individuals may not recognize or want to acknowledge their needs. Lack of awareness of "true" needs may exist in contrast with what an individual wants. For example, because of a preference for "junk food," teenagers may not consume the balance of nutrients necessary in a diet, regardless of awareness that a balance is needed to prevent a deficiency. Compulsive cocaine users feel the need for daily intake of cocaine though they may deny any addiction or interference with performing work or other tasks.

Despite the limitations of felt needs, identifying and understanding felt needs can provide very useful information about a population's readiness to change. Identifying felt needs can indicate areas in which education may be warranted to increase awareness about community problems that are not recognized. Considering the views of the target population is also justified in terms of learning theory and ethics (which are discussed in a later section). Thus, while relying exclusively on felt needs is not recommended, including an analysis of felt needs as one component of needs assessment is often essential.

Performance vs. Treatment

What are the problems that should be addressed through a health education program? Achieving a lower prevalence of automobile accidents, a higher rate of completed childhood immunization levels, or a lower incidence of unplanned teenage pregnancies are all examples of what Scriven and Roth would refer to as performance needs. Clearly, the need for a sixth grade student to reach a specified reading level is different from a need for entering a school-based remedial reading program. In this latter example, the reading level is the performance need while the remedial reading program is referred to as the treatment or intervention need.[10] The nature and scope of a planned intervention require careful analysis of performance needs, as well as an analysis of alternative interventions available.[11] The child may need eye glasses, more sleep, or a different reading instructor instead of placement in a remedial reading program.

The distinction between performance needs and treatment needs has implications for the design of a needs assessment. If the intent of the needs assessment relates to identifying, describing, and prioritizing performance needs (i.e., problems that can be addressed through health education programs), the end product might be formulating goals and objectives that are top priorities. If, on the other hand, the intent is to focus on treatment needs, the results would describe the types of health education strategies and methods that should be employed. In order to conduct an assessment of treatment needs, performance needs (or priority goals and objectives) must be specified first.

Basic vs. Incremental Needs

Basic needs are ongoing and stable, while incremental needs are based on changing circumstances. An elderly person needs to maintain an adequate daily intake of nutrients in order to avoid nutritional deficiencies and illness precipitated by poor nutrition. In contrast, certain needs are incremental. A series of short-term stressful life events such as retirement, moving to an apartment or nursing home, death of a spouse or close friend all require social and emotional support. The needs for a range of supports will be different the first month as compared with five years after retirement or moving into a new living arrangement.

DIMENSIONS OF NEEDS

Three conceptual dimensions of need are useful to consider when planning programs: (1) importance, (2) feasibility, and (3) desirability.[12] Importance is represented by the nature and extent of health problems and their predisposing risk factors found in a defined population. Feasibility is concerned with the resources necessary and available to meet selected needs, and includes finances, personnel, facilities, equipment, time, resources of the target population, and technical sophistication. Desirability focuses on the extent to which the target population, decision makers, and other stakeholding audiences are interested in, committed to, and willing and ready to address alternative needs. Failure to consider any one of these dimensions may produce results that do not make good use of available resources.

How Important Is the Need?

The importance of health education needs may be assessed by studying health problems in a community in terms of:

- distribution
- prevalence
- severity of consequences for individuals (e.g., disability, suffering)
- severity of consequences for the community (e.g., economic, social)
- urgency (e.g., predicted incidence)

Importance can be estimated through population data that are useful in making inferences about illness problems in a defined population. Some of these data are relatively accessible, such as age- and sex-specific mortality rates. However, data about morbidity are often less accessible unless access privileges to individuals' medical records, insurance claims, or hospitalization data can be obtained. Even if access to confidential records is possible, inconsistent definitions and reporting formats may present problems for arriving at a reliable and valid description of problems.

Conducting a thorough descriptive epidemiological analysis of a defined population may not be necessary or possible for most health educators. A less thorough and less specific analysis of morbidity and mortality may be performed by drawing upon existing demographic or epidemiological data bases. Knowing one characteristic about the defined population, such as age distribution, can suggest what kinds of problems are likely to be most prevalent.[13] Other general characteristics about population distributions, including sex, race, occupation, marital status, and religion, can also be informative with respect to opportunities for disease prevention.[14] Thus analysis of the sociodemographic composition of the community and current and anticipated patterns of injuries, illnesses, and deaths in the defined target population is one way of justifying importance.

Identifying the incidence and prevalence of physiologic risk factors that may provide early warning signals of illness, such as high blood pressure or high serum cholesterol, is another way of describing which needs are most important. Risk factors vary according to population subgroups. For example, inner-city preschool children may be at risk for high levels of lead in their blood; black males over age 35 often have hypertension; women over age 55 are at greater risk of breast cancer than younger women. Several sources provide guidelines for the kinds of physiological characteristics that warrant screening or examination in various high risk groups and at various stages in the life cycle.[15] Principles and ethical issues related to establishing screening programs for determining risk factors should be considered prior to initiating such programs as a component of a needs assessment.[16]

Relying exclusively on mortality, morbidity, and symptomatology as indicators of the importance of community health problems has limitations, particularly if the focus of the program to be designed will be on primary prevention—reducing susceptibility and exposure to problems and promoting optimum health. Because behaviors that are within individuals' discretion have been established as important determinants of health status, a thorough assessment of which needs are most important includes an analysis of the incidence and prevalence of certain behavioral health risk factors in the community. Examples of the kinds of behavioral (and other) risk factors that may be most relevant to preventing various health problems are shown in Table 3-1.

Table 3–1 Major Causes of Death in 1977 and Associated Risk Factors

Causes	Percent of all deaths	Risk factors
Heart disease	37.8	Smoking,* hypertension,* elevated serum cholesterol* (diet), lack of exercise, diabetes, stress, family history
Malignant neoplasms	20.4	Smoking,* work-site carcinogens,* environmental carcinogen, alcohol, diet
Stroke	9.6	Hypertension,* smoking,* elevated serum cholesterol,* stress
Accidents other than motor vehicle	2.8	Alcohol,* drug abuse, smoking (fires), product design, handgun availability
Influenza and pneumonia	2.7	Smoking, vaccination status*
Motor vehicle accidents	2.6	Alcohol,* no seat belts,* speed,* roadway design, vehicle engineering
Diabetes	1.7	Obesity*
Cirrhosis of the liver	1.6	Alcohol abuse*
Arteriosclerosis	1.5	Elevated serum cholesterol*
Suicide	1.5	Stress,* alcohol and drug abuse, gun availability

*Major risk factor.

Source: U.S. Department of Health and Human Services, *Health, United States, 1980,* DHHS Publication No. PHS 81-1232, Washington, D.C.: U.S. Government Printing Office, 1980, p. 274.

Thus assessment of the importance dimension may include numerous kinds of data: demography, current and predicted disease incidence, distribution and severity patterns of health problems, prevalence of physiological and behavioral risk factors. Even though some problems may be very important, based on the extent of disease, disability, and death they cause or are expected to cause, some may not be feasible to address. In such cases, scarce health education resources would be used more effectively to address problems that are less important but more feasible to resolve through health education.[17]

What Is Feasible?

Feasibility assessment focuses on resources that are required to deal with problems identified. Resources may include the time, money, personnel, facilities, equipment, materials, and technical support that are available within an organization, a community, and the target population. For a target population resources may include time and money to participate in programs, the kinds and level of skills members have, and their social support systems. Technical resources in this context refers to the extent to which the state-of-the-art educational, behavioral, clinical, or other technology exists that has demonstrated ability to effectively address a given problem.

Feasibility assessment should distinguish resources that are available to address a given need and are being used for that purpose from those that are available but not allocated. For example, feasibility of addressing the problem of low levels of fitness in a community might be improved since schools usually have gymnasiums, showers, various types of recreational equipment, and personnel specially trained in physical education. Workplace health promotion programs may be feasible in relatively large corporations that can afford to build recreational facilities, but small companies may have difficulty establishing such programs because of inability to support a staff and provide facilities. Even though a particular school, business, or hospital may not have many resources, the community or region in which it is located may have a variety of resources that can be utilized.[18] Local voluntary agencies, K–12 schools, colleges, and other public and private organizations sponsor various educational and service programs and provide a wealth of facilities and human resources that can be tapped.

An effort may also be made to study resources of the target population. This effort may be cursory and focus on the amount of time and money they have available to participate in programs. Or it may be more in-depth and consider the target population's levels of literacy, skills, and social support. Knowledge about the resources of a target population will help to assess the feasibility of addressing certain needs, and may also be useful in discovering situations in which improving the resources of a target group may be the focus of programs to be designed.

A different aspect of feasibility assessment relates to technical resources necessary to bring about change. Has educational, behavioral, clinical, or other technology progressed to the point of being able to resolve a particular problem? Even though feasibility may be low, for example, because of scarce resources or unavailable technology, in some cases needs may be so important (e.g., high incidence rate and high virulence of Acquired Immune Deficiency Syndrome) that they warrant being a top priority in order to improve feasibility. A problem may be very important and addressing it may be feasible, but if community members or leaders do not legitimize the need, the success of any programs that are developed will be hampered. Thus assessment of the desirability of alternative needs provides information necessary for developing priorities.

What Is Desirable?

Assessment of desirability is intended to identify problems that the target population is most interested in and supportive of based on members' feelings and opinions. This represents a more affective dimension of need as compared with importance and feasibility. Many health education programs have relied on felt needs as the primary or even the sole basis for needs assessment. As mentioned previously, relying exclusively on felt needs has been criticized as being merely assessment of wants. Although individuals may not truly be aware of their needs, they are likely to perceive that they do know what they need. A practitioner (often an "outsider") may not be able to see the world as the target group sees it. Thus it may be debated whether a practitioner's assessment of community needs reflects "true" needs. Considering the target group's views in needs assessment is consistent with the ethical and philosophical principles of health education practice.[19] From a practical learning theory perspective, familiarity with the target group's views will maximize the chances that programs are planned in ways that they will be implemented, maintained, and sustain a high level of participation.[20]

The dimension of desirability is particularly important for assessment of health education needs because the health problems that are often identified as priorities involve behaviors within the area of the individual's freedom of choice. Hochbaum argues that the best way to bring about change in personal health-related behaviors is to convince the individual or group of individuals that one choice is more advantageous to them than another in order to achieve what *they* want.[21] Those who could benefit most from programs are often least likely to participate. Thus a relevant question that can be answered by assessing desirability is: How can we adapt ideas, programs, and services to the interests, concerns, values, vocabulary, and customs of our target group?[22] According to Nix, "The most effective way is to involve the people themselves in defining their own health (or other) problems or needs, and then to involve them in a study-planning-action process to solve their identified health problems."[23] Three stakeholding audiences—those with vested interests—for whom desirability (i.e., felt needs) should be assessed are (1) representatives and leaders from the target population, (2) leaders from the community, and (3) organizations and staff members who are most likely to be responsible for program implementation. Health care providers and significant others in the lives of the target population may also provide useful input in desirability assessment.

In assessing desirability, health educators may be able to apply some of the strategies and methods used in marketing research. The analysis of wants certainly appears to play a major role in the marketing of programs, products, and ideas. The advertising industry has utilized marketing analysis as a tool to manipulate human behavior.[24] Perhaps one reason why marketing research has been applicable is that it assists the management and creative people in advertising agencies to see the world as the target audience see it. This information can then be utilized as a tool for planning advertising strategies.

The value of applying marketing to health education practice as well as to the health services and social causes has been described in the literature.[25] We should remember that unlike marketing and advertising agencies, which are most effective at affecting brand preferences, have extensive resources, communicate simple messages, and are satisfied with changes in small segments of the population, health education programs may be intended to affect well-established and valued behaviors, may have limited resources to work with, may seek to communicate complex messages and may be expected to influence large segments of the population.[26]

DATA COLLECTION METHODS FOR ASSESSING HEALTH EDUCATION NEEDS

Needs assessment will, in most cases, call for the use of multiple methods of data collection. By using multiple methods we are able to maximize benefits and minimize limitations. The following data collection methods are useful for assessing health education needs:[27]

1. reviewing secondary sources of population data
2. reviewing service utilization records
3. conducting a community survey
4. utilizing key informants
5. conducting a community forum

Reviewing Secondary Sources of Population Data

A review of secondary sources of data can include published statistical reports, census data, and other research results. These data bases describe social and health-related characteristics of a population. At the national level, many data systems have been established to document the health status of population subgroups and these can provide data for a specific locale. For example:

1. National Vital Registration System, which includes natality—births and birth rates by place of birth and mother's age, sex, race, parity and place of residence; and mortality—deaths by age, sex, race and cause
2. National Case Reporting System, which includes reported cases of sexually transmitted diseases

3. National Morbidity and Mortality Reporting System, which includes data about reportable communicable diseases.[28]

The National Health Survey, which includes the Health Interview Survey, the Health and Nutrition Examination Survey, and the National Family Growth Survey, is a national population-based survey that is not intended to collect information about specific localities but may be useful for drawing inferences about various population subgroups. Other national data bases are the Vital Statistics Registration System, the National Death Index, and the Professional Activity Study System. There are also ongoing national surveys conducted for specific health-related behaviors, such as drug use among certain population subgroups.[29]

State- and local-level sources of population information are also useful. The state health department and planning agencies are likely to have a variety of background data about the population. Some states may have disease registers to facilitate monitoring and follow-up of certain diseases. Surveys of health-related risk behaviors in the population are currently conducted by many state health departments in cooperation with the Centers for Disease Control. The Department of Health, Department of Education, Department of Motor Vehicles, and the central office of the State Police also maintain records that relate to various health problems. State-level professional organizations, such as hospital associations, medical societies, and public health groups, may also provide archival data about disease incidence and prevalence and about availability of resources. Note, however, that it may be difficult to obtain access privileges to these data, and even if access can be obtained it may be difficult to abstract the relevant data in a usable form. The quality of these data varies widely.

At the local level, government agencies, hospitals, clinics and practitioners, school systems, police, counseling centers, businesses and industries, health-related voluntary agencies, planning groups, and insurance companies are examples of possible sources of demographic and health-related data about a local population. Local data may be provided to practitioners in the form of numbers of cases rather than rates. If this is so, census data can be used to estimate the population at risk (which in some cases may be difficult) and calculate rates. Local data may be very useful when conducting needs assessment because, despite evidence to the contrary, community members may not believe that state- and national-level statistics accurately depict their locality.

An advantage of health and social statistics is that they help describe communities regarding income, population density, housing, unemployment, crime, health care utilization and distribution, and types of morbidity and mortality. Using rates, comparisons can be made about the extent of a given illness or accident problem relative to state or national rates. These kinds of data are useful for identifying the importance and feasibility dimensions of local needs.

Health and social statistics in some cases represent large units of analysis (e.g., regions). Practitioners should recognize that these data are indirect measures of need, they may be unreliable and invalid, and they may not be in a usable form.[30] Cautions and caveats about using health and social indicators based on large populations for assessing needs have been discussed and should be considered when designing studies.[31] If the scale of the needs assessment is on a macro level or there is reason to believe that the data can be generalized to local populations, these approaches are potentially very useful, particularly for identifying high-risk groups.

Reviewing Service Utilization Records

Data from service utilization records describe the nature and extent of medical care and related services being utilized. Data may also come from internal audits or service accreditation reports. The assumption is that patterns of utilization to some degree reflect community problems or demands and may reveal significant educational needs. Management information systems may be used to collect data on an ongoing basis for monitoring patterns of service utilization.[32] Secular, cyclical, seasonal, and short-term trends in various health problems can become more evident and would be useful indicators for program planning.

In conducting needs assessment, the availability of data sources (e.g., clinic records), relatively low cost and timeliness, potential to predict future demands, and ability to analyze differences for different community segments underlie advantages of using service utilization records. A major drawback of this technique is that those individuals or groups that have the greatest needs may be isolated, poor, and lack skills to obtain services. The transient nature of some population segments in the community, as well as groups that overutilize services, can result in a skewed representation of needs. The reliability and validity of these records may vary widely and they may be incomplete, inaccurate, and illegible.[33]

Conducting a Community Survey

A community population survey involves collecting new data about a defined population. While surveys are conducted frequently, it seems that adequate attention to reliability and validity is often lacking. Community survey approaches seem most relevant for collecting data about the importance and desirability dimensions of needs. Data can be obtained by observations, interviews, or self-administered questionnaires. Community survey methods that seem to be used often are mailed questionnaires, telephone interviews, and personal interviews. The detailed advantages and disadvantages of alternative data collection methods and the type of information that can be most appropriately obtained with each have been described in detail elsewhere.[34]

The major advantages of community survey techniques for obtaining data about a target group's knowledge, attitudes, behaviors, and experiences are their ability to: collect many different kinds of information; provide anonymity (in some cases); utilize probability sampling designs and thus obtain representative samples and estimate sampling error; involve the target populations; and, potentially, to obtain reliable, valid, and direct information about needs. The disadvantages include the relatively high cost, difficulties in acquiring or designing appropriate instruments and procedures for sampling, as well as difficulties related to data collection and analysis.[35]

One type of survey tool useful in conducting community surveys for health education needs assessment is the health risk appraisal. This tool is designed to estimate probabilities of morbidity and mortality by analyzing information about an individual's personal and health characteristics. Estimates of risk are derived from statistical probabilities based on population parameters. Individuals' responses to a questionnaire, and, for more elaborate appraisal systems, clinical measures (e.g., anthropometric characteristics, blood pressure, blood lipids, etc.), are used to produce a personal health profile report indicating ways in which an individual can modify his or her behavior to reduce the risk of various illnesses or injuries.

Health hazard appraisals have been used to motivate individuals to become interested in changing certain health-related behaviors, for example, using seatbelts or eliminating cigarette smoking. Although these tools are generally used to motivate individuals to modify behaviors, when they are administered to an entire population or a representative sample, the aggregated data set may provide very useful information about the health-related problems and risk factors within that population. Research and methodological issues related to risk estimation and limitations of health hazard appraisal tools have been reviewed elsewhere.[36]

Utilizing Key Informants

The key informant approach involves collecting information from individuals who are considered to be experts or representatives of certain groups and who can identify and define community needs relevant to a given topic area. An extension of this technique is to convene a meeting of several key informants to discuss health problems and identify health education needs.

The key informant approach often uses a nonprobability sampling design. Nonprobability sampling designs possess a number of inherent problems. Identifying individuals who are truly representative or expert may be difficult. Those selected may be biased depending on their personal or organizational perspective. Key informants may not be aware of the spectrum of needs of particular subgroups. Data obtained from discussions are impressionistic.

Table 3–2 Examples of Key Informants by Dimensions of Need and Setting

Dimensions of Need	Setting			
	School	Workplace	Medical	Community
Importance	School nurse Pediatricians Emergency department personnel Students	Medical directors Insurance agent OSHA expert NIOSH expert Personnel director Employees	Hospital administrator Medical director Nursing director Epidemiologist Patients Physicians	Physicians Emergency department personnel Health department officials Epidemiologists Community members
Feasibility	School superintendent School principals Teachers Technical experts	CEO Mid-level managers Personnel directors Technical experts	Hospital administrator Medical director Nursing director Technical experts	Positional leaders (e.g., mayor, bank president, etc.) Human services agency director Community leaders Technical experts
Desirability	Students Parents School board members PTA members Teachers School administrators	Employees Union representatives Mid-level and high-level administrators	Patients Patient subgroups Nurses Physicians Staff Students Mid-level and high-level administrators	General population Leaders and representatives of solidarity groups (e.g., PTA, Lions, etc.) Positional leaders and those with social influence

This approach involves low to moderate costs, is relatively easy and quick, and enables different perspectives (e.g., administrators, staff, target population, etc.) to be voiced. The process of conducting discussions with key informants also establishes the potential for fostering collaborative efforts during program planning and implementation.[37]

The key informant approach may be used to obtain information about all three dimensions of need—importance, feasibility and desirability. Selecting informants may be difficult, depending on the setting, culture, language, and other social factors. Specific techniques for identifying key informants and other aspects of implementing this method have been described elsewhere.[38] Table 3-2 lists examples of key informants in different settings that can provide input about each of the three dimensions of need.

Conducting a Community Forum

The community forum approach to needs assessment involves arranging one or more meetings where community members are invited to attend to express their views about certain issues or health problems. These forums should be adequately publicized and held in an accessible and a secure location. Questions prepared in advance allow a group leader to focus discussions around the selected topics. Community forums are useful for assessing the desirability of alternative needs. A forum may also be an effective means to obtain input from various population segments and, more important, it may be a useful means of identifying local individuals who are most interested in the topic and may be excellent resources for planning, implementing, and evaluating programs, as well as identifying local individuals that may be major opponents to future efforts. Conducting a community forum is relatively easy and inexpensive. Difficulty in obtaining representative attendance and the inability of some individuals to articulate their views in a public meeting are some disadvantages. Also, if not planned well, a forum can develop into a grievance session or raise awareness about needs that may not be feasible to address.

INTEGRATING PERCEPTIONS OF NEEDS AND DATA IN AN ORGANIZATIONAL CONTEXT

Few authors have dealt with the challenging problem of integrating the different kinds of data obtained in order to establish priorities. Consensus methods have been used for solving problems and defining levels of agreement related to a wide variety of topics.[39] An advantage of these methods is their ability to integrate information. Fink and her colleagues have described advantages, limitations, and guidelines for use of four consensus methods: (1) the delphi technique, (2) the nominal group technique, (3) NIH consensus development, and (4) Glaser's state-of-the-art approach.[40] Critical incident technique[41] and Q-sort technique[42] could also be grouped appropriately into this family of methods. These methods are compared and contrasted in Table 3-3.

Another approach to integrating many different kinds of data collected in needs assessment is decision analysis. There are many techniques that can be applied to analyze decisions regarding needs assessment.[43] These techniques facilitate weighting the importance of various data and standardizing results in a way that permits deciding on priorities using different evaluative criteria. These techniques do not deny the interplay between facts and values but rather they may be used to make explicit the value judgments that are guiding decisions.

Decisions about needs and goals take place within a political context.[44] There will often be stakeholders that try to prioritize problems and goals to meet their agenda. Needs assessment results are only one of many forms of input that go into a political decision-making process to allocate scarce resources; other factors may be who knows and likes whom and who owes a favor or who may want a favor in the future.

Conducting a needs assessment involves technical knowledge and skills, but it is essential that decisions about priority needs and goals in a community not be left to technicians. Involvement of those with vested interests to integrate the data obtained and reach consensus about priority needs and goals is a key feature of successful needs assessment. Assisting individuals to pursue their own goals distinguishes health education from other fields that may aim to manipulate individuals' behaviors through coercive or involuntary means.[45] The goal of community organization, one of the major methods of health education, is to empower people to identify and solve their own problems.[46] If practitioners can assist community members to identify problems by using systematic methods of needs assessment, they will have improved the chances for developing programs that will be supported and maintained. As noted previously, people who are involved in programs from their inception will be more likely to feel ownership of the program and will be more likely to participate and learn.

PLANNING A NEEDS ASSESSMENT

The framework proposed in this chapter emphasizes defining needs utilizing three dimensions, importance, feasibility, and desirability, and measuring these dimensions of needs by applying multiple data collection methods. This framework is consistent with well-established principles of measurement.

Table 3-3 Characteristics of Methods for Collecting Data from Small Groups

Description	Possible Applications	Advantages	Disadvantages
Delphi			
Respondents work independently but are informed of consensus among the total group. Responses are obtained for several rounds until an acceptable level of agreement or a point of diminishing returns is reached.	Rate alternative scenarios depicting a problem; predict problems that will increase in the future; prioritize goals, objectives, needs; assign weights of importance to different data sources; develop new information and integrate information.	Flexible regarding numbers of respondents and rounds, and possible range of topics; relatively inexpensive; potential for anonymity; potential to sample from wide geographical area; ability to determine agreement about complex issues for which definite answers are not known; may be used with specific community segment.	Reliability related directly to group size and number of rounds; may be time consuming; may be difficult to identify most appropriate respondents.
Nominal Group			
A structured group process activity in which respondents work on a topic independently and then share, discuss, clarify, and critique the total pool of responses.	Generate alternative definitions of a problem; prioritize goals, objectives, needs; develop new information about desirability and importance of needs; integrate information.	Timely; relatively inexpensive; applicable to diverse topics; generating new ideas and new ways of viewing problems; group spontaneity may lead to serendipitous findings; usable with specific community segments.	Requires trained discussion leader; geographical constraints; onus on facilitator and respondents to collaborate with one another for technique to work.

(continues)

Table 3–3 continued

Description	Possible Applications	Advantages	Disadvantages
NIH Consensus Development The National Institutes of Health (NIH) has attempted to gain consensus about emerging health problems and the safety, efficacy, and appropriateness of clinical procedures and medical technology by bringing together individuals from various perspectives (e.g., practitioner, researcher, consumer, etc.) to jointly evaluate existing technology.	Obtain alternative definitions of problems; use various perspectives represented to make decisions about priorities; generate new information and integrate existing information; collect data about importance, feasibility, and desirability of needs.	Obtains input from diverse perspectives; applicable to wide range of topics; timely; facilitates publicity of finding, which, in turn, may promote policy change.	May be difficult and costly to coordinate recruitment and meeting of respondents; requires trained leader.
Glaser's State-of-the-Art-Approach Technique for describing the state-of-the-art in a given topic area. A small group of respondents highly respected in their areas of study are selected who, with the assistance of a group facilitator, develop an initial position paper that is distributed for comments to other individuals who are knowledgeable about the given topic. Then the small group and the facilitator redraft the initial position paper into a form that is generally acceptable. Final revisions may then be undertaken based on the small group's remaining concerns.	Define the state-of-the-art of resource technology and assessing feasibility of needs.	Including prominent individuals improves visibility of results and may be perceived as credible by various audiences; timely; promotes participation among representatives of solidarity groups, such as professional associations; may help gain support for findings; reaches consensus about areas that contain many unanswered questions and are important to resolve.	Very skilled facilitator and knowledgeable respondents are required; relatively expensive; results may be biased by selection of initial small group; relatively large burden on initial small group.

Critical Incident Respondents describe situations from their personal experience relating to a given topic or problem. Stories and anecdotal reports and observations can be considered collectively or in a segmental fashion to gain insight from various respondents' experiences.	Collecting in-depth information about context may be used to learn about the experience of community members in their own words and gain understanding about how they perceive problems.	Can use authorities to describe situations with a specific focus; can provide a direct measure of personal experience rather than relying on indirect measures; and specific information may be obtained.	Requires a population capable of understanding what is being asked and able to articulate their response verbally or in writing; may be time consuming and complicated to analyze results; relies on personnel trained in content analysis; relatively high burden on judges, thus it may be difficult to identify interested and qualified judges; may be difficult to obtain reliability in isolation of key concepts and categorization of events.
Q-Sort Technique Numerous possible values for a given variable, such as possible program objectives, needs, problems, or interest areas, are written on separate cards. Then respondents place cards into categories indicating the position of one variable value relative to others on a scale, for example, highest priority to lowest priority.	To prioritize problems, needs, and objectives. To integrate existing and newly developed information.	May be timely; can be used to obtain consensus; relatively easy to analyze results and inexpensive.	May be difficult to administer; difficult to obtain information requiring many different types of response scales; may be difficult for respondents.

Source: Portions of material on pp.67 and 68 are based on "'Consensus Methods: Characteristics and Guidelines for Use," by A. Fink, J. Kosecoff, M. Chassin, and R. Brook, *American Journal of Public Health* 74 (1984): 979–983.

There is no single best approach to conducting needs assessment. The process may be small in scale and informal or it may require substantial resources. The questions listed below are useful to consider when planning a needs assessment:

- Does it make sense to conduct a needs assessment given the amount of time and money available and the likelihood that
  the information obtained will be utilized for decision making?
- When must the needs assessment be completed to be useful for decision making?
- How can vested interest groups and community decision makers be involved in the needs assessment?
- Who are trusted individuals that can serve as go-betweens to reach compromise among competing factions?
- What is the purpose and scope of the needs assessment with respect to the target population and the kinds of needs to be identified?
- What information about the importance, feasibility, and desirability dimensions of needs will be collected, and how will this information be used?
- Are there any existing data sources that can be used in the needs assessment?
- Which methods will be used to collect data about the various dimensions of needs?
- Who will be responsible for the various tasks in the needs assessment?
- What are the salient values of those conducting the needs assessment and the target population and how will these values influence the process and outcome of the effort?
- What are the greatest anticipated barriers to conducting a useful needs assessment and how can they be overcome?
- What are the limitations of the data collected in the needs assessment?
- How will the data obtained be integrated to prioritize needs and make decisions?
- What are the ethical issues involved in conducting the needs assessment (e.g., privacy, raising expectations, unanticipated adverse side effects, etc.) and how will these be dealt with?
- How can needs assessment be planned to reflect changing needs, opportunities, and constraints?

NOTES

1. Reginald D. Archambault, "The Concept of Need and Its Relation to Certain Aspects of Educational Theory," *Harvard Educational Review* 27 (1957): 40.

2. Michael Scriven and Jane Roth, "Needs Assessment: Concept and Practice," *New Directions in Program Evaluation* 1 (1978): 1–11; Jonathan Bradshaw, "The Concept of Social Need," *Ekistics* 220 (March 1974): 184–187; and Ronald Walton, "Need: A Central Concept," *Social Service Quarterly* 43 (1969): 13–17.

3. Larry M. Siegel, C. Clifford Attkission, and Linda G. Carson, "Need Identification and Program Planning in the Community Context," in *Evaluation of Human Service Programs,* ed. C. Clifford Attkission et al. (New York: Academic Press, 1978), 216, 220.

4. H.L. Blum, *Planning for Health: Development and Application of Social Change Theory* (New York: Behavioral Publications, 1974); George J. Warheit, Roger A. Bell, and John J. Schwab, *Needs Assessment Approaches: Concepts and Methods,* DHEW Publication No. 79-472 (Washington, D.C.: Government Printing Office, 1979); Roger A. Kaufman, "Needs Assessment," in *Fundamental Curricular Decisions: ASCD 1983 Yearbook,* ed. F.W. English (Alexandria, Va.: Association for Supervision and Curriculum Development, 1983), 53–67; Edna Kamis, "A Witness for the Defense of Needs Assessment," *Evaluation and Program Planning* 2 (1979): 7–12; and Michael Scriven, *Evaluation Thesaurus,* 3rd ed. (Iverness, Calif.: Edgepress, 1981).

5. Joan Hayes and Betty Mathews, "Human Values: Implications for Health Education Practice," *International Journal of Health Education* 17 (1974): 266–273.

6. Lawrence W. Green et al., *Health Education Planning: A Diagnostic Approach* (Palo Alto, Calif.: Mayfield, 1980), 73.

7. Egon G. Guba and Yvonnea S. Lincoln, "The Place of Values in Needs Assessment," *Educational Evaluation and Policy Analysis* 4 (1982): 311–320.

8. Scriven and Roth, "Needs Assessment," 1–11.

9. Archambault, "The Concept of Need," 38–62; Scriven and Roth, "Needs Assessment," 1–11; Bradshaw, "The Concept of Social Need," 184–187; Scriven, *Evaluation Thesaurus;* Guba and Lincoln, "The Place of Values," 311–320.

10. Scriven and Roth, "Needs Assessment," 1–11.

11. Ibid.; Stuart J. Cohen, "Potential Barriers to Diabetes Care," *Diabetes Care* 6 (1983): 499–500; Donna M. Howard. "Health Education Needs Assessment in an HMO: A Case Study," *Health Education Quarterly* 9 (1982): 23–41; Judith H. Nicklason, Molla S. Donaldson, and John E. Ott, "HMO Members and Clinicians Rank Health Education Needs," *Public Health Reports* 98 (1983): 222–226; H.A. Goddard and M.J. Powers, "Educational Needs of Patients Undergoing Hemodialysis: A Comparison of Patient and Nurse Perceptions," *Dialysis Transplant* 11 (1982): 578–583; and P. Lauer, S.P. Murphy, and M.J. Powers, "Learning Needs of Cancer Patients: A Comparison of Nurse and Patient Perceptions," *Nursing Research* 31 (1982): 11–16.

12. Siegel, Attkission, and Carson, "Need Identification," 215–252.

13. Office of the Assistant Secretary for Health, *Healthy People: The Surgeon General's Report on Health Promotion and Disease Prevention,* DHHS Publication No. (PHS) 79-55071 (Washington, D.C.: Government Printing Office, 1979).

14. Judith S. Mausner and Shira Kramer, *Epidemiology: An Introductory Text* (Philadelphia: W.B. Saunders, 1985).

15. Katherine G. Bauer, *Improving the Chances for Health: Lifestyle Change and Health Education* (San Francisco: National Center for Health Education, 1980); Lawrence W. Green and C.L. Anderson, *Community Health,* 4th ed. (St. Louis: C.V. Mosby, 1982); Council on Scientific Affairs, "Medical Evaluations of Healthy Persons," *Journal of the American Medical Association* 249 (1983): 1626–1633; and Jonathan E. Fielding, "Risk Reduction Goals Throughout Life," in *Promoting Health Through Risk Reduction,* ed. Marilyn M. Farber and Adina M. Reinhardt (New York: Macmillan, 1982).

16. Mausner and Kramer, *Epidemiology.*

17. Green et al., *Health Education Planning.*

18. Charles E. Basch, Sharon Zelasko, and Barbara Burkholder, "An Alternative Approach to Worksite Health Promotion: The Consortium Model," *Health Education* 15, no. 7 (1985): 22–24.

19. Godfrey Hochbaum, "Ethical Dilemmas in Health Education," *Health Education* 11, no. 2 (1980): 4–6; Lawrence W. Green, "Health Education Models," in *Behavioral Health: A Handbook of Health Enhancement and Disease Prevention,* ed. J.D. Matarazzo et al. (New York: John Wiley, 1984), 181–198; and Lawrence W. Green. "Determining the Impact and Effectiveness of Health Education as It Relates to Federal Policy," *Health Education Monographs* 6 (1978, Suppl. 1): 28–66.

20. Jeannette Simmons, "Making Health Education Work," *American Journal of Public Health* 65 (1975, Suppl.): 13; and Harold L. Nix, *The Community and Its Involvement in the Study-Planning-Action Process,* DHEW Publication No. (CDC) 78-8355 (Washington, D.C.: Government Printing Office, 1977).

21. Godfrey Hochbaum, "How Do You Want to Live the Rest of Your Life?" (Paper presented at the Nutrition-Health Education section session of the Fiftieth Annual Meeting of the Florida Public Health Association, Orlando, Florida, October 5, 1978).

22. Simmons, "Making Health Education Work."

23. Nix, *The Community and Its Involvement,* 73.

24. Michael Schudson, *Advertising, the Uneasy Persuasion: Its Dubious Impact on American Society* (New York: Basic Books, 1984).

25. Richard Manoff, *Social Marketing: New Imperative for Public Health* (New York: Praeger, 1985); John Bonaguro and George Miaoulis, *Marketing and Health Promotion* (Athens: Ohio University, 1982); Karen Fox and Philip Kotler, "The Marketing of Social Causes: The First 10 Years," *Journal of Marketing* 44 (Fall 1980): 24–33; Philip Kotler, *Marketing for Nonprofit Organizations,* 2nd ed. (Englewood Cliffs, N.J.: Prentice-Hall, 1982); and W.A. Flexner, J.E. Littlefield, and C.P. McLaughlin, "Discovering What the Health Consumer Really Wants," *Health Care Management Review* 1 (1977): 43–49.

26. Godfrey Hochbaum, "Selling Health to the Public," in *Consumer Behavior in the Market Place,* ed. I.M. Newman (Lincoln: University of Nebraska, 1976).

27. Warheit, Bell, and Schwab, *Needs Assessment Approaches;* and National Institute of Drug Abuse, *A Needs Assessment Workbook for Prevention Planning,* vol. II, DHHS Publication No. (ADM) 81-1061 (Washington, D.C.: Government Printing Office, 1981).

28. Office of the Assistant Secretary for Health, *Promoting Health, Preventing Disease: Objectives for the Nation* (Washington, D.C.: Government Printing Office, 1980).

29. Mausner and Kramer, *Epidemiology;* and Lloyd D. Johnson, Patrick M. O'Malley, and Jerald G. Bachman, *Drugs and American High School Students,* DHHS Publication No. (ADM) 85-1374 (Rockville, Md.: National Institute on Drug Abuse, 1984).

30. Warheit, Bell, and Schwab, *Needs Assessment Approaches.*

31. Roland N. Pippin, "Assessing the Needs of the Elderly with Existing Data," *Gerontologist* 20 (1980): 65–70; Steven B. Withey. "On the Wide Open Options for Social Indicators," *Evaluation and Program Planning* 2 (1979): 5–6; Laurence T. Cagle, "Using Social Indicators to Assess Mental Health Needs," *Evaluation Review* 8 (1984): 389–412; George G. Warheit, Joanne M. Buhl, and Roger A. Bell, "A Critique of Social Indicators Analysis and Key Informant Surveys as Needs Assessment Methods," *Evaluation and Program Planning* 1 (1978): 239–247; Joan E. Sieber, "Critical Appraisal of Social Indicators," *Evaluation and*

Program Planning 2 (1979): 13–16; and Nancy Cochran, "On the Limiting Properties of Social Indicators," *Evaluation and Program Planning* 2 (1979): 1–4.

32. J. Philip Shambaugh, Harold F. Goldsmith, David J. Jackson, and Beatrice M. Rosen, "The Mental Health Demographic Profile System," *Journal of Health and Social Behavior* 6 (1979): 215–237.

33. Warheit, Bell, and Schwab, *Needs Assessment Approaches.*

34. Lynn Morris and Carol Fitz-Gibbon, *How to Measure Program Implementation* (Beverly Hills, Calif.: Sage, 1978); Sir Claus Moser and Graham Kalton, *Survey Methods in Social Investigation* (London: Heinemann, 1979); Fred N. Kerlinger, *Foundations of Behavioral Research* (New York: Holt, Rinehart, & Winston, 1973); and R. Zemke and T. Kramlinger, *Figuring Things Out* (Reading, Mass.: Addison-Wesley, 1985).

35. Warheit, Bell, and Schwab, *Needs Assessment Approaches.*

36. Jeffrey J. Sacks, W. Mark Krushat, and Jeffrey Newman, "Reliability of the Health Hazard Appraisal," *American Journal of Public Health* 70 (1980): 730–740; Edward H. Wagner, William L. Berry, Victor J. Schoenbach, et al. "An Assessment of Health Hazard/ Health Risk Appraisal," *American Journal of Public Health* 72 (1982): 347–352; Axel A. Goetz, Jean F. Duff, and James E. Bernstein, "Health Risk Appraisal: The Estimation of Risk," *Public Health Reports* 95 (1980): 119–126; and T.M. Vogt, "Risk Assessment and Health Hazard Appraisal," *Annual Review of Public Health* 2 (1981): 31–47; and William Beery, Victor J. Schoenbach, Edward H. Wagner, et al., "Health Risk Appraisal: Methods and Programs with Annotated Bibliography," DHHS Publication No. (PHS) 86-3396 (Rockville, Md.: National Center for Health Services Research and Health Technology Assessment, 1986).

37. Warheit, Bell, and Schwab, *Needs Assessment Approaches.*

38. Ibid.; Nix, *The Community and Its Involvement;* and National Institute of Drug Abuse, *A Needs Assessment Workbook.*

39. Arlene Fink, Jacqueline Kosecoff, Mark Chassin, and Robert Brook, "Consensus Methods: Characteristics and Guidelines for Use," *American Journal of Public Health* 74 (1984): 979–983.

40. Ibid.

41. John C. Flanagan, "The Critical Incident Technique," *Psychological Bulletin* 51 (1954): 327–358.

42. Douglas R. Berdie and John F. Anderson, *Questionnaires: Design and Use* (Metuchen, N.J.: Scarecrow Press, 1974).

43. Ward Edwards, Marcia Guttentag, and K.A. Snapper, "A Decision Theoretical Approach to Evaluation Research," in Elmer L. Struening and Marcia Guttentag, eds., *Handbook of Evaluation Research* (Beverly Hills, Calif.: Sage, 1975); and Ward Edwards, "Use of Multiattribute Utility Measurement for Social Decision Making," in *Conflicting Objectives in Decision,* ed. Roger A. Bell et al. (New York: John Wiley, 1977).

44. Carol Weiss, "Where Politics and Evaluation Meet," *Evaluation* 1 (1973): 37–45.

45. Green, "Determining the Impact," 28–66.

46. Murry G. Ross, *Community Organization: Theory and Principles* (New York: Harper & Bros., 1955).

Chapter 4

Marketing for Health Educators

Elizabeth F. Dunn, PhD

The words "marketing" and "health" are no longer incompatible. Once considered a purely "business" function—and therefore unacceptable in the health care field—marketing today has a recognized and respected role to play in the provision of health-related services. Hospitals, for example, are creating such positions as Director of Marketing, Marketing Manager, or Vice President for Marketing and Planning. Such new organizations as the American College of Healthcare Marketing are springing up. College courses entitled "Health Care Marketing" and "Marketing for Health Care Professionals" are now being offered. The new emphasis can be seen in all the health-related professions, from hospital administration to medicine and surgery, dentistry, nursing, and consumer health care advocacy. The profession of health education is no exception.

The purpose of this chapter is to provide a brief overview of marketing. The chapter is divided into three major segments. The first segment—"Why Marketing?"—describes the reasons why marketing is such a "hot" issue among health educators today. The second segment—"Marketing Fundamentals"—presents some concepts that are common to any marketing effort. The third segment—"Your Strategy for Success"—explains the components that are required to create and deliver a successful health education program.

WHY MARKETING?

Why is marketing such a "hot" issue among health educators today? There are several reasons. Among the more important are:

- the reduction in outside funding for health education programs
- new consumer attitudes
- the changing role of health educators

Let's look at these in turn.

75

Reduction in Outside Funding

In the 1960s and 1970s, health education programs received a steady flow of federal, state, and local dollars. For the most part, all that was needed to obtain funding was a well-thought-out grant proposal. This is no longer true. The federal government's present attitude toward social program funding means that health education budgets are tight—indeed, many programs are struggling just to survive. Health educators must therefore try to increase the cost efficiency of their programs. They must get the most possible out of every dollar they spend. Sound marketing can be a powerful tool for doing this.

New Consumer Attitudes

Consumers are becoming more knowledgeable, sophisticated, and demanding about the health care products and services they purchase. No longer do they automatically accept physicians' recommendations; in fact, they are likely to switch to a new provider if they are dissatisfied with the present one. They are eager to acquire health care information; the sale of medical books and pamphlets has become a multi-million dollar industry.

Such consumers offer both an opportunity and a challenge to health educators. On the one hand, their thirst for knowledge makes them eager participants in health-related educational programs. On the other hand, their expectations are higher than those of consumers ten years ago. They demand top quality and will not be satisfied with less. The marketing techniques we will review in this chapter enable health educators to develop an understanding of the needs and desires of these consumers and to use this understanding to build programs that will appeal to them.

The Changing Role of Health Educators

In the past few years, health educators have moved into many new and diverse fields. Today, for example, they are:

- designing and implementing prevention programs for HMOs
- creating and communicating employee health care cost-containment programs
- designing programs for hospitals to increase patient referrals
- marketing wellness programs as consultants to private industry
- conducting patient relations programs for hospitals.

In these and similar jobs, the need for marketing expertise is clear. Health educators are finding that a knowledge of marketing tools and methodologies has become a requirement of even such traditional jobs as developing community education programs—in part, at least, because of the reduction in outside funding and the changing consumer attitudes discussed above.

MARKETING FUNDAMENTALS

Although different marketers may advocate different approaches, most would agree that the following steps are fundamental to any effective marketing effort:

1. Determine your objectives.
2. Select your target market.
3. Analyze the needs and preferences of potential consumers.
4. Study your competition.

Once you have taken these steps, you are ready to devise a strategy for designing a successful health education program.

Step 1. Determine Your Marketing Objectives

Let's suppose that you plan to offer a diabetes education program in your community. In doing so, you may be trying to fulfill a number of objectives in addition to the fundamental one of educating the public about this disease. Some examples:

- to have at least 200 community members attend the course
- to generate 10 referrals for the hospital (or group practice or HMO) that is sponsoring the program
- to generate $500 in contributions if the program is being sponsored by a fund-raising organization
- to project a quality image for the sponsoring organization
- to generate $400 in revenue by charging a fee for the workshop.

When determining the objectives your program is to meet, it is important to ensure that they are consistent with those of your sponsoring organization. For example, let's say that *your* objective is to attract 200 people to one diabetes workshop. Given your limited budget, you decide to accomplish this by renting the high school gymnasium, filling it with folding chairs, and packing everybody in. However, one of your *organization's* primary objectives is to create a professional image in the community. Your plan to "pack them in at the gym" will certainly not help your organization achieve its goal!

Once you are sure that your objectives support those of your organization, state them *precisely*. The more explicit your objectives, the easier your planning will be. Where possible, be quantitative. For example, "to attract a large audience to the workshop" is a less explicit objective than "to attract 200 individuals to the workshop" and it is far less useful for planning. The second statement will help you make sound decisions when you are confronted with such issues as how to design the program or where to hold the workshop.

Even when your goals cannot be stated quantitatively, they can and should be stated as precisely as possible. Consider these two objectives:

- to project a good image to the community
- to project an image as a highly professional, caring hospital to the community

The second statement will provide much clearer guidance for you than the first as you make decisions about program content, location, and publicity.

Step 2. Select Your Target Market

Based on your objectives, you must next select your target market. Do you want to market your program to the entire community or do you want to market it to some specific group in the community?

Translated into marketing terminology, this question reads, Do you want to *broad-market* your program or do you want to target a certain market *segment?*

A market segment can be defined in any number of ways. You could choose, for example, to design your program for those in a certain age group—say, those who are between 30 and 55 years of age. Or you could use health status as the determinant—your program could be designed especially for those who are at risk for diabetes. Still another market segment could be based on education—you could design a program specifically for people who have not attended college. Other possibilities might be market segments based on geography, income or lifestyle.

In many cases, segmenting your market makes it easier to plan and promote an effective program. Let's say that the target market for diabetes education program A is community members aged 50 and older; Program B is designed for the total community. You would select the content of

Program A in accordance with the needs and interests of older people; you could choose a setting that is accessible and attractive to the 50-plus segment, and you would design promotional materials to appeal to this group, as well as an appropriate way to deliver them. In contrast, your broad-market Program B would have to be interesting to both 19-year-olds and 65-year-olds—a very difficult requirement. And your setting, promotional materials, and fees would also have to be suitable for all age groups.

Remember that targeting a particular market segment does not mean excluding other groups from receiving your services. What it does mean is that you will have to adjust your basic program to meet the different needs of different groups. For example, your first diabetes workshop might be targeted toward the 50-and-over segment. A month later, you could use the program again for a different age group, as long as you modified it to be appropriate for your new audience.

Step 3. Analyze the Need and Preferences of Potential Consumers

The key to successful marketing is understanding the needs and preferences of the consumers in your target market. The most frequently used "tools" for developing that understanding are imagination, informal market research, and formal market research.

Imagination

You can gain many insights into what consumers need and want simply by using your imagination and adopting their perspective. Ask yourself, "What would I want if I were the consumer?"

To really get an understanding of what it feels like to switch from your own perspective to someone else's, try the following exercise:

Write out a shopping list as you normally would; then give it to a friend and ask her to do your shopping for you.

The result? Frustration on her part and dissatisfaction on yours. The problem, of course, is that you knew what you wanted when you put "bread, milk, and eggs" on your list. She didn't. What would have been a simple purchase for you was an ordeal for her. Did you want white, whole wheat, or rye bread? Sliced or unsliced? How many loaves? Almost certainly, the two loaves of unsliced rye bread, quart of skim milk, and three dozen large eggs she finally decided on were not at all what you had in mind.

Obviously, had you known from the start that you were writing your list for a friend to read, the list would have been very different. It probably would have read something like: "one loaf of Argo's whole wheat bread, two quarts of skim milk, one dozen extra large brown eggs." You would have prepared the list from your friend's perspective rather than your own. The question for a marketer is always, "What does the consumer need and want?" To answer it, you must consciously discipline yourself to step out of your own shoes and into the consumer's.

In the case of our diabetes workshop, your imagination and your common sense will tell you that most consumers are unlikely to be attracted by a lengthy discussion of the history of the medical profession's various approaches to treating diabetes over the last 20 years. (Unless, of course, the market segment you have targeted has a particular interest in medical history!) Nor would most people care about the chemical formula for insulin. Most consumers in most communities will be interested in receiving practical information about diabetes that may be useful to them in their daily lives.

At this point, you may well be thinking to yourself, "I would *never* prepare a community program and talk about chemical formulas. I am more sensitive than that!" But how many times have you been thoroughly bored by a classroom lecture, a community program, or even a television commercial? The most likely reason for your boredom is that the person who designed the lecture or program or commercial failed to do so from your perspective—he or she ignored your needs and preferences.

Informal Market Research

Another way to gather useful information about the consumers in your target market is to conduct informal market research. To do this, hold face-to-face or telephone conversations with nine or ten people who represent your target market, asking potential workshop participants what *they* would like to hear. (Be sure you select respondents who *do* represent the target market—who have the same characteristics as the market segment you are trying to reach. Otherwise, the information they give you will not be useful.) Begin by briefly explaining that you are seeking advice from a few selected people in order to make the program as interesting as possible. When talking with the respondents, try to avoid asking broad, formless questions; be as specific as you can. For example, it is relatively easy for people to respond to a question like "Would you be interested in a presentation on the new drugs being used to treat diabetes?" But a question such as "What topics would you like to hear about?" may well leave respondents frustrated and at a loss for words.

Remember, when conducting informal market research, it is essential to approach the respondents with "kid gloves." They must be treated with the utmost courtesy and respect. These people are often the first in the community to hear about your program; if they are not treated with courtesy and respect, you will have negative publicity about your program before you have even designed it!

Formal Market Research

Probably the best way to learn about consumer wants and needs is through formal market research, where researchers use sampling methodology, unbiased interviewing techniques, and statistical analysis to obtain information. If the research is conducted appropriately, the information from the sample can be projected to the entire population under study. For example, during United States presidential elections, pollsters frequently make such statements as "Forty-seven percent of voters favor the Democratic candidate, forty-three percent favor the Republican candidate, and the rest are undecided." This does not mean that the pollsters have actually interviewed the millions of adults who are registered to vote in the United States. In fact, they typically interview only about 1,000 respondents; the findings are then projected from this sample to the population (all adult voters in the United States).

The following is an example of formal market research relevant to health education: A large urban HMO conducted telephone interviews with 500 local consumers to determine the consumers' habits and attitudes concerning preventive health practices. The HMO used the results of the research to design preventive health and lifestyle programs. The cost of the research was $15,000.

Formal market research is an expensive undertaking. Depending on the methodology used and the size of the sample, typical market research studies conducted by professional research organizations cost between $10,000 and $50,000 or more, with many such studies costing about $20,000.

Step 4. Study Your Competition

Once you know who your potential consumers are and have examined their needs and preferences, it is time to take a look at your competition. If you can meet consumer needs by designing and delivering a program that is different from anyone else's, your chances of success are good. But if your program is no different from competitive programs, consumers will have no reason to choose it. Find out what your competitors are offering, and then try to make your program distinctive—more entertaining, for example, or more educational, more convenient, less expensive, better publicized. This will give you a decided "competitive edge."

If, for example, you are marketing wellness programs to corporations, you need to find a way to make your wellness program different from your competitors' programs. You might offer your programs at a more convenient time of day than your competitors. Or you might find a way to offer them more inexpensively than your competitors. The key is to learn what the competition is offering and then find a way to make your program somehow different and better.

It is important, but not difficult, to learn what the competition is offering. A good way to do this is to set up a "competitive clipping file" to collect flyers, newspaper ads, or other published information on programs similar to your own. Don't forget to include information you hear on the radio or television or in conversation; jot it down and add it to your file. Be sure to collect reports on past programs as well as events to come. You want to learn as much as you possibly can about competitive programs so that you can make yours distinctive.

YOUR STRATEGY FOR SUCCESS

Now that you have determined your objectives, selected your target market, learned about the needs and preferences of potential consumers, and studied competitive offerings, you are ready for the final step—devising a strategy for success. This strategy should cover what marketers term the "4 Ps"—Program, Place, Price, and Publicity.

Program

During Steps 3 and 4, you will have answered the most fundamental question of all: whether consumers have any need or desire for the program you plan to offer. It is possible, for example, that your particular community has little or no need for a program on diabetes. Let's say that from your study of the competition, you have learned that three organizations similar to yours have recently offered such programs and that the third was poorly attended. Or perhaps you have learned from your informal market research that a popular television program has just finished a series on diabetes. In other words, your community has been supplied with such a large quantity of information about diabetes so recently that the need or desire to learn more just is not there. If that is the case, you do not want to use your limited budget on such a program.

But suppose you find that only one of your competitors has conducted a program on diabetes in the past six months and that it was a well-attended workshop on the prevention of the disease. You have learned two things:

first, the subject of diabetes is of interest to your community; second, your program should focus on something other than prevention. Perhaps it should be directed toward helping diabetics and their families cope with the disease. Or, from your discussions with your representative sample, you may have learned that your audience would be most interested in learning how to identify symptoms of diabetes or finding out what community resources are available to help diabetics.

Whatever the case, the work you have done to date is paying off now. You have enough information to design a program that will:

* meet your objectives and those of your organization
* be responsive to the needs and preferences of the audience you have targeted
* give you a competitive edge

The first "P" has been accounted for.

Place

In determining the best location for the program or service you plan to offer, remember your organization's objectives (you may be able to cram more people into a high school gym, but if your organization's goal is to present an image of quality, the gym probably won't be a suitable location). Remember, too, that the location you select can give you a competitive advantage—it can be one thing that distinguishes your program from similar ones.

Perhaps your diabetes workshop would have most credibility if you held it in the hospital auditorium. However, the hospital may be inconvenient for consumers to travel to; they might be more likely to attend if the workshop were held in a neighborhood community center. Go back to Steps 2 and 3— what are the needs and desires of the consumers in your target market segment? Is the place you have chosen accessible to them? Will they regard it as safe and secure? Does it offer special features they need (e.g., a child care center for an audience of young married couples, a wheelchair ramp for an audience of retired people)? If your potential consumers will be driving, does the place you have selected have ample parking? If your program is being offered in a city, have you found a location convenient to public transportation?

If the best place you can find presents certain problems, you may be able to devise appropriate solutions. For example, if accessible transportation is a problem, you could use a community van to transport participants. If consumers believe that the neighborhood is not safe, you could provide for "valet parking" or arrange to have someone meet attendees at the bus stop. Such extra efforts add cost because they require additional personnel. But they can go a long way toward increasing attendance. Moreover, if they are well publicized, they can help to distinguish your organization as one that really cares about the needs of the people it serves.

Price

Assuming that one of your objectives is to cover the cost of your program, you will need to charge an attendance fee. There are two ways to determine what the fee should be—cost-based pricing and consumer-based pricing.

The first step in cost-based pricing is to project all the expenses for the event you plan to offer. By adding up the estimated costs of personnel time, facility rental, program materials, publicity, and any extras you need (such as valet parking or security guards), you will arrive at a total projected cost for your event. Say that you expect your total cost to be $200. Your next step is to estimate the number of people who will attend your workshop— you expect an audience of 50. By dividing your expected costs by the number of attendees, you arrive at a program fee of $4.00 per person.

You can also determine program fees through consumer-based pricing techniques. The first step is to use your informal market research to determine the price consumers would be willing to pay for the program. Put yourself in the consumer's shoes—what would such a program be worth to you? Include questions on price in your conversations with your representative sample. Again, be sure that the individuals in your sample (the 10 people you call) are representative of the individuals in the total population (all people who are likely to attend the event). Do not, for example, select the 10 names from your list of major contributors if you are also trying to attract less affluent people to the workshop!

Once you have established what appears to be a reasonable price, multiply it by your estimated number of attendees. Now you know at least approximately how much you have to work with; this will help you make realistic decisions on how much to spend for speakers, the hall, publicity, and the like.

To summarize, with cost-based pricing, you determine what your program expenses will be and then calculate how much you need to charge to cover them. Conversely, with consumer-based pricing, you determine how much consumers are willing to pay, and then calculate how much you will have for program expenses.

In most situations, consumer-based pricing is the preferred approach. When you determine your fees without any consumer input, the price you arrive at may be too high or too low. Suppose you decide to rent an expensive hall and serve an elaborate luncheon; the program fee needed to cover these costs could be high enough to discourage attendance. The result is that your revenues are insufficient to cover your costs. Conversely, you may decide to keep your expenses—and therefore your program fee—low. You set a fee of $2 and put on a low-budget program when, in fact, attendees would have gladly paid a $4 fee for a better program.

Publicity

You can have the best designed program in the world, but if potential consumers are not aware of it, attendance will be low. Look at the consumers in your target market—how can you best reach them with publicity about your program? What kind of publicity will be most attractive to them? Ask yourself:

- What would be the most effective *content* for my promotional materials?
- What would be the most effective *medium* for the promotion (e.g., radio, television, the community newspaper, pamphlets)?

Large corporations with million-dollar marketing budgets answer the first question by copy-testing. They give a number of versions of the same advertisement—different in size, color, graphics, and/or verbal content—to a large sample of consumers to evaluate. Then they ask the consumers a variety of questions about the different versions, including:

- Which version do you remember the best?
- Which was the most attractive to you?
- Which would be most likely to motivate you to purchase the product?

Corporations use the results of these interviews to design what consumers indicate will be the most successful ad.

Although formal market research concerning promotional content is clearly impractical and far too expensive for organizations with small budgets, you can use the informal techniques we have discussed to learn what is most likely to attract consumers to your program. The research you have done on your competitors also comes into play here. What gives you your "competitive edge"? What is it about your program that uniquely differentiates it from similar programs? Is it the different content, lower fees, such special features as child care? Whatever it is, feature it prominently in your publicity. Put it in large letters in your pamphlets or newspaper ad; repeat it several times in your radio announcement.

Determining the most effective medium for your publicity depends on defining your target market clearly and on determining how that target market is most likely to be reached. If you want to promote an arthritis education program for consumers aged 50 and older, you will use different media from what you would use to promote a sex education program for adolescents. When marketing to adolescents, you can sometimes obtain access to classrooms through the local school district. A personal presentation to students is more effective in building support for a teen program than putting ads in the community newspaper, which adolescents are not likely to read, or securing radio or television public service announcements, which are frequently aired at 6:00 a.m.

In general, the key to effective media decisions is to think carefully about the people who are your target audience and decide (1) where they are most likely to be exposed to publicity and (2) which medium can be expected to impress them favorably.

A CLOSING WORD

The fundamentals of marketing covered in this chapter can be summarized as follows:

1. Determine your program objectives as precisely as possible.
2. Learn as much as you can about your potential consumers and your competitors.
3. With your program objectives always in mind, use what you know about your consumers and competitors to decide on program, place, price, and publicity.

Although we have discussed these fundamentals primarily as they might apply to the design of a community education program on diabetes, they can be applied to any marketing situation. If you use them faithfully, you will significantly increase your chances of meeting your program objectives.

SUGGESTED READINGS

Kotler, Philip. *Marketing for Nonprofit Organizations.* Englewood Cliffs, N.J.: Prentice-Hall, 1975.

_____. *Principles of Marketing.* Englewood Cliffs, N.J.: Prentice-Hall, 1983.

Lovelock, Christopher H., and Weinberg, Charles B. *Marketing for Public and Nonprofit Managers.* New York: John Wiley, 1984.

Chapter 5

Ethics and Health Education: Issues in Theory and Practice

Marc D. Hiller, DrPH

In recent years, there has been a remarkable growth in the popularity of health education and health promotion. The contributions of assuming and maintaining a healthy lifestyle and reducing personal health risks have been realized in all sectors. Fuchs has argued that "the greatest potential for improving health lies in what we do and don't do for and to ourselves."[1] McKeown, Illich, Wildavsky, and Knowles are only a few other notables who have articulated the limits of curative medicine and the benefits of individuals assuming more of a personal responsibility for their health.[2]

In responding to this heightened attention and its concomitant demands, the field of health education has expanded beyond its more traditional mission during the first half of the century. Previous concerns of accident avoidance, hygiene, and physical education have been replaced by efforts directed at prevention and early detection of chronic diseases and risk-taking behaviors.

Increasingly, health educators are struggling with thorny ethical dilemmas. "Conflicts of interest, whistle-blowing on corruption, obligations to clients or patients versus duties to society, and the consequences of deception versus truthtelling"[3] are among the common sources precipitating ethical questions. While there are certain ethical dilemmas that arise more frequently in health education, the majority of concerns affecting most professions are surprisingly similar.

This chapter has several objectives. It explores some fundamental concepts concerning ethics, values, and morals. It examines the process of applying ethical principles to guide rational resolution of complex value-laden issues and moral dilemmas. Collectively, these provide health educators with a basic understanding of ethics and how ethics may be used to facilitate sound decision making. In addition, it identifies several critical ethical issues confronting the field of health education with which individual health educators must wrestle during the course of their careers. It purposefully avoids prescription; rather, it challenges health educators to consider the ethical issues and implications associated with certain practices or advances in the field of education.

CAN WE MOVE FORWARD?

Clearly, one might say health education is on the move. Its potential impact has only begun to be realized in terms of improving health status (e.g., lowering morbidity and mortality rates, increasing life expectancy), containing health care costs, increasing workforce productivity, and extending a higher quality of life.

Throughout the United States, government and private organizations, including hospitals, schools, corporations, and businesses among a wide array of other civic and community groups, already have introduced a variety of health education and promotion initiatives aimed at preventive health care.

People engaged in the formulation of public health policy, those professionally involved in the delivery of health education and promotion services to groups and individuals, and individual citizens are concerned about ethical issues in Health Education and Health promotion. Why? Are the issues new or simply a magnification of old ones? How can people be doing "good" things and be considered unethical?

Health educators yield considerable influence in terms of choosing where they direct their attention and the manner in which they do so. How are they to wrestle with their individual morals and personal values that may obstruct or affect their decisions or unduly influence their actions regarding other individuals or groups? How do they balance conflicting priorities? Engaging in public-oriented efforts is known to risk violating individual rights or limiting what can be done for individuals. Increasingly, health educators are being forced to challenge their values and to concede tradeoffs in reckoning with difficult ethical dilemmas. The following questions illustrate these points:

- To what extent should health educators intervene in efforts to change a client's behavior or lifestyle?
- To what extent is coercion or deception ethical in promoting an improved health status of a client?
- What distinguishes a purely informational and educational program from a persuasive appeal?
- What is a fair balance between efforts to benefit society and those that respect individual liberty; how is such a balance achieved?

- To what extent is the disclosure of confidential client data to various third parties ethical? When, if ever, does the public interest (to know) supersede an individual interest (for privacy)?
- To what extent is marketing health promotion for personal profit and gain ethical? Is it ethical to employ health promotion or health education as a tool to market goods and services?
- Who should bear the financial burden for individuals requiring costly medical care who have consciously practiced a risk-oriented lifestyle?

Throughout American history, the dominant theme in government has been individualism, with minimal restrictions on property and personal lifestyles.[4] With the mounting documentation of morbidity and mortality associated with risk-taking behaviors and the heavy social and economic tolls produced by these practices, hard questions are being asked forcing a confrontation of ethical values among those involved in both government and health care delivery.[5] For example, to what degree should individual liberty be sacrificed in promoting the public's health? Wikler asks, "what should be the government's role in promoting the kinds of personal behavior that lead to long life and good health?"[6] While resolution of such questions falls upon public officials in the policy arena, they raise equal ethical dilemmas for health educators as well.

Amid the expanding field of health education and promotion, both in terms of its continuing development as a profession and its "practice" employing modern advances in the behavioral sciences and communications, health educators are increasingly confronting serious ethical quandaries. However, no consensus exists as to a single "code of ethics" for persons working in health education. The absence of such a formal code, which, according to experts, constitutes a required attribute of an established profession, results in health education practitioners having no common frame of reference in wrestling with ethical issues.[7]

Practitioners do have certain basic ethical obligations:

1. Recognition of ethical issues in the provision of health education and promotion services;
2. Awareness of potential ethical implications that may arise in seeking solutions;
3. Application of sound ethical reasoning in clarifying values and resolving moral dilemmas.

Health educators must be sensitive to ethical issues associated with the services they provide to each individual client. Further, they must recognize the implications of various organizational/management decisions that might affect the services they provide. For example, certain financial decisions made to improve the organization's economic condition may generate a variety of ethical issues holding significant implications for one's clients (e.g., implementing a management information system in a clinic may facilitate more accurate billing and immediate data entry into a client's medical record, but, without imposing adequate safeguards to ensure confidentiality, it may pose added risk of the disclosure of confidential information shared with the health educator). In other words, health educators must have a working knowledge of what constitutes an ethical issue and know how to employ ethical principles in their decision making in appropriate situations.

Toward facilitating such ends, this section offers several basic concepts and fundamentals related to ethics in health education.

ETHICS, VALUES, AND MORALS

In commencing a discussion of ethics and health education, certain terms must be understood. Most likely, persons engaged in health education have heard the terms "ethics," "morals," and "values" before. Often, such terms have been viewed as vague, interchangeable, and confusing. Further, many distinctions that have been made among these terms are more artifactual than substantive. Yet, clarification among them is important to ensure maximum understanding and application by health educators.

What Is Ethics?

Ethics is a branch of philosophy that deals with systematic approaches to understanding morality. Its roots date back to ancient Greece and the teachings of Plato and Aristotle. It is the disciplined study of the nature and discussion of moral principles, decisions, and problems. It does not reflect particular moral or value positions. Rather than attempting to explain why one values one thing over another, ethics as applied in health care assumes a normative role.

As a result of engaging in an ethical analysis, a health educator is better equipped to rationally, and more objectively, respond to the question "What should I do?" This question is arising more often as health education practitioners are dealing with issues such as alcohol and other substance abuse, including mandatory screening and reporting programs, and the highly emotionally charged topics of sex education, adolescent pregnancy, and abortion. Just what should health education practitioners do in general; how should they respond in specific situations? And what happens when professional expectations or personal beliefs conflict with institutional (agency) or social policies or obligations?

Ethics are involved in an assessment of whether or not there are norms, standards of behavior (or practice), or guidelines that have some form of general application in judging human acts. The intellectual tools of ethics permit the analysis of cases of conflict and a better comprehension of why certain types of acts or behavioral characteristics are considered "morally" better than others.[8]

Normative ethics focuses on concrete issues and attempts to address the hard questions of conduct and practice. For example, it might guide health educators in wrestling with questions of confidentiality and information disclosure. Normative ethics seeks to determine what "ought" to be done rather than what "is" actually practiced. While normative ethics does not "dictate" specific answers to difficult questions or situations, it is nonetheless prescriptive in nature.[9]

Beauchamp and Childress have attempted to illustrate a model of ethical reasoning that is instructive in understanding the application of ethical theories, principles, and rules to problems confronting health educators.[10] They identify four levels in a hierarchy of ethical reasoning, as exhibited in Figure 5-1.

For example, utilitarian theories argue for surrendering individual goods or desires for the common, or collective, good of society (i.e., many). Public (or community) welfare is prioritized regardless of the individual welfare. Utilitarians would argue in support of health education initiatives that would benefit the largest number, even at the expense of sacrificing certain programs that are more directed at a small number of persons (or individuals).

Alternatively, deontological theories argue that an adequate ethical position ought to be duty-based rather than consequential as in utilitarian theories. Deontologists hold that there are certain rigid principles that are always in force, regardless of the outcomes they may engender. For example, libertarians demand that absolute liberty ought to always prevail, no matter

---

Figure 5–1 Hierarchy of Ethical Reasoning

- Theories   Systematically related bodies of principles and rules; used to resolve conflicts between principles
  ⬇
- Principles   Serve as a foundation or source for justifying rules
  ⬇
- Rules   State that actions of a certain kind ought (or ought not) to be made because they are "right" or "wrong"
  ⬇
- Judgments or Actions   A particular decision, verdict, or conclusion

Source: Adapted from *Principles of Biomedical Ethics*, 2nd ed., by T. L. Beauchamp and J. F. Childress, with permission of Oxford University Press, © 1983.

what; similarly, certain devout religious groups argue obeyance to divine commands regardless of anything else.

On the basis of such very general theories, fundamental ethical principles may be derived to guide decision making. While the precise nature of the distinction between principles and rules is often debated, the former are usually viewed as being more general and fundamental.[11] For example, the principle of respect for persons, therefore, supports many ethical rules such as "it is wrong to lie," "disclosure of confidential information is wrong," and "coercion and deception are wrong." In turn, adherence to such rules facilitates making certain judgments or engaging in particular actions in specific situations. Fundamental ethical principles serve as the foundation of most of the more specific rules that ought to be employed in the decision making of health educators when confronted with an ethical dilemma.

What Are Morals?

In contrast with ethics, morals reflect traditions of beliefs about right and wrong often associated with a particular religion or social consensus. Morals represent a social institution with a history and code of learnable rules by which people govern their actions. That is, morality exists, and people are taught as they mature to mold to its rules and traditions. Morality is a product of social consensus, and it often differs from actions grounded in emotion, prejudice, or personal interest.[12]

While actions governed by morals do not necessarily differ from those based on ethical principles, it is possible that an act which is judged ethical may not concur with the morals of certain individuals. For example, providing birth control information to a sexually active minor may be judged ethical based on respecting that adolescent's privacy (e.g., derived from the principle of respect for persons), but not deemed moral based on the practitioner's religious teachings or the prevailing values of a particular community. In other religions or communities, the provision of this service might be viewed as both ethical and moral.

In other words, while morals often direct one's decisions and determine one's actions, they risk imposing one person's beliefs on another regardless of any consideration of ethical reasoning. Actions solely based on an individual's moral behavior fail to recognize that while some morals may be shared (or even more or less universally agreed upon), not everyone subscribes to a singular set, given the pluralistic nature of our society.

What Are Values?

One of the most important axiological questions that an individual needs to ask is "why do I value some things more than others, and should I?" A general consensus exists that certain groups of values exist, such as moral, political, esthetic, religious, and intellectual. Further, there is general agreement that genetic, biological, and cultural influences produce many of these values. However, little agreement exists with respect to their nature, their relative importance, or their relationship to one another.[13]

Among the major factors affecting values is morals. Hence, values may or may not heavily reflect an individual's moral or religious leanings. Other factors strongly contributing to an individual's personal value formation include his or her personal experiences, culture (e.g., race, ethnicity), and peer group (e.g., members of one's chosen profession, others in one's socioeconomic class). Hence, there is a wide range of potentially significant contributing sources of the values to which one consciously or subconsciously subscribes.

For example, if one's experience has included being a patient, there is likely to be a greater sensitivity to a patient-oriented perspective or concern, or even to "patient rights." If an individual's culture is one that pays homage to one's elders (e.g., most Asian cultures), then greater attention and sensitivity may be given to the elderly.

At bottom, while values may be common or shared, they remain highly personal. They contribute significantly to behavior and decision making, both consciously and subconsciously. They may or may not contribute to ethical actions or outcomes.

Thus, it is important for all health professionals to clarify their values periodically throughout their careers. Values clarification provides insight regarding an individual's values and valuation process. It provides no set standards, principles, or norms for value formulation but simply offers a descriptive means of identifying and illuminating one's values. Hence, it permits a critical analysis of how values affect making judgments.

Values clarification for health educators is very important since as individuals they hold a range of personal values that both consciously and unconsciously influence their behavior and practices. It is essential for them to become more aware of their values prior to engaging in decision making. Subsequently, this awareness will allow for making more analytical and objective decisions. Obviously, while values clarification will not preclude their influencing decision making, it does limit their impact. According to German and Chwalow, when health educators impose their own values on patients—particularly, when dealing with sensitive subjects—it results in "ambivalence in the presentation of specific interventions, defensive postures with resistant patients, and possible vitiation of the effectiveness of the health education strategy."[14]

At a collective level, values clarification can assist in ensuring that those values to which a field, such as health education, subscribes do not unduly color decision making. For example, the high value placed on "health" and "healthy lifestyles" may affect decisions regarding program design and clients. Allowing this value to overly affect decisions may lead to insensitivity regarding clients' interests, needs, or problems.

ETHICAL PRINCIPLES IN HEALTH EDUCATION

Central to the resolution of ethical dilemmas is the application of fundamental ethical principles. To better comprehend the application of these principles, consider the following short vignette.

> You are a health educator employed by a local community health agency. The administrator of your agency is interested in marketing health education services to local businesses. Your agency has been contracted to provide health education services to the employees of a nearby manufacturer of computer parts. The owner of the company is concerned about his employees using alcohol and other drugs. While his concern is expressed in terms of their welfare, he also expresses some hostility concerning lost productivity (less than maximum efficiency and above-average employee sick days). What are the issues before you and what should you do?

Prior to considering specific ethical principles, the health educator must first ask "To whom do I bear my primary obligation: to my employer (agency); to the company owner, who may seek the disclosure of worker/ client information; to the field of health education, which may subscribe to certain informal ethical positions; to my client, who is the prime recipient of my services; or to myself in adherence to my personal values (or morals)? If a client had a problem that was either infectious or produced risk to others, what obligation might the health professional have to society (or his or her co-workers)?

Clearly, the prioritization of responsibilities is important and may affect the application of ethical principles. While no clear-cut resolution is mandated, for a direct provider of health care services most established ethical codes (e.g., the Hippocratic Oath, the Code of Ethics of the American Medical Association) direct principal accountability to one's individual clients/patients, except when their actions may place others in society at risk. Beyond addressing this issue, several fundamental principles exist that must be considered and applied as appropriate by health education practitioners (Table 5-1). Each bears thoughtful consideration in ensuring ethical decision making and actions that transcend individual moral beliefs and personal values.

Since most situations pose ethical dilemmas to which more than one principle is applicable, in most cases complete analysis requires consider-

Table 5–1 Fundamental Ethical Principles Relevant to Health Education

• Beneficence	The obligation to benefit one's client.
• Nonmaleficence	The obligation to bring no harm to one's client.
• Respect for Persons	The obligation to respect the autonomy (right to self-determination) of one's clients.
• Justice	The obligation to treat one's client fairly in terms of burdens (e.g., risks, costs) and benefits.
• Utility	The obligation to balance the above principles to maximize the greatest utility.

ation of several principles in tandem. Viewed collectively, they assist in resolving conflicting ethical claims.

As this often produces a conflict between, or among, different ethical principles and eventually leads to a prioritization of applicable principles in a given situation, it ensures a more adequate and complete examination of all possible alternatives and their respective implications.

No single ethical principle possesses sufficient weight to outweigh or overwhelm all other potential conflicting ethical claims. Health educators must appreciate the pluralism of several fundamental principles as a basic feature of moral life while concurrently recognizing that the weight, or priority, allocated to specific ones may vary according to the uniqueness of given situations. When collectively applied to thorny ethical issues arising in health education, the use of these principles orchestrates a well-balanced approach toward reaching rational solutions.

Through their application, sound ethical judgments may be distinguished from weak moral claims, personal attitudes, or intuitions, i.e., unreflective and nonobjective principles. Accordingly, Beauchamp and McCullough have stated that "one must have defensible moral reasons for holding a position, and neither the position nor the reasons that underlie it can be justified if they rest solely on prejudice, emotion, false data, the authority of another individual, or claims of self-evidence."[15]

Nonmaleficence and Beneficence

The principle of nonmaleficence dictates: inflict no harm. It reflects the popular medical ethos *primum non nocere* (first of all, do no harm) and instructs health educators not to engage in activities known to risk or cause harm to clients or a target population.

Beneficence is a more active principle. Dating back to the oath of Hippocrates, this action-oriented directive instructs health educators to benefit clients by preventing or removing harm and promoting good. It obligates action in the best interest of clients in promoting their health and welfare.

Whereas nonmaleficence holds that it is the health educator's responsibility to bring no harm to an individual, beneficence further extends this obligation to benefit the individual whenever possible.

With respect to the vignette, the principle of beneficence obligates the health educator to provide services aimed at benefiting the company's employees. As a health professional engaged in clinical care, the educator's primary moral obligation is to care for his or her clients above and beyond what might otherwise be in the best interest of other parties (e.g., company management, which seeks increased profitability or productivity). In terms of nonmaleficence, the health educator is obligated to ensure that, at a minimum, his or her actions do not cause any harm to come to the clients involved. Adherence to this principle might be viewed as disallowing any disclosure of client information that might result in harm (e.g., loss of employment, termination of benefits). On the other hand, if a client is viewed as being self-destructive or harmful to others, appropriate third-party disclosure (e.g., to a mental health agency) would be appropriate.

Respect for Persons

The principle of respect for persons, also referred to as autonomy, self-determination, and liberty, serves as the foundation for "patient's rights." Many specific ethical rules and legal doctrines based on this principle have emerged, such as those related to informed consent, confidentiality and privacy, and truth telling.

Health care professionals should honor the self-respect and dignity of each individual, as an autonomous, free actor. All competent individuals have an intrinsic right to make decisions for themselves on any matter affecting them, at least so far as such decisions do not bring harm to another party. If an individual possesses a diminished capacity to exercise this right because of a physical or mental condition, this obligation should still not be ignored. Respect for persons offers a clear directive to health educators despite its frequent unavoidable clash with the principle of beneficence. For example, health educators may be inclined to induce "healthy" lifestyle practices through behavior modification or other modalities. In attempting to benefit their clients (i.e., in adherence to beneficence), through programs designed to stimulate healthy diets, reduce drug and alcohol consumption, and eliminate smoking, they risk becoming paternalistic, deceptive, or even coercive. While such ends may be desirable from the health educator's perspective, employing such means violates respect for persons.

According to Dworkin, restricting a competent individual's liberty—even for his or her own good—should be done only when attempting to prevent far-reaching, potentially dangerous, and irreversible outcomes.[16] Dworkin contends that those who impose paternalistic interventions on others should clearly demonstrate why such actions were taken and ensure that they were the least restrictive measures necessary to reduce the risks. In contrast, Beauchamp argues that "public health offers a community justification for paternalistic measures that, for example, discourage smoking or require seatbelts."[17]

In practice, respect for persons promotes the recognition that individuals (e.g., patients or clients) should bear the principal role in decision making. Health educators are obligated to disclose all known risks associated with their clients' "unhealthy" behaviors and practices. Based on known empirical studies, clients should be informed as to the probability that such behaviors or practices may affect their health status. Further, in suggesting possible alternatives (interventions) designed to improve health status, health educators bear an obligation to be honest and objective in acknowledging potential risks. To choose what is to be done or not done should be considered an inalienable moral right of individuals.

In the case of the above vignette, the health educator is ethically obligated to several actions grounded on the principle of respect for persons. For example, the educator is bound to obtain a voluntary informed consent from each employee prior to initiating any individual services. The educator is equally bound to respect that employee's refusal to participate in the program without any reprisal or denial of benefits to which the employee might otherwise be entitled, without any coercion. As mentioned above, respecting the autonomy of any employee might precipitate other ethical conflicts should it dictate a sacrifice of beneficence.

Alternatively, the health educator's actions might be viewed as being paternalistic, which in some cases may be deemed justifiable on moral grounds. Other issues affected by this principle include ensuring the confidentiality and privacy of the workers in dealing with this highly sensitive issue. While employee assistance programs may be sponsored and paid for by employers, worker participation in them should not be disclosed to employers unless the safety or health of others is threatened.

Justice

What is fair or "just"? While various concepts of justice exist based on a variety of criteria, each demands fairness and impartiality in determining that which each individual deserves—be it a burden (or risk) or a benefit.

While many rival theories of justice exist, all major ones share a common element: all cases should be treated similarly, i.e., equals should be treated equally and unequals unequally.

Each theory of justice subscribes to a different set or combination of material (substantive outcome) or procedural (process) criteria. Beauchamp and Bowie have identified six "material principles of justice" used as a basis for many of the theories.[18] While there is no need to accept more than one of these material principles to systematically defend one's interpretation of fairness, often a combination or prioritization is used in defending just decisions.

Interpretations of justice vary according to one's social, economic, and political values. For example, differences of egalitarian, Marxist, libertarian, or utilitarian perspectives influence ethical decision making. Egalitarians emphasize equal access to health care. Health educators holding this material principle would defend programs that were available to anyone—access for all practical purposes must be unlimited, thus ensuring equity. However, should such an approach ever be economically feasible, services obviously would have to be less than extensive, given the realization that resources are limited.

Marxists tend to emphasize need as the primary basis for allocation. Health educators holding this position advocate that most of the resources available for health education should be allocated to those bearing the greatest need for them. Advocates of a triage theory would hold that services should first be allocated to those for whom they are most likely to benefit; those determined to be beneath an established minimum threshold (i.e., those beyond meaningful recovery) would be denied services. Libertarian theories emphasize that services ought to be rendered based on the criteria of contribution and merit. Criteria vary, from the degree of one's community contributions, to the number of one's dependents, to one's ability to pay the price charged for a particular service. Utilitarians support a mixed use of such criteria so that both public and private utility are maximized.

Dilemmas frequently arise in terms of what proportion of the health care budget ought to be allocated to health education and promotion. Of the resources allocated for health education, how should they be distributed (e.g., for primary or secondary prevention)? What types of procedural mechanisms can be imposed to ensure a fair distribution avoiding bias and prejudice? Who should decide?

Regarding the vignette, several issues related to justice arise, not the least of which is assessing how to ensure that all employees are treated in a similarly fair manner. In addition, the principle of justice dictates the use of a common set of criteria in judging the allocation of the scarce, or limited, resources (e.g., the program's budget, the health educator's time, benefits associated with the program).

Utility

The principle of utility is unlike the principles discussed thus far. As a procedural principle, it instructs health professionals to "balance" both the good and bad outcomes associated with the various alternatives arising in individual cases. It recognizes that none of the other principles are mutually exclusive and that often they directly conflict with each other (e.g., when doing what is in the client's best interest conflicts with what the client seeks). The "utility" or "usefulness" of an action is determined by the extent to which it produces the most desirable outcome.

For utilitarians, there is one and only one basic principle in ethics, namely that of utility. Utility determines the order of activities in a manner that maximizes benefits and minimizes harm. In contrast, for those not holding utility as their sole guide to behavior, it instructs a balancing of the unavoidable conflicts resulting from the application of the other principles.

With regard to the vignette, the principle of utility dictates that the health educator must carefully weigh the preceding principles regarding which holds priority over others amid their inevitable clashes (e.g., to do what will benefit one employee the most will demand sacrificing fairness in treating others, to do what is best in promoting the health of a worker will require denying his or her expressed wishes, to do what will maximize institutional efficiency will force sacrificing that which is in the best interest of an individual employee).

LEVELS OF ETHICAL ANALYSIS

Specific ethical problems should be analyzed at multiple levels. At what level does an ethical question lie? While they may exist at only one level, ethical dilemmas become more complex when they require analysis at multiple (i.e., two or three) levels concurrently. Serious conflicts often arise when a sound ethical argument to do one thing (reflecting the application of one principle at one level) is juxtaposed with an equally strong case to do another (using the same or another principle at another level).

At the *macro* level, the focus is on societal, or community, concerns. Issues at this level typically involve problems or options affecting large numbers of individuals, such as communities or society at large, and tend to be of a public policy nature. At the *meso* level, the orientation is on the organization or a given profession. Among the priority concerns arising at this level are those maximizing that which is good for the institution (e.g., a hospital or health education center) to facilitate carrying out its designated mission. In contrast, issues arising at the *micro* level focus on individual interrelationships and tend to be most concerned with doing good for the individual (e.g., the client or patient).

When applying the above ethical principles, it is equally important to ensure recognition of each of the three levels. This ensures that all possible alternatives are identified and applicable principles employed. Additional conflicts often become more apparent on prioritizing one level versus another.[19]

Thorny ethical dilemmas often arise when one must choose among alternatives that bear incompatible positive consequences—one that will produce a social good (i.e., a macro-oriented benefit) and another that will produce a client good (i.e., a micro-oriented benefit), and a single choice must be made. Similarly, conflicts often arise between meso and micro levels when favoring one option will maximize an institution's objective while opting for another may be in an individual's best interest.

Referring back to the vignette, identifying and disclosing those employees who may be using alcohol or drugs in the workplace may contribute to the company's objective of ridding itself of such workers and thereby increasing its productivity (meso level), but such action is clearly not in the best interest of the affected employees (micro level).

Another, more clearcut example would involve implementing an automated medical record system, which would contribute to a health center's efficiency (meso level). Given increased efficiency, the health center may even realize additional resources to provide more community services (macro level). Such a move appears ethical from a utilitarian standpoint. However, such centralization would require granting various authorized (and potentially unauthorized) personnel access to confidential client information. This may increase the risk of disclosure of sensitive patient information to undesired parties (micro level). At this level, the principle of respect for persons would be sacrificed.

Often such clashes cannot be avoided regardless of the application of ethical principles. In these cases, ethical decision making becomes more value-laden and may simply be resolved on the basis of which level is most valued or awarded greater priority. Such prioritization might reflect the mission of the institution or the personal values of the decision maker.

For health educators practicing at the micro level (i.e., engaged in the direct delivery of client services), wrestling with multiple-level dilemmas may not occur often. However, practitioners holding administrative or health education planning responsibilities may have to combat a conflict between what makes the most sense for the agency (or department) versus what might be in the best interests of individual clients.

USING ETHICS IN HEALTH EDUCATION

Health educators are often forced to choose what services they will provide and which segments of the population will most likely benefit from them. Hence, they bear an obligation to fairly distribute the benefits that are available.

Understanding and applying fundamental ethical theories and principles to complex problems provide a strategy and a means for promoting increased professional responsibility and for increasing individual reasoning capacity. For problem situations, five goals have been identified by Callahan:[20]

1. Stimulating the moral imagination—Health educators need to be able to appreciate the fact that each ethical decision they make holds implications for others; each act they commit bears consequences for someone. Hence, they are not free to simply dismiss all decisions as "strictly professional."

2. Recognizing ethical and value-laden issues—Health educators need to learn to appraise their immediate responses. Such responses commonly bear hidden assumptions and values. Hence, they must ask whether a visceral response alone provides sufficient reasonable justification for making a moral judgment. They need to be able to make an ethical response rather than one grounded in politics or economics. In part, this requirement is predicated on the ongoing clarification of one's values.

3. Developing analytical skills—Health educators need to comprehend major ethical theories and principles and apply them in a consistent and coherent manner to the problems they confront. When sponsoring or designing a health education program, the practitioner should be able to both challenge and defend the chosen actions and their consequences on ethical grounds rather than simply accepting them as givens.

4. Eliciting a sense of ethical responsibility—The freedom for clients to make moral choices should be ensured. Professional, and personal, conduct should always be ethical.

5. Tolerating—and resisting—disagreement and ambiguity—Problems generate ethical conflicts and are not always resolved by reaching a single conclusion. Yet, even when such dilemmas generate ethical uncertainty, the reasoning that led to a particular conclusion needs to be precise. Differences in choice (e.g., among administrators, colleagues, clients) should be tolerated without labeling the choices of others as unethical or immoral. Practitioners need to be able to engage

in ethical discourse with those holding opposing positions—through an honest attempt to extract the exact points of difference, to objectively examine the reasoning used by others, and to resist false distinctions and evasions—with the aim of solving disagreements rationally.

"DOING ETHICS" IN HEALTH EDUCATION: SIX STEPS

When health educators encounter ethical questions, they need to be able to employ an adequate problem-solving methodology for analyzing and justifying their decisions, a process that may be described as "doing ethics."

In their effort to successfully resolve ethical problems, health educators need to be able to engage in ethical analysis. While multiple models of ethical decision making have been developed,[21] no single one guarantees the elimination of all ethical quandary. The six-step process presented by Harron, Burnside, and Beauchamp considers each of the critical elements needed to make an ethically sound decision.[22] It maximizes a rational, systematic examination of alternative courses of action based on the application of fundamental ethical principles. Professional and personal values may be considered during the course of decision making, assuming that practitioners have previously undergone a clarification of them. Their influence should be acknowledged and limited.

Step 1: Identification

Identification represents three activities: the existence of an ethical problem must be perceived, the problem must be identified, and it must be confirmed. Beyond the initial perception of an ethical problem, health educators face two tasks. First, they must ensure that a real choice exists among possible courses of action in resolving the problem. During this effort, the gathering of relevant information is essential. Secondly, they must be able to attribute a significantly different value upon each possible action, or upon the consequences of each.

In fulfilling the above two tasks, health educators establish the existence of the two essential ingredients of an ethical problem. However, the mere presence of these ingredients does not categorically confirm an ethical problem. Situations, for example, that pose acting in an ethical manner on the one hand (i.e., one choice) or acting in self-interest or in an illegal manner on the other (i.e., another choice) would not constitute ethical problems.

Step 2: Analysis

The next step is to list all possible courses of action that may be employed in addressing the problem. Unfortunately few lists exhaust every alternative. In confronting a decision, one too often opts for considering only two. This risks further assuming that one may be weighed against the other.

Human conditioning prefers limiting choice between two alternatives; it is easier to think in terms of "either-or" than to deal with the complexities of multiple alternatives that require juggling or some form of matrix-like analysis. However, there are usually more than two, and often it is the third or fourth that provides the most optimal solution. Hence, it is essential to delineate all possible alternatives, even those that may appear to be somewhat remote.

Step 3: Weighing

This step involves assessing the consequences that would most likely result from considering the respective implications, such as the strengths and weaknesses, associated with each alternative. It dictates that the implications posed by various alternatives be contrasted and balanced individually and comparatively.

Before initiating the actual weighing process, the more immediate and dramatic consequences of particular alternatives—those quick to come to mind—must be examined. A further investment of time and effort is required to generate a list of long-range consequences associated with specific alternatives.

While it is common to think of individual or independent consequences, the degree to which effects may be interrelated or aggregated must be assessed. At times, resolving conflicting alternatives and consequences requires minimal compromise; in other instances, considerable sacrifice is required at one level or for one party. Among the most difficult realities that must be reckoned with is the fact that the process will inevitably produce a degree of uncertainty. At some point, however, the weighing must give way to justification.

Step 4: Justification

The justification process permits an accurate determination of the type of ethical dilemma that has emerged. Potentially acceptable alternatives and their respective implications are examined on the basis of application and analysis of relevant ethical principles.

After analysis of ethical principles (and rules), a sound, justifiable argument should be constructed to defend a particular choice of action. Significant effort must be made in attempting to examine any competitive choices in terms of their respective ability to withstand similar ethical inquiry.

In a genuine ethical dilemma, this justification process forces a prioritization of alternatives based on acknowledged ethical principles. This step frequently reflects either a utilitarian view (i.e., being most concerned with the consequences associated with particular alternatives) or a deontological posture (i.e., ranking a certain principle(s) above others independent of the consequences it might precipitate).

Up to this point, the process has maintained a considerable avoidance of values and morals. However, since most decisions, particularly those involving health care issues, employ a value element, values must be considered at this phase. A conscious and sensitive reflection of applicable values, including moral teachings, may at this point bear some influence on the pending choices. Having undergone a values clarification process, one must ascertain, control, and defend the extent to which values affect the decision-making process. To the extent that personal values conflict with prior ethical deliberations, further wrestling with the problem at hand may be in order before making an actual choice.

Step 5: Choice

Making an actual choice brings a degree of closure to the process. In noting, however, that other "ethical" choices could have been made, one can see that the process does not ensure unanimous agreement of a particular choice.

Inevitably, some, if not most, choices mirror professional and personal value judgments. Hence, the importance of values clarification cannot be overemphasized.

Step 6: Evaluation

The final step in "doing ethics" calls for a reexamination of one's choice and its justification, an identification of any unresolved questions, and a comparison of the choice made in this case with decisions made in similar cases elsewhere at other times.

This step, imposed between making a decision and implementing it, ensures a retrospective analysis prior to immediate action. It may be characterized as a sort of "ethical safety net," demanding reconsideration. It ensures that before committing an action that may be irrevocable, one can firmly support a choice and justify it on sound ethical grounds.

SUMMARY

As illustrated throughout this chapter, issues demanding ethical considerations abound in contemporary health education. Moreover, as the technologies associated with communication, media, and the behavioral sciences advance, their application will undoubtedly generate a plethora of ethical issues heretofore not even considered.

Given a meaningful appreciation of fundamental ethical principles and the ability to use them in critical decision-making situations, health educators need to be fully prepared to meet the challenges presented by the growing popularity of health education and health promotion. Their ability to engage in ethical analyses, particularly amid thorny dilemmas involving conflicting alternatives, constitutes an essential professional responsibility. Further, being able to justify decisions on solid ethical grounds contributes to an improved sense of both professional and personal competency.

Finally, the application of a generic set of ethical principles permits sound decision making without having to generate a limited, and too-often restraining, code of ethics specifically for the profession of health education—particularly, given the multiple number of other health care professions (e.g., medicine, nursing, social work) called upon to deliver health education services.

****

ORGANIZATIONS TO CONTACT FOR FURTHER INFORMATION

The Institute of Society, Ethics and the Life Sciences
(The Hastings Center)
360 Broadway
Hastings-on-Hudson, NY 10706
***Daniel Callahan, PhD, Director

Joseph and Rose Kennedy Institute of Ethics
Georgetown University
Washington, DC 20057
***Edmund D. Pellegrino, MD, Director

NOTES

1. Victor R. Fuchs, *Who Shall Live? Health, Economics, and Social Choice* (New York: Basic Books, 1974), 151.

2. Thomas McKeown and G. McLachlan, eds., *Medical History and Medical Care: A Symposium of Perspectives* (New York: Oxford University Press, 1971); Ivan Illich, *Medical Nemesis* (New York: Pantheon, 1976); Aaron Wildavsky, "Doing Better and Feeling Worse: The Political Pathology of Health Policy" in *Doing Better and Feeling Worse: Health in the United States,* ed. John H. Knowles (New York: W.W. Norton, 1977), 105–123; and John H.

Knowles, "The Responsibility of the Individual" in *Doing Better and Feeling Worse: Health in the United States,* ed. John H. Knowles (New York: W.W. Norton, 1977), 57–80.

3. Daniel Callahan, "Applied Ethics: A Strategy for Fostering Professional Responsibility," *Carnegie Quarterly* 28, no. 2–3 (Spring-Summer 1980): 2.

4. Daniel E. Beauchamp, "Community: The Neglected Tradition of Public Health," *Hastings Center Report* 15, no. 6 (December 1985): 28; and R.P. Shafer, "Government Control of Individual Behavior: Its Right and Its Proper Role," *American Journal of Public Health* 56, no. 3 (April 1974): 390–393.

5. Jonathan D. Moreno and Ronald Bayer, "The Limits of the Ledger in Public Health Promotion," *Hastings Center Report* 64, no. 6 (December 1985): 37–41.

6. Daniel I. Wikler, "Persuasion and Coercion for Health: Ethical Issues in Government Efforts to Change Lifestyles," *Milbank Memorial Fund Quarterly/Health and Society* 56, no. 3 (1978): 297.

7. E. Greenwood, "Attributes of a Profession," *Social Work* 2 (July 1957): 44–45.

8. Ruth B. Purtilo and Christie K. Cassel, *Ethical Dimensions in the Health Professions* (Philadelphia: W.B. Saunders, 1981), 27–29.

9. Tom L. Beauchamp and Norman E. Bowie, *Ethical Theory and Business,* 2nd ed. (Englewood Cliffs, N.J.: Prentice-Hall, 1983); and Tom L. Beauchamp and James F. Childress, *Principles of Biomedical Ethics,* 2nd ed. (New York: Oxford University Press, 1983).

10. Beauchamp and Childress, *Principles of Biomedical Ethics.*

11. Ibid., 5.

12. Beauchamp and Bowie, *Ethical Theory and Business,* 1.

13. Vincent Barry, *Moral Aspects of Health Care* (Belmont, Calif.: Wadsworth, 1982), 22.

14. P.S. German and A.J. Chwalow, "Conflicts in Ethical Problems of Patient Education," *International Journal of Health Education* 19, no. 3 (July-September 1976): 195.

15. Tom L. Beauchamp and Laurence B. McCullough, *Medical Ethics: The Moral Responsibilities of Physicians* (Englewood Cliffs, N.J.: Prentice-Hall, 1984), 11.

16. Gerald Dworkin, "Paternalism," in *Morality and the Law,* ed. Richard Wasserstrom (Belmont, Calif.: Wadsworth, 1971), 107–126.

17. Beauchamp, "Community," 28.

18. Beauchamp and Bowie, *Ethical Theory and Business,* 42.

19. Marc D. Hiller, "Ethics and Health Administration: Issues in Education and Practice," *Journal of Health Administration Education* 2, no. 2 (Spring 1984): 147–192.

20. Callahan, "Applied Ethics," 3–4.

21. Purtilo and Cassel, *Ethical Dimensions,* 27–29; Howard Brody, *Ethical Decisions in Medicine,* 2nd ed. (Boston: Little, Brown, 1981), 9–15, 353–357; and Frank Harron, John Burnside, and Tom Beauchamp, *Health and Human Values: A Guide to Making Your Own Decisions* (New Haven, Conn.: Yale University Press, 1983), 4–5.

22. Harron, Burnside, and Beauchamp, *Health and Human Values,* 4–5.

SUGGESTED READINGS

Bassford, H.A. "The Justification of Medical Paternalism." *Social Science and Medicine* 16 (1982): 731–739.

Beauchamp, Tom L., and Leroy Walters. *Contemporary Issues in Bioethics,* 2nd ed. Belmont, Calif.: Wadsworth, 1982.

Belcastro, Philip A. "Health Education . . . Don Quixote's Ethics, Not Tilting, Captured Our Hearts." *Health Values: Achieving High Level Wellness* 6 (March-April 1982): 36–67.

Childress, James F. *Who Should Decide? Paternalism in Health Care.* New York: Oxford University Press, 1982.

Faden, Ruth R., and Alan I. Faden. "The Ethics of Health Education as Public Health Policy." *Health Education Monographs* 6, no. 2 (Summer 1978): 180–197.

Hiller, Marc D. "Ethical and Legal Issues Confronting College Health." *Health Policy and Education* 3 (1982): 133–155.

Pollard, Michael R., and John T. Brennan. "Disease Prevention and Health Promotion Initiatives: Some Legal Considerations." *Health Education Monographs* 6, no. 2 (Summer 1978): 211–222.

Part II

Program Tools

Chapter 6

Humor As a Health Education Tool

William Carlyon, PhD, and Pauline Carlyon, MS, MPH

No human emotion is as familiar yet as little understood as humor. That it is purposeful, adjustive, and, for the most part, life affirming is unchallenged. But exactly what it is and how it works is still largely unknown. Its diversity and subjectivity make it an elusive research target. Valid generalizations are rare.

Humor, it seems, connects with some of the less accessible dimensions of our selves—our deeper more powerful fears, longings, and conflicts, parts of our selves that we are reticent to examine and that do not yield to conventional ways of knowing. We have trouble, for instance, with the apparent paradox in the close parallels between humor and sorrow, laughter and tears, joviality and anger. Perhaps we need research into conceptualizations of humor as much as we do into how to make more people laugh. Our concept of humor, how we think about it, determines everything we do in its name.

Take, for example, the concept of humor as a health education tool. That notion is based in our technical interventionist cultural mindset and its extension in the medical model. It is an axiom of that mindset that we invent tools with which to build or fix things. This outlook has yielded astonishing material progress and the most technologically sophisticated medical care in history.

But this outlook may or may not be an appropriate way to view humor. We may be casting as a tool a phenomenon not amenable to such manipulation and standardization. If humor is a tool, perhaps it needs to be custom made by the user as needed. Perhaps our job is to encourage custom humor toolmaking by patients and clients, rather than to contrive a standard humor tool with which we can "fix" them. It is their tool, not ours, except when we invent one to meet our own needs.

These preliminary cautions need not lessen enthusiasm for humor's health-engendering possibilities. It appears created for that purpose. The question is, How can health educators help themselves and others profit from humor's seemingly infinite potential for good?

The purpose of this chapter is to explore that potential by examining the nature of humor, assessing its usefulness in patient care and health promotion, and taking a quick look at how some people are using humor in health and patient education.

THE COUSINS CONNECTION

Sparked by Norman Cousins' 1976 account of his dramatic recovery from an assumed-to-be-fatal collagen disease, the subject of humor and health has received increasing attention in recent years.[1] In *Anatomy of an Illness,* Cousins describes in detail how he checked out of the hospital and into a hotel where he spent his days watching old Groucho Marx movies and listening to recordings of comedy routines—and doing a lot of laughing.[2] His ensuing complete recovery appeared miraculous.

He used his unique approach to therapy successfully a second time following a serious heart attack in 1980. That experience is described in *The Healing Heart.*[3]

Since then, the "laughter is good medicine" idea has become extremely popular in and outside the health care field. It has also become distorted and oversimplified.

Noting this, Cousins took pains to correct the widespread notion that he simply laughed himself out of serious illness. "Careful readers . . .," he said, "knew that laughter was just a metaphor for the entire range of positive emotions. Hope, faith, love, will to live, cheerfulness, humor, creativity, playfulness, confidence, great expectations . . . all these I believe had therapeutic value."[4]

It is Cousins' belief that negative emotions, such as fear, panic, and depression, set the stage for illness, and that disease can be forestalled and healing enhanced by replacing those negative emotions with positive ones.

THE NATURE OF HUMOR

Humor and its physical expression, laughter, are ubiquitous in humans. There is no known human group that does not display individual or group humor. But somehow, the literature seems to grow in inverse proportion to understanding of why people laugh. Until recent years, explanations have been left to philosophers and naturalists. Medical investigators have largely ignored the subject, except as it is related to some medical condition such as "giggle incontinence," brain dysfunction, or as it holds promise as an aid to healing.[5]

The range of stimuli that evoke laughter seems endless. There is no subject or life situation about which humor is not possible, including dying. Humor can be subtle, witty, and comic, or gross, tasteless, and vulgar. It can ease tensions, create tensions, flatter, or insult.

Depending upon what we find comic, funny, farcial, ridiculous, or hilarious, we may grin, titter, simper, snort, cackle, chuckle, guffaw, chortle, or hee haw! All while splitting our sides, laughing our heads off, and rolling in the aisles. Less charitably, we might smirk or snicker our ridicule at someone and finish them off with a horse laugh.

Humor is indeed everywhere in our language and lives. And it always feels good—at least to the laugher.

Darwin's observations on laughter are still valid. Darwin viewed laughter as a continuum from mere cheerfulness to a gentle then broader smile and finally to laughter of varying degrees. He observed that in laughter the mouth is open, corners drawn back and up. The upper lip and cheeks are raised. The upper front teeth are exposed and wrinkles (laugh lines) form under the eyes. The eyebrows are slightly lowered and there is trembling at corners of the mouth and eyes, which are bright and sparkling, the face flushed. During excessive laughter, the whole body gets involved, thrown backward shaking almost to convulsions. Respiration is much disturbed. The head and neck become gorged with blood and tears are freely shed.[6]

Black observes that immediately following laughter, muscles become flaccid, pulse rate elevates, probably due to increased catecholamine levels "that vary directly with laughter intensity and reflect activation of the hypothalamus—pituitary—adrenal axis."[7]

No laughter center has been identified in the brain and its possible location is a subject of much speculation.

Pathological laughter due to brain damage or functional mental illness is real laughter but unmotivated (to the viewer), uncontrolled, and inappropriate. Irrepressible contagious giggling and laughter that strikes children and occasionally adults at inopportune moments may be embarrassing, but probably should not be considered pathological.

According to William Fry, laughter is essentially a respiratory act. While there are many laughing styles, laughter is characterized by expiratory predominance. There is pulmonary ventilation beyond that with normal breathing. However, "despite this expiratory predominance," says Fry, "peripheral blood oxygen concentrations are not greatly disturbed and maintain stability even during prolonged laughter of pronounced intensity."[8]

Heart rate and systolic and diastolic blood pressure increase in direct proportion to intensity and duration of laughter. There is a short-lived drop below normal of blood pressure at cessation of laughter.

The musculoskeletal system gets a workout in proportion to laughter intensity; from modest facial/scalp and shoulder involvement with chuckling to involvement of most skeletal muscles in "convulsive" laughter.

There are few laboratory studies that support the presumed activation of the central nervous system during laughter. Assumptions about the effects of laughter on the endocrine system, including the endorphins, as yet find little laboratory substantiation.

The role of emotions in some disease has been established. Anger and fear may precipitate heart attacks or contribute to the accumulation of emotion that sets the stage for an attack. "It is proverbial," says Fry, "that humor minimizes the intensities of both fear and anger." Those two emotions cannot exist in full force while mirth is experienced. And in many instances, fear and anger are completely dissipated by a cultivated sense of humor."[9]

Laughter and Exercise

Fry also notes a similarity in the benefits of laughter and exercise. Both provide increased heart rate, blood pressure, and circulation, as well as increased frequency and depth of respiration with expulsion and replacement of residual air in the lungs and coughing out of mucous accumulations. Both provide musculoskeletal activity and a sense of well-being and pain relief, possibly attributable to increased levels of endorphins, the body's natural opiates. "Indeed," says Fry, "laughter can be said to give the body a miniworkout and has been compared to stationary jogging."[10]

Because of its universal human presence, humor is considered a genetic disposition shaped by an individual's environment. Because each individual's environment is unique, no two people—not even twins—have identical humor repertoires.

Origins of Humor

Fry observes that the biological origins of humor are related to inherited capacities for play and ambivalence. "The spirit of play," he points out, "establishes a context for interpreting and responding to forms of communication—verbal or non verbal—intended to be humorous. Without this context or frame, the communication presumably intended as humorous would appear inconsequential, bizarre or incongruous."[11] Without the human ability to hold two or more conflicting attitudes or feelings at the same time (ambivalence), humor would be perceived as inconsistent or conflictual.

These observations are of great importance to anyone intending to use humor as a tool. The standup comedian "dies" in front of an audience not yet in a playful mood—or not attuned to the comic's unique brand of playfulness.

Contrariwise, playful rapport, say, between teachers and students, can escalate to the point that everything said is funny and no serious work can be done. One has to listen for cues to a patient's/client's/student's frame of playfulness and help that individual shape it into dimensions he or she finds exciting, fun, and useful.

Kinds of Humor

The richness and variety of humor defies categorization. For convenience, some researchers have identified five basic types: nonsense, sick, ridicule, hostile, and sexual. Humor most often appears as some combination of these. The television series *M.A.S.H.* masterfully used them all in nearly every episode.

Such varieties of humor serve many purposes: to wound, relieve tension, assert power, reduce fear, or make unbearable situations tolerable. It is crucial to remember that it is the listener's perception of purpose that gives meaning to humor. This is why using humor as a health education tool can be tricky.

Using Humor As a Health Education Tool

The following are some useful guidelines:

- Remember, humor is not just a joke. It is one of a range of positive emotions you want to evoke.
- Do not assume that others share your sense of humor and its underlying social attitudes.
- Beware of satire and irony. They are easily misread as sarcasm or ridicule.
- Do not tell jokes, unless they are "on you." Save your standup comedy for your family and friends, who are familiar with your eccentricities.
- Avoid ethnic humor and dialect imitations particularly. You will almost always sound insulting.
- Do listen to your clients/patients/students and encourage their humor by participating in its enjoyment. Only they know the humor that's best for them.

HUMOR IN PATIENT CARE

Probably no "normal" cultural experience carries more befuddlement, fear, and indignity than being a patient in a hospital. Interrogated, stripped, probed, poked, hurried, and ignored, a person is reduced to childlike status at the hands of strangers.

In such a milieu, damaging negative emotions flourish—guilt, rage, shame, and, most important, fear and panic followed by depression. These feelings cause changes in body chemistry that are inimical to healing. There's something about fearing the worst that moves the body in that direction.

Cousins observes that, although there may be a dearth of "hard" evidence that laughter has specific significant therapeutic value, what is clear is that laughter is an antidote to apprehension and panic. An optimistic outlook that expects the best can move the body in that direction, too.

"Gallows" Humor

Gallows humor, the macabre "laughing at death" kind, occurs in all patient care settings. Gallows, or Black, humor tends to be ironic and satiric. It is a form of hostile and sick humor aimed primarily at alleviating the anxieties of the person who is speaking rather than amusing others. But the anxieties of patients are different from those of health care professionals. So there are really two kinds of gallows humor in patient care: first, that which helps the patient deal with fear and rage and second, the in-group "medical" humor that serves as the professional's defense against being overwhelmed. Death, disfigurement, grief, and despair are stark realities of the professional's daily life, not to mention feelings of inadequacy in dealing with it all. And, too, there are hostilities toward the patients and "the system," which are sometimes dealt with through acerbic witticism, ridicule, and derogating slurs.

This is not the kind of humor that can engender positive emotions in patients.

Humor As a Communications Tool

Humor facilitates communication in any setting. It breaks the ice in a waiting room, classroom, or cocktail party. It is a form of small talk. It decreases social distance. Vera Robinson observes, "The messages which need to be communicated within the hospital or other health setting are usually very serious and emotion laden: anxiety, fear, embarrassment, anger, tragedy, concern, hope and joy. Yet their direct expression is not always acceptable or comfortable. Humor serves to convey these in an indirect fashion, and, because of its play frame, provides a vehicle for moving easily in or out of the 'serious' as the situation warrants."[12] Humor helps diffuse awkward and embarrassing situations, asserts individuality, and preserves self-respect.

Jokes about the bad food, being awakened for a sleeping pill, shots, toilet indignities, the bill, all help reduce tension and socialize the patient into the hospital culture. Patients joking with each other about such common experiences gives a sense of cohesiveness—and shared misery.

The best humor in patient care happens spontaneously to meet the needs of the moment as perceived by the patient. It can be encouraged by participating in it, thus giving permission for it to happen. If one must initiate humor, it might best be a bit self-deprecating—let the joke be on you. This signals your own appreciation of the comic and your openness to it. No two people think the same things are funny. Ethnic appreciation of humor and what is permissible varies widely and holds booby traps for those who try too hard to be funny.

Using Humor in Patient Care

The following are some useful guidelines:

- Remember, your major goal is to forestall negative emotions, especially fear and panic. Humor is just one tool for that purpose.
- Keep professional "gallows" humor in the in-group. Patients would be devastated by such apparent callousness and indifference to their suffering.
- Don't try to be funny. Nothing is more obvious, falls as flat, or is resented as contrived cheerfulness in a hospital or clinic.
- Do work with other staff to create an atmosphere that is warm, friendly, caring, reassuring, and respectful of individual dignity.
- Smile a lot. It warms the atmosphere and is a universal sign of reassurance.

HEALTH PROMOTION

Humor courses are increasing in popularity in health promotion settings. They are almost always well attended, vary widely in scope and content, and tend to be superficial.

A major purpose of such courses is to provide a "safe" opportunity to loosen up, laugh, and get in touch with the humorous side of life. Audience participation is encouraged. Activities include recollecting "my most embarrassing moment," tossing marshmallows, putting on funny costumes, and just plain acting silly.

Most limit their goals to the fun of the moment, which led one health educator to observe "It feels good at the time but it doesn't last. They have to keep coming back to get their funny bones retickled."

Such humor sessions are good as far as they go, but there needs to be more than one-shot humor courses, especially those designed primarily for agency marketing or public relations purposes. Humor in health education needs to be more than a tool for entertainment. People come to humor courses in health promotion programs for more than a few laughs. They come because they hurt somewhere in their lives and they want to do something about it, to feel better.

The prevalence of such a malaise is not surprising, considering the condition of our modern civilization. We are under constant pressure to compete, to win, to get ahead. Madison Avenue keeps reminding us of our shortcomings with unrealistic images of how we are supposed to look, act, and feel. We must push harder and harder—"no pain, no gain."

All this against a world background that includes the nuclear arms race, international terrorism, a rotting environment, economic calamities, mass starvation, and endless slaughter. Optimistic images of the future are getting scarce. We mal-cope with stoic masks and increasing amounts of noise, trivia, violence, and drugs. No wonder we are feeling blue.

We have named this malaise "stress," and it sounds a lot like those negative emotions that Norman Cousins says can set people up for illness. Perhaps the function of humor is the same everywhere—as a natural defense against the stress, sadness, and absurdity of human living and dying. Comedy and tragedy, laughter and tears, are never far apart.

Perhaps our job as health educators is to encourage humor wherever and whenever we can, to bring balance to our personal and professional lives.

Using Humor As a Health Promotion Tool

The following are some useful guidelines:

- Remember, humor is one tool for evoking a wide range of positive emotions.
- Build on the initial humor offering by incorporating humor into courses on stress-related topics such as child rearing, relationships, employment, self-esteem, loneliness.

- Offer a mindstyle retraining course. Much stress results from faulty perceptions of reality. Help clients identify and change thoughts and images that bring on negative emotions.
- Encourage daily humor breaks at work, home, and school, particularly when stress begins to build.

SUMMARY

Humor clearly has a bright future as a health education tool. It fits well with health educators' humanistic approach to their work. However, humor is a delicate tool that must be used with great astuteness and sensitivity. Its possibilities and limitations need to be thoroughly understood before its implementation. Curriculum guides and course materials need to be developed for preservice and inservice education.

***

SUGGESTED RESOURCES

•The Humor Project, 110 Spring Street, Saratoga Springs, New York 12866. Joel Goodman, Director. Major clearinghouse networking agency for resources and activities in all aspects of humor and health. Offers the following: speeches, programs, conferences and seminars, hospital staff training, professional preparation, graduate courses. Publishes *Laughing Matters,* a quarterly magazine focusing on the positive power of humor. Includes practical tips and examples of how to apply humor personally and on the job.

•Vera Robinson, RN, EdD, Chairman and Professor, Department of Nursing, California State University, Fullerton, California 92634. Author of *Humor and the Health Professions.* Additional material is available along with other resources.

•William F. Fry, MD, Associate Clinical Professor, Stanford School of Medicine, Stanford University, Stanford, California 94305. The premier humor researcher offers current research data on physiology of laughter, essays, books, and bibliographies.

•Nurses for Laughter, a national organization of 1,100 members. California State University, Fullerton, California 92634. Deborah Leiber, President, Vera Robinson, Vice President. Promotes use of laughter in patient care. Regional groups collect and share educational materials. Offers workshops, speeches, materials, sources.

•Andrus Volunteers, University of Southern California, University Park, Los Angeles, California 90089-0191. Polly McConny, Director of Volunteers. A group of older adults who serve the University Gerontology Center and the community. Information on Humor As Enrichment for Older Persons. Conducted a nursing home demonstration project to explore therapeutic use of humor in long-term care. Book: *Humor: The Tonic You Can Afford,* foreword by Norman Cousins, $6.50 plus $1.00 for shipping and handling. California residents add 42 cents state tax.

•University of California, Santa Barbara, Student Health Service, Santa Barbara, California 93106. Sabina A. White, Health Educator. Conducts laughter and humor workshops for college students. Conducts funded research into effectiveness of laughter in stress reduction. Offers training program for humor workshop leaders. Offers a how-to-do-it handbook, "Laughter and Stress," $10. Videotape also available that includes workshop excerpts and interviews. Write for price.

•Ravenswood Hospital Counseling and Education Department, 4545 N. Damen, Chicago, Illinois 60625. Laurieann Chutis, A.S.C.W., Director. Offers both six-week and one-night courses to the public on "How to Get in Touch with Your Humorous Side." Places humor within broad context of positive emotions and creativity. Write for course outline and materials.

•World Humor and Irony Membership (WHIM), English Department, Arizona State University, Tempe, Arizona 85287. Contact Don Nilsen. Pursues four strands of humor: British literature, American literature, popular culture and religion, and psychology and health. Sponsors annual interdisciplinary conference during April's first weekend. Publishes conference proceedings as *World Humor and Irony Membership Serial Yearbook* (WHIMSY), $10 per copy. Past three available.

•Health at Work, Center for Health Promotion, Group Health Cooperative of Puget Sound, 1625 Terry Avenue, Seattle, Washington 98101. Wendy Graff, Corporate Health Promotion Specialist. Promotes humor at work as guerrilla warfare to make work more humanistic and productive. Write for descriptive materials.

•Gesundheit Institute, 404 N. Nelson Street, Arlington, Virginia 22203. Patch Adams, M.D. A totally unique live-in, commune-type of approach to healing, living, and growing. Uses humor and laughter extensively in all activities. Offers courses and seminars especially to medical students, medical schools, allied health professionals.

NOTES

1. Norman Cousins, "Anatomy of an Illness (As Perceived by the Patient)," *New England Journal of Medicine* 295, no. 26 (1976): 1458–63.

2. —, *Anatomy of an Illness As Perceived by the Patient* (New York: W.W. Norton, 1979).

3. —, *The Healing Heart* (New York: W.W. Norton, 1983).

4. *Ibid.*

5. M.P. Rogers, R.F. Gittes, D.M. Dawson, and P. Reigh, "Giggle Incontinence," *Journal of the American Medical Association* 247, no. 10 (1982): 1446–48; Donald W. Black, "Pathological Laughter," *The Journal of Nervous and Mental Disease* 170, no. 2 (1982): 67–71; Roma Safranek and Thomas Schill, "Coping with Stress: Does Humor Help?" *Psychological Reports* 51 (1982): 222; and Victor N. Hirsch and Walter E. O'Connell, "No Laughing Matter: The Lack of Humor in Current Psychotherapists," in *Does Psychotherapy Really Help People?* ed. Josseph Hariman (Springfield, Ill.: Charles C Thomas, 1984), 102–11.

6. Charles Darwin, *Expression of the Emotions in Man and Animals* (Chicago: The University of Chicago Press, 1986), 196–219.

7. Donald W. Fry, "Laughter," *Journal of the American Medical Association* 252, no. 21 (1984): 2995–98.

8. William F. Fry, "Laughter and Health," in *Medical and Health Annual* (Chicago: Encyclopaedia Britannica, 1970), 261.

9. *Ibid.*, 262.

10. *Ibid.*

11. *Ibid.*, 260.

12. Vera M. Robinson, *Humor and the Health Professions* (Thorofare, N.J.: Charles B. Slack, 1977), 41.

SUGGESTED READINGS

Fry, William F., Jr. *Sweet Madness: A Study of Humor.* Palo Alto, Calif.: Pacific Books, 1963.

Fry, William F., Jr., and Melanie Allen. *Make 'Em Laugh: Life Studies of Comedy Writers.* Palo Alto, Calif.: Science and Behavior Books, 1983.

Fry, William F., Jr., and Waleed A. Salameh, eds. *Handbook of Humor and Psychotherapy: Advances in Clinical Use of Humor.* Sarasota, Fla.: The Professional Resource Exchange, 1986.

McGhee, Paul E., and Jeffrey H. Goldstein, eds. *Handbook of Humor Research.* Vol. II, *Applied Studies.* New York: Springer-Verlag, 1983.

Powell, B.S. "Laughter and Healing: The Use of Humor in Hospitals Treating Children." *Association for the Care of Children in Hospitals Journal* (November 1974): 10–16.

Chapter 7

The Use of Computers in Health Education

Laurel Burch-Minakan, MPH

The purpose of this chapter is to discuss the many uses of computerized health education for health educators and other health professionals. This chapter attempts to demystify the ever-growing world of computers and software and help the program manager avoid some costly pitfalls. Various types of health education software and their advantages and disadvantages are discussed. The chapter concludes with the assertion that computerized health education has tremendous potential as an educational tool in health care settings.

Until recently, the design and development of computer hardware and software has been primarily for business (payroll, customer orders, inventory control, etc.) and scientific (statistical analysis) applications. However, with the advent of smaller business computers and home computers, software companies are now beginning to offer programs for the education market. This phenomenon has lead to the growth of "personal" software firms offering word processing, home finance programs, educational programs for children, etc. Now, with the public's and major corporations' renewed interest in health issues and fitness programs, software companies and enterprising health professionals are specializing in software for fitness and health education.

HARDWARE

The computer is an invaluable tool. However, before you go out and buy sophisticated software and a personal computer, be careful not to become too entranced with computer capability and develop unrealistic expectations. The computer is neutral; how we use it determines the degree of its success or failure. Prior to your journey into the computer jungle, it would be a good idea to read *The Silicon Jungle,* by David Rothman[1] (especially the afterword). It will help you develop a necessary sense of humor and maybe avoid some costly, embarrassing mistakes.

Computer hardware is not as important as the software that makes it useful. A computer is hardly more than a box of miscellaneous electronic parts. These parts are connected into a useful machine only through software—the array of languages, programs, data, and special internal operating procedures.

There are so many computers on the market—how do you know which is best? To begin, you must assess what hardware already exists at your workplace. For example, maybe your company uses a mainframe that you could have access to, or someone thought it would be a good idea to purchase an IBM PC and it is sitting in a corner collecting dust because no one has taken the time to figure out how to use it. Even if your company has a mainframe, you may want to purchase a microcomputer so you will have total control of your system. After reviewing software for health education, it appears that most of it is being created for the Apple II series and the IBM PC. However, never buy a computer without seeing for yourself that it, and the software will together serve your needs.

HOW TO CHOOSE THE RIGHT SOFTWARE

What are your needs? Shopping around for the right software package is not easy. "With press agents and flashy boxes for disks, the software market is going Hollywood."[2] You will need to analyze your health program and determine exactly what you need a computer to do. You must have a clear idea of your goals, be realistic, and choose your software package accordingly.

There are many packages available, each with its own approach and particular emphasis—health risk appraisals, software on health topics, and self-instructional fitness and nutrition programs. Before selecting a software package you will have to assess the program's capabilities and limitations and then compare these facts against your program objectives. Ask the prospective vendor to prove that the software can meet your minimum needs. See if you can use the package on a trial basis for review and evaluation.

Questions that should be addressed: What are the software capabilities? Does the program prescribe action, analyze it, or merely provide record keeping? What is the print capability of the software? Can you get a hard copy of the data analysis? How much data can you file? Can you compare records from one time period to another? How versatile is the software? Can you edit or add to available data bases to meet individual needs? Is the documentation (instructions) easy to follow?

Inspect the documentation to assess the difficulty in setting up and using the program. Depending on the package, it shouldn't take more than a few hours to learn and operate the program. Is the software credible? This should be a major factor in choosing your software package. Examine the documentation and support material. Learn about the program's author(s) and designer(s) and if they are well-known writers or experts, read their books and/or articles. Also, read software reviews (*Infoworld* is an excellent computer magazine), examine advertisements and product literature, and consult with a professional in the field in which you are interested.

SOFTWARE FOR HEALTH

Software for health education available on microcomputers is still in its infancy. Health professionals and software manufacturers are just waking up to the fact that there is a need and a market for self-instructional computer programs on various health topics and issues. On the other hand, mainframe computer-generated health risk appraisals have been offered for some time by outside consulting agencies who provide the questionnaire, process the data, and then send aggregate and individual computerized reports to the client. Although use of a consulting firm requires minimal effort on your part, it is relatively expensive ($10-$40 per evaluation) and you give up control of the data and the capability to track employees. Another factor to consider is the potential danger of unnecessarily alarming a person who is appraised at an above-average risk or reassuring another person who is appraised at below-average risk. It is important that users understand the limitations of this type of software.[3] Some examples are *Health Risk Profile*,[4] *Personal Health Profile*,[5] *Health Risk Questionnaire*,[6] *Healthline*,[7] *Innerview Health Assessment*,[8] and *Life*.[9] The Centers for Disease Control in Atlanta, Georgia, offers health risk appraisal software that you can purchase for mainframes.[10]

INTERACTIVE MICROCOMPUTER-BASED HEALTH RISK APPRAISAL SOFTWARE

Fairly new on the scene are user-friendly, interactive (see Definitions in Appendix 7-A) health risk appraisals (HRA) designed for microcomputers to be used by the person whose risk is being evaluated. The program involves its user in a personalized question, answer, and feedback format. The user learns which behaviors to change to reduce his or her health risks and a summary printout is provided to reinforce motivation. An example is The University of Minnesota's *Health Risk Appraisal*[11] (see Appendix 7-B), based on the Centers for Disease Control health risk questions and calculations. This interactive HRA asks the user 35 lifestyle and physiological questions to determine the user's risks for 10 leading causes of death. A one-page summary of the user's risks is also provided. Another example is *COMPUTE-A-LIFE I*[12] by the National Wellness Institute, an interactive HRA, which uses high-resolution color graphics to make the appraisal process more interesting and informative. The Institute also offers *COMPUTE-A-LIFE II,* a batch-processed version of the same program, which allows the health professional to distribute the questionnaire to employees and then have the data entered into the computer at a later time.

The Hospitalization Risk Assessment Program,[13] by Tulane University Medical Center, is designed to assess hospitalization risks that an individual can modify. There is a short (5–10 minute) and a long (15–20 minutes) version with questions covering alcohol consumption, smoking, weight, blood pressure, cholesterol levels, driving habits, and depression. Interestingly, the user can ask why some information is requested and receive explanations. Each risk factor contributes to the risk score, which is adjusted for age and sex, and there are suggestions for modifying risks. Another interactive HRA is *Personal Health Inventory,*[14] which asks questions concerning health habits, lifestyle, medical care, and women's health. A five-minute, color, graphic analysis displays the participants' risk of dying from the ten most frequent causes of death. The results can also be printed—not all HRA software has print capability.

SOFTWARE ON HEALTH TOPICS

Computer-assisted instruction/education programs on health are just now being developed. This type of software has the greatest potential for enhancing the health education process. It should be used in conjunction with other health education techniques and materials, and promises to become one of the best educational tools for motivation. This software provides answers via a user-friendly menu of questions on different medical and health topics such as alcohol, smoking, weight control, cancer prevention, etc. An example of this type of software is *Personal Health II,*[15] designed for young adults and health-conscious adults. It is an interactive, educational computer program containing specific topics on health habits, health costs, immunizations, and specific health problems. There is also a quiz section to test one's knowledge of health facts and myths. *Positive Lifestyling*[16] is designed to educate the individual in the areas of nutrition, exercise, stress management, chemical dependence, and weight control. This program can monitor a person's daily progress for up to four years, and uses graphics to show this progress. The National Wellness Institute[17] developed *TESTWELL,* a computerized test that measures the wellness of the individual in the areas of physical fitness, nutrition, self-care, social and emotional awareness, drugs and driving, and intellectual, occupational, and spiritual dimensions. In addition, the Institute has developed software on stress, STRESS ASSESS, which evaluates current stress resources, distress symptoms, and lifestyle behaviors, and *WHY SMOKE,* an interactive program designed to help individuals discover why they smoke cigarettes.

HEALTH AND FITNESS SOFTWARE

Health and fitness software has been called "life-enrichment" or "self-help" software. Future Computing, a market research firm, estimates earnings in the area of 57 million.[18] There are dozens of software packages available to help keep you trim and stick to your fitness regimen. These packages fall into three general categories: exercise, nutrition, and combined exercise and nutrition software.

Fitness programs track your running, aerobics, and other exercise activities. Nutritional-analysis programs break down your meals into their components for menu planning and dieting. The combined fitness and nutrition programs offer the nutrient makeup of meals, weight, calorie intake, and other nutritional factors, in addition to monitoring fitness activities.

Fitness Software

Fitness programs on the market are designed primarily for individuals and families to use on their home computers. However, this software can be used in the corporate environment as an addition to, or if you have limited resources, as an alternative to a costly in-house fitness facility or program. You would have to inquire into the capability of the software to accommodate many users and would have to station the computer in an area that would be accessible to a majority of employees.

Before purchasing the software, consult with an exercise physiologist to get an opinion on the content of the package. Also, make it clear, through written instructions, that participants should check with their health professional before beginning an exercise program—especially if they are over 35.

Fitness software packages vary a great deal and, generally, the higher the cost ($19–$350), the more sophisticated the package. Software programs range in capability from simple recording and updating to analyzing exercise, to prescribing a conditioning program based on individual abilities and needs. An example of fitness software already available for small business and home computers is *Aerobics*,[19] the first program to make use of an animated instructor that leads you through your aerobic workout. *The Aerobics Master*[20] is primarily geared for runners to log their progress and has no significant analysis capabilities. Other programs for runners who need only a method of charting their running progress are *The Running Log*,[21] *Running Coach*,[22] *Be Your Own Coach*,[23] and *The Running Program*.[24] *In Shape*[25] and *Healthpath*[26] feature nutrition and exercise components that can be tailored to meet individual fitness goals.

NUTRITION SOFTWARE

Nutrition-only programs vary widely in sophistication and price but are basically specialized data bases with hundreds of food and nutrient breakdowns. The majority of the programs follow the U.S. Department of Agriculture's charts on protein, carbohydrates, fats, and calories, and the Recommended Daily Allowances (RDA) for vitamins and minerals established by the Food and Nutrition Board of the National Academy of Sciences.

Simple diet-analysis programs, such as *Eating Machine*,[27] *Evrydiet*,[28] or *Nutri-Pack*,[29] provide a data base of a few hundred foods and the ability to add more foods and to create and analyze daily menus. *Total Health*[30] provides simplified nutrition analysis with a data base of 150 food items as well as looking at calories, sodium, fat, protein, and carbohydrates. *Nutri-Calc*,[31] by PCD Systems, Inc., has a data base of 900 foods, which can be expanded to 1,000 on the Apple. Dietary patterns are analyzed and the caloric intake to maintain or lose weight during a specific period of physical activity (walking, sitting, sleeping, standing, vigorous work) is given. The *Nutritionist/The Nutritionist II*,[32] by N-Squared Computing, includes a data base of 730 food items and analyzes your diet for 19 nutrients. *The Nutritionist II* has a larger data base, analyzes more nutrients, and factors in exercise into the nutrition analysis. *Nutri-Byte*[33] stores the breakdowns of more than 1,200 foods, guides you through a five-week weight program, and also asks where and with whom you eat, your hunger level, physical activity, and moods.

COMBINED EXERCISE AND NUTRITION PROGRAM

The more well-rounded approach to health is software that contains both exercise and diet components. Generally, this software emphasizes diet and nutrition more than it does exercise. Among the most sophisticated programs are *The Original Boston Computer Diet*,[34] which gives greater weight to nutrition, and *The James F. Fixx Running Program*,[35] which focuses more on fitness.

The Boston Diet includes a 50-page instruction booklet, 97 pages of educational information, a data base of 700 foods and their calories, and a master disk and a "daily" disk. The disks are copy-protected with no provision even for back-up, so, for more than one person to use the program, you must purchase additional daily disks for a nominal fee. There are three personalities from which to choose as your "counselor"—one is sympathetic, one is stern, and the third is easygoing. Users are supposed to report to the computer once a day giving the date, hour, mood, food item, and portion size of every food eaten. After entering the day's meals, a summary of the week's meals and the counselor's comments are provided. Also, each daily session ends with a reading assignment containing information on nutrition and human physiology.

The *James F. Fixx Running Program* evaluates the user's current fitness level before advising a training regimen. In addition to asking about age, sex, height, weight, and frame size, the program guides the user through the Harvard Step Test and a timed two-mile run/walk. Next, the user chooses a training goal from four ready-made models, entering information about distance and time goals. Workouts are entered on a daily basis along with the user's weekly mileage goal and the number of weeks desired to train. Besides keeping exercise logs, the user also maintains nutrition logs and the program calculates the daily intake of calories, grams of protein, fat, carbohydrates, and serum cholesterol level.

An example of a highly sophisticated and expensive software package is *FITCOMP*,[36] a nutrition and exercise assessment system that is used at Southern New England Telephone. *FITCOMP* was designed and developed by Frank and Victor Katch and can provide individualized reports that take into account body size, body composition, age, sex, current fitness status, and aerobic activity preference. *FITCOMP* was developed from detailed measurements of body composition on a variety of world-class athletes and diverse groups of young and old men and women. It offers the user a choice of measurement techniques including fatfolds, girths, bone diameters, and hydrostatic weighing. Following American Dietetic Association guidelines, menu plans for breakfast, lunch, and dinner are generated to provide an optimal blend of nutrients for achieving ideal body mass and fat percentage. The individual can select an aerobic exercise program from nine different activities, including walking, jogging, running, cycling, and swimming. To reduce cost, the software is leased and SNET's IBM 360 mainframe computer with a laser printer is utilized to generate the typical 16-page computer report. The authors are currently in the process of making the FITCOMP program interactive with home computers, which will significantly lower the cost of both hardware and software.

PSYCHOLOGICAL SOFTWARE

A very recent product on the market is psychological self-care software. An example of this software is *Eliza*.[37] The user types in his or her problems as though speaking to a therapist and then *Eliza* responds on the computer screen using nondirective statements.

Another recently developed psychological program is *Mind Prober*,[38] which differs from *Eliza* in that it asks the user to pick a person and then decide whether a list of objectives suits the person. A psychological profile is then printed out. More sophisticated versions of these software packages will certainly be available in the near future.

INTEGRATED SOFTWARE

Computer-based technologies, in addition to informing and assisting individual users to change their health behaviors, can also be utilized as a management information system. The purchase of appropriate integrated software can improve the management of health data. An outstanding example is *SAS* (Statistical Analysis System)[39] for data base management, record keeping, and report generation.

SAS was developed to provide data analysts with one system to meet all their computing needs instead of having to learn programming languages, several statistical packages, and utility programs. Users can add tools for graphics, forecasting, data entry[40] and interface other data bases to the basic *SAS* system and create one total system. The basic *SAS* system provides tools for information storage and retrieval, data modification and programming, report writing, statistical analysis, and file handling. SAS is easy-to-learn and cost-effective compared with other complex software packages. It is extremely powerful, a real number cruncher, and user friendly.

A good example of utilizing *SAS* is Kimberly-Clark's Health Management Program.[41] *SAS* was already being used throughout the Kimberly-Clark Corporation on the company's IBM mainframe computer before being passed on to the Medical Department. The Kimberly-Clark health promotion program, initiated in 1977 by Kimberly-Clark Corporation, consists of four components: a medical screening, health education, aerobic exercise and cardiac rehabilitation, and an employee assistance program. *SAS* has enabled the Medical Department to computerize its medical data base, appointment scheduling for high risk individuals, individual health screening profile, heart attack risk profile, and Exercise Facility sign-in sheets and attendance reports. *SAS* eliminated the cost of an outside vendor for individualized health risk appraisals. *SAS* is also used to monitor participation rates and evaluate lifestyle risk factors over time.

A similar situation was experienced by the health promotion staff at Southern New England Telephone. In the search for management information software, it discovered that the Information Systems Department already had *SAS* up and running. *SAS* is utilized to generate individual health risk profiles, to interface with other *SNET* data bases, to process accounting data, and produce statistical reports on the demographic and health status of employees. All pre- , post- , and follow-up evaluation data from health education and fitness programs are being entered and, in the future, health data will be merged with *SNET* utilization claims data in order to evaluate the impact the health promotion program has had on health care utilization.

FUTURE IMPLICATIONS OF INTERACTIVE COMPUTER SOFTWARE PROGRAMS AND HEALTH EDUCATION

It was said that television would become a revolutionary educational tool and yet this did not become a reality—are we too optimistic about the potential of computers and education? Probably not. Today's computer technology allows the individual to *interact* with the computer—to be an active participant. Television is passive. In addition, there is a new attitude toward computers that views them as "knowledge processors."[42] This recent development has had practical implications in the design and use of computers and software—small business computers and home computers—and the development of "self-care" software.

In the next ten years, we are going to see an increased application of interactive technologies to health education and the determination of individual health behaviors. The software will become less categorical, much more comprehensive, cheaper, and available everywhere. Health professionals, especially physicians, will begin to integrate this technology into their practices to develop behavior plans and educational programs for their patients/clients.

At the moment, interactive computer software programs offer certain advantages and disadvantages. The primary advantages of a computer-administered program include the ease of handling data and immediate reporting of results to individuals participating in the session. Immediate feedback improves the level of motivation of participants. Furthermore, the use of a computer alters the dynamics of the instructional situation in a way that provides a nonthreatening challenge to the user, which thereby may encourage participation. The major disadvantages of computer programs are the cost and availability of equipment as well as the difficulties in choosing the right software and/or microcomputer.

Control Data's STAYWELL Program, a worksite wellness program, found computer-delivered programs to be positive in the following ways: (1) they are individualized; (2) people are able to have a direct dialogue with the author of the program; (3) they represent a more efficient way to enable people to set goals and track their progress; (4) people can focus their learning on the material that is most relevant to them; (5) they provide positive reinforcement of desired behaviors; (6) they are more patient, flexible, less expensive, and available at more convenient times than human instructors; (7) they are available in the home so that the programs can be used more conveniently, more often, and by other family members; and (8) they are capable of providing support groups of similar people by linking them via computer.[43]

There is sparse information on computerized health education and even less research on this subject. However, a recent study by William Deardorff compared the computerized health education format with face-to-face and written methods and found that computer conditions were comparable to a face-to-face format in terms of participant satisfaction and superior to the face-to-face format in terms of recall of the text. The study pointed out that there is a potential for very different reactions to the computerized format, from boredom to increased anxiety, and therefore care must be taken in choosing a computerized health education program that is accessible, interesting, and applicable to the general population.[44]

To conclude, computers and software could turn out to be a health educator's best friend. The potential of computer technology in the health education field is tremendous, and is limited only by the creativity of software designers and the willingness of health educators to learn this new health education tool.

NOTES

1. Rothman, David H., *The Silicon Jungle* (New York: Ballantine Books, 1985).

2. Ibid., 3.

3. Beery, W., et al., *Description, Analysis and Assessment of Health Hazard/Health Risk Appraisal Programs* (Springfield, Va.: National Technical Information Service, 1981); Faber, M.M., and Reinhardt, A.M., eds., *Promoting Health Through Risk Reduction* (New York: Macmillan, 1982); Hyner, G.C., and Melby, C.L., "Health Risk Appraisals: Use and Misuse, *Journal of Family and Community Health* 7, no. 4 (February 1985): 13–24; Proceedings of the annual meetings of the Society for Prospective Medicine (Suite 700, 1101 Connecticut Avenue, N.W., Washington, DC 20036); Wagner, E.H., "An Assessment of Health Hazard/Health Risk Appraisal," *American Journal of Public Health* 72, no. 4 (April 1982): 347–352.

4. Control Data Corporation, Benefit Services Department, *Health Risk Profile,* P.O. Box O-HQCO2P, 8100 34th Avenue South, Minneapolis, MN 55440.

5. General Health, *Personal Health Profile,* 3299 K Street, N.W., Washington, DC 20007.

6. Health Enhancement Systems, *Health Risk Questionnaire,* 9 Mercer Street, Princeton, NJ 08540.

7. Health Logics, *Healthline,* P.O. Box 3430, San Leandro, CA 94578.

8. National Computer Systems, *Innerview Health Assessment,* 1100 Prairie Lake Drive, Eden Prairie, MN 55344.

9. Wellsource, *Life,* 15431 Southeast 82nd Drive, Suite F, Clackamas, OR 97015.

10. Centers for Disease Control, *CDC Adult HRA-Large Computer Version.* Health Risk Appraisal Activity, CDC, Building 3, Atlanta, GA 30333. (FORTRAN IV, Level 6, designed for batch processing on medium to large mainframes.)

11. University of Minnesota Media Distribution, *Health Risk Appraisal,* Box 734, Mayo Building, 420 Delaware St., S.E., Minneapolis, MN 55455. (Available for Apple II and/or IIe; $97.)

12. National Wellness Institute, *COMPUTE-A-LIFE I and II,* University of Wisconsin-Stevens Point, South Hall, Stevens Point, WI 54481. (Available for IBM PC; $449.)

13. Department of Health Systems Management, Tulane University Medical Center, School of Public Health and Tropical Medicine, *Hospitalization Risk Assessment Program,* 1430 Tulane Avenue, New Orleans, LA 70112. (Available for IBM PC; $75.)

14. American Corporate Health Programs, *Personal Health Inventory,* 85 Old Eagle School Road, Strafford, PA 19087. (Available for Apple II (personal version), $34.95; (corporate version) $200; IBM-PC (corporate version—without graphics), $200; IBM PC with paper-and-pencil questionnaire, $495.)

15. RAM Resources, Inc., *Personal Health II,* 100 Lynn Street, Peabody, MA 01960. (Available for Apple II, Apple IIe, Apple III (requires 48K, DOS 3.3); $49.)

16. Softworld, Inc., *Positive Lifestyling,* San Diego, CA. (Available for IBM PC and XT; $145.)

17. The Institute for Lifestyle Improvement, *TESTWELL* $300.00; *STRESS ASSESS* $75.00; *WHY SMOKE* $349.00. University of Wisconsin—Stevens Point Foundation, Stevens Point, WI 54481. (Available for IBM PC.)

18. Don, Joel C., *"Use Your Computer to Keep In Shape," Popular Computing* 4, no. 9 (July 1985): 68–72.

19. Spinnaker Software, *Aerobics,* One Kendall Square, Cambridge, MA 01239. (Available for Atari 400/800, Commodore 64; $34.95.)

20. Free Lance Ink, *Aerobics Master,* 1806 Wickham, Royal Oak, MI 48073. (Available for Apple II series, 48K (disk); $24.95.)

21. Marathon Software, *The Running Log,* Box 26 Pinecrest, Clancy, MT 59634. (Available for IBM PC, 64K (disk), $39.95.)

22. Software Publishing Corp., *Running Coach,* POB 306, 125 Main St., Half Moon Bay, CA 94019. (Available for Apple II series, IBM PC, XT, PCjr; $69.95.)

23. Avant-Garde Publishing Corp., *Be Your Own Coach,* 37B Commercial Blvd., Novato, CA 94947. (Available for Apple II series, IBM PC, XT, PCjr; $49.95.)

24. Micro Educational Corporation of America (MECA), *The Running Program,* 285 Riverside Ave., Westport, CT 06880. Available for IBM PC and PCjr (enhanced), $79.95.

25. DEG Software, Inc., *Inshape,* 11999 Katy Freeway, Suite 150, Houston, TX 77079. (Available for IBM PC, 64K (disk) and 96K (with DOS 2.0; double-sided disk), $95.)

26. Healthpath Associates, *Healthpath*, 68 Olive St., Chagrin Falls, OH 44022. (Available for the IBM PC, 64K (disk), under $100.)

27. Muse Software, *Eating Machine*, 347 North Charles St., Baltimore, MD 21201. (Available for Apple II series; $49.95.)

28. Evryware, *Evrydiet*, 1950 Cooley Ave. #6208, Palo Alto, CA 94303. (Available for IBM PC, XT, PCjr, and compatibles; $62.95.)

29. Microcomp Inc., *Nutri-Pack*, 2015 NW Circle Blvd., Corvallis, OR 97330. (Available for Apple II series; $39.95.)

30. Computer Software Associates, *Total Health*, 65 Teed Drive, Randolph, MA 02368. (Available for Commodore 64, disk $29.95, cassette $24.95.)

31. PCD Systems Inc., *Nutri-Calc*, P.O. Box 277, 163 Main St., Penn Yan, NY 14527. (Available for IBM PC, XT, PCjr, Apple II series, TRS-80 Models II, III, 4, 12, 16, Epson QX-10; $129.)

32. N-Squared Computing, *Nutritionist I*, 5318 Forest Ridge Rd., Silverton, OR 97381. (Available for Apple II series, IBM PC, XT, PCjr, TI Professional; $145.)

33. ISC Consultants Inc., *Nutri-Byte*, Suite 602, 14 East Fourth St., New York, NY 10012. (Available for IBM PC, XT, and Apple II series; $79.95.)

34. Scarborough Systems Inc., *Original Boston Computer Diet*, 55 South Broadway, Tarrytown, NY 10591. (Available for Apple II series, IBM PC, XT, and PCjr; $79.95. For Commodore 64, $49.95.)

35. Micro Education Corporation of America, *The James F. Fixx Running Program*, 285 Riverside Ave., Westport, CT 06880. (Available for IBM PC, XT, PCjr (with 256K bytes of RAM); $79.95.)

36. Katch, Frank I., and Katch, Victor L., "Computer Technology to Evaluate Body Composition, Nutrition, and Exercise," *Preventive Medicine* 12 (1983): 619–631.

37. Artificial Intelligence Research Group, *Eliza*, 921 North LaJolla Avenue, West Hollywood, CA 90046. (Available for most home computers; $45.)

38. Artificial Intelligence Research Group, *Mind Prober*, 921 North LaJolla Avenue, West Hollywood, CA 90046. (Available for most home computers; $40.)

39. SAS Institute, Box 8000, Cary, NC 27511, *SAS User's Guide: Basics*. (Available for the IBM PC XT and PC AT, recommends 640K.)

40. SAS Institute, Box 8000, Cary, NC 27511, *Full Screen Product* (SAS/FSP).

41. Dedmon Robert, Smith Tom, Swanson Audrey, "Data Base Management in a Corporate Health Promotion Program," *Corporate Commentary*, no. 1, 1984: 34–39.

42. Papert, Seymour A. "Computers and Learning," in *The Computer Age: A Twenty-Year View*, ed. Michael L. Dertouzas and Joel Moses (Cambridge, Mass: MIT Press, 1979), 73–86.

43. Naditch, Murray, "Computer Assisted Worksite Health Promotion: The Fit between Workers and Programs," *Corporate Commentary* XX, no. 1 (1984): 39–49.

44. Deardorff, William W., "Computerized Health Education: A Comparison with Traditional Formats," *Health Education Quarterly*, 13, no. 1 (Spring 1986): 61–72.

SUGGESTED READINGS

National Health Information Clearinghouse (NHIC). *Healthfinder*, 1–7. (P.O. Box 1133, Washington, DC 20013-1133.)

Newsweek. "The PCjr's Sudden Death," April 1, 1985, 65.

Appendix 7–A

Some Useful Definitions of Computer Terminology

Application Package—Specialized programs for a particular industry or discipline, marketed for widespread customer use.

Batch Processing—A technique in which data to be processed or programs to be executed are collected into groups and then processed.

Bit—A "1" or a "0." Patterns of bits form *bytes*.

Bytes—A letter or a number.

Cathode-Ray Tube (CRT)—An electronic vacuum tube containing a screen on which information can be stored or displayed.

Hard Copy—A permanent record of machine output in human-readable form; generally, reports, listings, and other printed documents.

Hardware—Physical equipment such as mechanical, magnetic, and electronic devices; i.e., computer, floppy disk, etc.

Input—Data to be processed by a computer.

Interactive Mode—Processing that permits frequent interchange between the user and the computer during the execution of a program. For example, when utilizing HRA software for a microcomputer, the user enters the answers directly on the microcomputer keyboard and sees the resulting profile immediately on the terminal's screen. Synonymous with *conversational computing*.

K—A scientific abbreviation for 1,000, e.g., 64K means a memory capacity of approximately 64,000 letters or numbers.

Magnetic Disk—A tape with a magnetic surface on which data can be written by selective magnetization of portions on the surface.

Microcomputer—A complete computer on a single miniature circuit board; also referred to as a personal computer, small business computer.

Minicomputer—A stored-program computer, generally having less memory and a smaller computer-word size than large machines; also referred to as a *small business computer*.

Output—The result of processing, usually in the form of a screen display or hard copy report.

Program—A sequence of instructions that directs the computer to perform specific operations to achieve a desired result.

Random-Access Memory (RAM)—Temporary computer memory. Data can be saved by transferring the information to floppy disks.

Soft Copy—A temporary, or nonpermanent, record of computer output; for example, a CRT display.

Software—A collection of programs that facilitate the programming and operation of a computer; may also include documentation and operational procedures.

Terminal—A keyboard device through which data can be input or output.

Appendix 7–B

Software

MICROCOMPUTER-BASED HRAs

American Corporate Health Programs, *PERSONAL HEALTH INVENTORY,* 85 Old Eagle School Road, Strafford, PA 19087. Available for Apple II (personal version), $34.95; (corporate version) $200; IBM PC (corporate version, without graphics), $200; IBM PC with paper-and-pencil questionnaire, $495.

Center for Corporate Health Promotion, *LIFESCORE M,* 11490 Commerce Park Drive, Suite 140, Reston, VA 22091. Available for IBM PC; $425.

Centers for Disease Control (CDC), *Adult HRA,* Health Risk Activity, CDC, Building 3, Atlanta, GA 30333. Available for IBM PC and its compatibles.

Department of Health Systems Management, Tulane University Medical Center, School of Public Health and Tropical Medicine, *HOSPITALIZATION RISK ASSESSMENT PROGRAM,* 1430 Tulane Avenue, New Orleans, LA 70112. Available for IBM PC; $75.

Medmicro, The Center for Medical Microcomputing, *PERSONAL HEALTH APPRAISAL,* P.O. Box 9615, Madison, WI 53715. Available for IBM PC (personal version $59.50, professional version $259.50).

National Health Screening Council for Volunteer Organizations, *HEALTH RISK APPRAISAL,* Volunteer Organizations, 9411 Connecticut Ave., Kensington, MD 20895. Available for IBM PC; $150.

National Wellness Institute, *COMPUTE-A-LIFE I and II,* University of Wisconsin-Stevens Point, South Hall, Stevens Point, WI 54481. Available for IBM PC; $449.

Planetree Medical Systems, *MICRO-HRA,* 870 East 9400 South, #104, Sandy, UT 84070. Available for IBM PC; $150.

University of Minnesota Media Distribution, *HEALTH RISK APPRAISAL,* Box 734, Mayo Building, 420 Delaware St., S.E., Minneapolis, MN 55455. Available for Apple II and/or IIe; $97.

Wellness Associates, *WELLNESS INVENTORY,* P.O. Box 5433, Mill Valley, CA 94942. Available for IBM PC, Apple, TRS-80, CP/M microcomputers; $29.

Wellsource, *HEALTH AGE,* 15431 Southeast 82nd Drive, Suite F, Clackamas, OR 97015. Available for Apple II, IBM PC, TRS-80, Model III; $200.

Wellsource, *HEALTHSTYLE,* 15431 Southeast 82nd Drive, Suite F, Clackamas, OR 97015. Available for TRS-80, Model III; $100.

FITNESS SOFTWARE

Avant-Garde Publishing Corp., *Be Your Own Coach,* 37B Commercial Blvd., Novato, CA 94947. Available for Apple II series, IBM PC, XT, PCjr; $49.95.

DEG Software, Inc., *Inshape,* 11999 Katy Freeway, Suite 150, Houston, TX 77079. Available for IBM PC, 64K (disk) and 96K (with DOS 2.0; double-sided disk); $95.

Free Lance Ink, *Aerobics Master,* 1806 Wickham, Royal Oak, MI 48073. Available for Apple II series, 48K (disk); $24.95.

Healthpath Associates, *Healthpath,* 68 Olive St., Chagrin Falls, OH 44022. Available for the IBM PC, 64K (disk); under $100.

Marathon Software, *The Running Log,* Box 26 Pinecrest, Clancy, MT 59634. Available for IBM PC, 64K (disk); $39.95.

Micro Educational Corporation of America (MECA), *The Running Program,* 285 Riverside Ave., Westport, CT 06880. Available for IBM PC and PCjr (enhanced); $79.95.

Software Publishing Corp., *Running Coach,* P.O. Box 306, 125 Main St., Half Moon Bay, CA 94019. Available for Apple II series, IBM PC, XT, PCjr; $69.95.

Spinnaker Software, *Aerobics,* One Kendall Square, Cambridge, MA 01239. Available for Atari 400/800, Commodore 64; $34.95.

Wm. C. Brown Publishers, *Running Your Best Race,* P.O. Box 539, 2460 Kerper Blvd., Dubuque, IA 52001. Available for Apple II series, Commodore 64, IBM PC, PCjr; $18.95.

NUTRITION SOFTWARE

Computer Software Associates, *Total Health,* 65 Teed Drive, Randolph, MA 02368. Available for Commodore 64 (disk $29.95, cassette $24.95).

Dietware, *Dietitian,* P.O. Box 503, Spring, TX 773773. Available for Apple II Series; $59.95.

Dietware, *Dietmac,* P.O. Box 503, Spring, TX 77373. Available for Apple Macintosh; $79.

Evryware, *Evrydiet,* 1950 Cooley Ave. #6208, Palo Alto, CA 94303. Available for IBM PC, XT, PCjr, and compatibles; $62.95.

ISC Consultants Inc., *Nutri-Byte,* Suite 602, 14 East Fourth St., New York, NY 10012. Available for IBM PC, XT, and Apple II series; $79.95.

Microcomp Inc., *Nutri-Pack,* 2015 NW Circle Blvd., Corvallis, OR 97330. Available for Apple II series; $39.95.

Micromedx, *Nutriplan,* 187 Gardiners Ave., Levittown, NY 11756. Available for Apple II series, IBM PC, XT, PCjr, Zenith 150; $75.

Muse Software, *Eating Machine,* 347 North Charles St., Baltimore, MD 21201. Available for Apple II series; $49.95.

Natural Software Limited, *NSL Diet Analyzer Program,* Suite 7E, 7 Lake St., White Plains, NY 10603. Available for IBM PC, XT, PCjr, and compatibles; $49.95.

N-Squared Computing, *Nutritionist I,* 5318 Forest Ridge Rd., Silverton, OR 97381. Available for Apple II series, IBM PC, XT, PCjr, TI Professional; $145.

Nutritional Data Resources, *Diet Wise,* P.O. Box 540, Willoughby, OH 44094. Available for Apple II series, IBM PC, XT, PCjr, CP/M-80 systems; $49.95.

Nutritional Data Resources, *Nutripak Professional,* P.O. Box 540, Willoughby, OH 44094. Available for IBM PC, XT, PCjr, CP/M-80 systems; $349.

PCD Systems Inc., *Nutri-Calc,* P.O. Box 277, 163 Main St., Penn Yan, NY 14527. Available for IBM PC, XT, PCjr, Apple II series, TRS-80 Models II, III, 4, 12, 16, Epson QX-10; $129.

Soft Bite Inc., *Heartwave,* P.O. Box 1484, East Lansing, MI 48823. Available for Apple II series, TRS-80 Models III, 4, IBM PC; $50.

Softsync Inc., *Model Diet,* 162 Madison Ave., New York, NY 10016. Available for Apple IIe, IIc; $49.95. Commodore 64, $34.95.

FITNESS AND NUTRITION SOFTWARE

Bantam Books, *Complete Scarsdale Medical Diet,* 666 Fifth Avenue, New York, NY 10103. Available for Apple II series, IBM PC, PCjr (color graphics required); $39.95.

Healthware, *Master Control Diet & Exercise Program,* Suite 209, 2300 Round Rock Ave., Round Rock, TX 78681. Available for IBM PC, XT, PCjr; $39.95.

Micro Education Corporation of America, *The James F. Fixx Running Program,* 285 Riverside Ave., Westport, CT 06880. Available for IBM PC, XT, PCjr (with 256K bytes of RAM); $79.95.

N-Squared Computing, *Nutritionist II,* 5318 Forest Ridge Rd., Silverton, OR 97381. Available for Apple II series, IBM PC, XT, PCjr, TI Professional, and CP/M-80 systems; $295.

Programming Technology Corp., *Health-Aide,* 7 San Marcos Place, San Rafael, CA 94901. Available for IBM PC, XT, Apple II series, Apple III, HP Portable; $79.95.

Scarborough Systems Inc., *Original Boston Computer Diet,* 55 South Broadway, Tarrytown, NY 10591. Available for Apple II series, IBM PC, XT, and PCjr; $79.95. For Commodore 64, $49.95.

Soft Bite Inc., *Balancing Act,* P.O. Box 1484, East Lansing, MI 48823. Available for Apple II series, TRS-80 Models III, 4; $65.00. *Balancing Act I* for IBM PC, XT; $349.

Katch, Victor L. *FITCOMP.* Department of Physical Education and Pediatric Cardiology, School of Medicine, University of Michigan, Ann Arbor, MI 48109.

PSYCHOLOGICAL SOFTWARE

Eliza and *Mind Prober,* Artificial Intelligence Research Group, 921 North LaJolla Ave., West Hollywood, CA 90046. Available on most home computers. *Eliza* $45.00, *Mind Prober* $40.

Chapter 8

Incentive Systems for Changing Health Behaviors

Larry S. Chapman, MPH

Most of us realize that health behavior is extremely difficult to change. A multitude of factors affect our behavioral choices. Incentives for health behavior change are intended to act as additional inducements to help people initiate and maintain selected health behaviors. They may be viewed as one important aspect of a comprehensive approach to health promotion programming.

The use of formal incentive systems is a relatively new development and therefore lacks an adequate sciences base. Further discussion and research on formal and informal incentive systems for use in community and workplace health promotion programs are necessary as additional means of assisting people in making health behavior changes through organized program efforts.

Incentives can be used to accomplish several objectives in the context of a health promotion program. Some of the major applications of incentives include:

- To promote learning
- To encourage participation in programs
- To encourage accomplishment of personal health enhancement objectives
- To encourage improvement in fitness test scores
- To encourage changes in health service use behavior
- To encourage compliance with professional health advice
- To encourage initiation and maintenance of specific health behaviors

This chapter will explore some fundamental definitions regarding incentives, why incentives are necessary, their advantages and disadvantages, a typology of types of incentives, how incentive systems should be designed, their relationship to other program components, and examples of incentive systems.

WHAT ARE INCENTIVES?

If we assume that most human behavior is purposeful, then incentives can be viewed as offering additional reasons or "purposes" for individuals to change their behavior. Some key definitions regarding incentives are as follows:

Definitions

Incentive
". . . An anticipated reward designed to influence the performance of an individual or group."[1]

Incentive Theory
". . . The theory that motivation arousal should be viewed as an interaction or relationship between environmental incentives (stimulus objects) and an organism's psychological and physiological state . . . what is emphasized is the role of both positive and negative incentives in arousing the organism and instigating behavior."[2]

Pay Value
". . . The perceived positive or negative reward associated with adherence to or avoidance of a specific behavior."[3]

System
". . . A set of elements that are organized to work together to perform a function."[4]

From these basic definitions it should be clear that incentives encompass a broad range of issues and items and that it requires some thoughtful analysis in order to construct incentive systems that utilize appropriate pay values and behavioral targets. The choice and strength of the pay value used will have a great deal to do with the extent to which the incentive helps induce or reinforce a specific health behavior.

Incentives can be viewed as formal or informal in nature. Formal incentives are those that are openly addressed in the design of a health promotion program. Informal incentives are usually not openly addressed and are implicit in the design of the program. An example of a formal incentive would be the announcement of a partial program fee rebate for completion of 80 percent of aerobic exercise sessions. An example of an informal incentive would be the opportunity to mix with members of senior management in the company's fitness facility. Incentives can use either positive or negative pay values. Positive pay values are viewed as desirable while negative pay values are not desirable. Incentive systems can also take a myriad number of forms, limited only by the constraints of a particular community or workplace setting.

WHY UTILIZE INCENTIVES?

Long-term health behavior change is difficult to achieve. The behavioral science literature offers a great deal of evidence concerning the difficulty of making long-term behavioral changes. However, underlying this difficulty is the reality that the vast majority of human behavior is purposeful in nature. We exhibit particular behavior for distinct and largely discernible purposes. We do not change our behavior without good reasons. Health educators or health interventionists who are attempting to help people change a specific health-related behavior need to determine what factors would aid the adoption of the new behavior. For example, would a cash rebate of 50 percent of the program fee for 80 percent attendance of multiple program sessions help participants attend the sessions? The commitment to attend is strengthened through the reason of a potential financial reward. Program attendance is usually increased with this kind of incentive.

The health promotion program designer needs to know why the target population would want to:

- wear seat belts?
- ask more questions of their doctor?
- get immunizations?
- exercise regularly?
- stop smoking?
- have surgery performed in an outpatient setting?
- use a community loan program for a child restraint device for their car?
- use a medical self-care reference book?

Questions such as these frequently provide a focus for selecting the appropriate pay value/s to use in the design of the incentive system.

ADVANTAGES AND DISADVANTAGES OF INCENTIVES

Incentives, in a generalized sense, have both advantages and disadvantages attached to their use. The potential advantages of using incentives are significant. They are related to the following factors:

- It is relatively easy to establish and operate incentive systems. The development of rules and their application can be specifically designed to operate using information that is produced as a by-product of an already existing activity. For example, a sick leave reduction incentive uses payroll data as its primary informational source.
- It is possible to adapt incentive systems to virtually any situation. Because incentive rules can be tailored to virtually any situation, they are extremely flexible.
- It is possible to combine several different kinds of formal and informal incentives into one incentive system. For example, a weight reduction program can include a financial rebate for sustained weight loss, a fee discount for registering a friend, a food scale as a door prize for attendance, and a recipe write-up in the employee newsletter for the best-tasting low-calorie recipe. The combination of incentives strengthens motivation for attendance, learning, participation levels and sustained weight loss.
- It is possible to provide a powerful source of motivation with incentives. If the desired behavior, the pay value, and the rules for the incentive system are well designed, it is possible to produce a very powerful and significant change in behavior.

Careful design of incentive systems can substantially eliminate their disadvantages, but it is important to recognize that incentives do have potential disadvantages. The disadvantages of incentive systems are related to the following factors:

- It is not easy to determine which pay values will function as effective inducements for behavior change. Some incentive system failures may be attributed to an inappropriate choice of pay values as the inducement for desired behaviors. For example, small amounts of cash as the incentive reward for wearing seatbelts may not change behavior in a relatively highly paid workforce.
- It is possible to reward inappropriate behavior if the incentive system is poorly designed. For example, a financial rebate competition that rewards short-term weight loss without any maximum limits on pounds lost per week may cause some participants to use hazardous weight loss techniques or diets.
- It is possible to produce unintended and undesirable artifacts from operation of the incentive system. For example, if the reward for not using sick leave is excessively valued by a workforce it may cause individuals to come to work with infectious conditions (e.g., upper

respiratory infections) and thus end up spreading the illness to many more people than would have otherwise gotten sick.

- It is possible for learned behavior to find a way around the rules established for the incentive system. For example, if a sun visor is handed out as an incentive for attending a "lunch and learn" educational session at the beginning of the session, the individual who wants the visor but doesn't want to attend will get the visor, then leave the session.

- It is possible for the incentive reward to create dependent behavior. In other words, no incentive—no behavior. For example, use of a subsidy for membership in a fitness club may cause participants to drop their membership when the subsidy is withdrawn, perhaps as a way of applying pressure to maintain the subsidy.

In summary, human behavior is multifactorial in nature, and it is extremely difficult for individuals to change their behavior without clearly perceived reasons to change. Incentives help provide those reasons to change. Therefore, it is important that we augment health promotion program efforts in community and workplace settings by including different types of incentives that will help individuals initiate and maintain specific health behavior changes.

WHAT KINDS OF INCENTIVE PAY VALUES ARE THERE?

A number of different kinds of pay values can be used in an informal or formal way as part of an incentive system focused on changing health behavior. Exhibit 8-1 is designed to provide an overview of some of the major types of formal and informal pay values that can be used as part of a health behavior oriented incentive system. Column "A" contains primarily informal types of pay values that are usually not explicitly addressed in the program's description of the incentive system. Column "B" contains primarily formal types of pay values that are usually explicitly addressed in any description of the incentive system given to participants. Some pay values can be either formal or informal depending on what is communicated to participants. Pay values are the driving force behind the incentive effect; therefore, they represent a critical issue in incentive system design.

HOW SHOULD INCENTIVES BE DESIGNED?

Health educators and health promotion program managers need to use a logical process for the design of incentives for health behavior change. The

Exhibit 8-1 Types of Incentive Pay Values

A
Informal Pay Values

Belonging: The personal sense of satisfaction from being a part of the program is the primary pay value. Membership in a fitness program group or Y is a primary example of this type of pay value. Belonging may not be formally communicated to participants or it may be informally discernible to program participants.

Mix with Important People: The informal pay value in this incentive utilizes the opportunity for employees in a work setting to meet and get to know senior managers who are using a fitness facility. Opportunity to improve career progression for participating employees is another way of viewing this type of pay value. In community settings the opportunity to run a race with a public figure may motivate some individuals to participate.

Humor: The pay value here is for the program participant to be able to share his or her humor with others or experience something humorous. Examples of this include the development of mock or humorous health newsletters for a school population, the development of fictitious fitness characters in a hospital fitness newsletter, bizarre fitness recipes, or cartoons with a health message on a Y bulletin board.

Fun/Lightness: This informal pay value includes providing the opportunity to experience play while engaging in a health-enhancing behavior. Use of "new" games at the start of a stress management workshop is one example of this type of pay value. Brainstorming from a humorous perspective is another way to add fun and lightness to the activity and will act as an inducement for some individuals to attend.

Self-Mastery: This type of informal incentive pay value emphasizes greater personal

B
Formal Pay Values

Belonging: The formal use of membership status and receipt of program T-shirts as inducements for selected behaviors are two examples of this kind of incentive. The pay value includes affiliation with others based on a common purpose or level of achievement. Earning T-shirts for belonging to a group that completes a community 10K run is another example of this kind of incentive.

Acceptance/Approval: Examples of this type of formal pay value include fitness program membership levels that denote fitness levels, charter membership status, acknowledgment of unusual health achievement, well-day incentive for employees not using sick leave within a six-month period, etc.

Recognition: Examples of this kind of pay value include use of aerobic points or "mile" conversion charts to track aerobic accomplishments of recreation center teams, use of write-ups of employees who make substantial health improvements, use of novelties for participation in runs, walks, etc.

Special Privilege: Examples of this kind of pay value include wellness employee of the month (based on health improvement), flextime provisions for employees who exercise, extended lunch hours for exercisers, use of a Y exercise facility for those who complete fitness testing, etc.

Gambling Urge: This pay value motivates by providing an opportunity to win a prize that is desirable. Examples of this include sick leave lotteries where employees not absent from work for a specific period of time have an opportunity to win a trip to Hawaii, drawings for various door prizes for attendance at a hospital health promo-

Exhibit 8–1 continued

A	B
Informal Pay Values	*Formal Pay Values*

control over one's behavior while helping individuals to increase their personal satisfaction levels by being able to more successfully control basic impulses and behaviors. This pay value can be formally acknowledged in program marketing materials. An example of this would be a Y-sponsored workshop on techniques for increasing self-control of eating impulses.

Creative Outlet: This type of pay value provides an opportunity to express personal creativity as the primary inducement for participation or behavior changes. Examples include health recipe contests, health limerick-of-the-month contest, development of program logos, program themes or creative writing opportunities for community health promotion newsletters.

Ability To Contribute: This type of pay value can be used to encourage participant involvement in program activities and can provide a pay value to those who like to see something change as a result of their personal involvement. Examples of this are using peer leaders in training sessions, using program monitors to assist in record keeping for a fitness contest, or setting up an advisory board by a voluntary community health agency.

Good Exemplars: This pay value includes the opportunity to function as a role model or example. The pay value also can provide a personal example of successful behavior change so that participants can perceive the feasibility of accomplishing a specific health behavior change. An example of this would be a "spotlight" column in a Y newsletter that would describe individuals who have made a substantial behavior change. This pay value can reinforce the individual who has made the

tion seminar, an extra days off lottery for school district staff who accomplish personal health objectives, or an opportunity for employees to play safety bingo as long as there are no lost-time work injuries.

Fun/Lightness: This type of pay value can be formally acknowledged and can emphasize lightness while not taking things so seriously. It may provide an opportunity to reduce some of the stress that is common in the workplace. An example would be a stretch break at a public hearing or corporate meeting or use of humorous titles on meeting agendas.

Time Reward: The pay value here is the ability to have more time to do the things we want to do. Examples of this include the award of "well" days for employees who have not submitted health insurance claims, additional annual leave hours for write-ups of unusual health achievements (i.e., triathlon completion, cross-country bike trips, etc.) or achievement of excellent fitness scores, or provision of employee release time for health promotion activities.

Material Goods: The pay value here is primarily seen as the utility of the material good linked to the accomplishment required to receive the item. Examples of this type of pay value include T-shirts, sweat shirts, sun visors, sweatbands, thermometers, gym bags, drink coolers, fitness equipment, desk-top air cleaners, colorimetric stress indicators, health board games, equipment catalogs, etc.

Financial Reward: The pay value here is a financial payment. The cash payment can then be converted into an item or activity that has the greatest utility to the recipient. Examples of this type of incentive include

Exhibit 8-1 continued

A
Informal Pay Values

change as well as encourage those who would like to make the change.

Personal Challenge: This type of pay value involves the challenge of personal accomplishment. Examples include 1,000-mile clubs, fitness achievement goals, accomplishment of personal wellness goals, or participation and completion of a triathlon.

Newness: This type of pay value involves offering something new as a relief to individual boredom. Examples include new program launch activities and communications campaigns that bring new topics and issues to community members' or employees' attention.

Personal Discomfort: This type of pay value usually involves avoiding personal discomfort. It may take the form of avoidance of the risk of chronic disease, injury, or physical impairment. Examples are the use of newsletter articles on personal health consequences of particular health behaviors, use of lung specimens for motivation of smokers to quit smoking, highlights of personal health situations, pictures of auto injuries associated with excessive alcohol use, etc.

B
Formal Pay Values

financial rebate systems, health insurance premium differentials for nonsmokers, a rebate of a portion of the program tuition for completion of a weight loss program workshop series, rebates for specific performance levels, sports equipment discounts, membership subsidies, etc. Contest points can also be given for particular behaviors and then be converted into money or material goods.

Financial Penalty: The pay value here is avoiding a financial penalty attached to certain behaviors. Examples of this are higher premiums for smokers, financial penalties for relapse of smoking behavior, forfeiture of program fees for weight gain, higher health plan cost sharing for those who do not receive a required second surgical opinion, etc.

Group Competition: The pay value here is group challenge and the opportunity to be part of a group that accepts a challenge. Team building often is associated with this type of pay value. Examples include corporate cup competitions, Y team participation competitions, departmental cups, etc.

High Visibility: This type of pay value involves high levels of personal recognition. The opportunity to be personally recognized can function as an inducement for particular behavior for some people. Examples include spotlight articles for those who have made a significant health habit change or have had a significant health accomplishment.

Ease of Access: This type of pay value involves the removal of personal obstacles that limit participation in a particular program activity. An example would be the provision of an aerobic exercise course that is moved from a Y to a local worksite to make it easier for employees to participate.

steps for designing formal incentive systems are fairly straightforward. In order to understand better the design process, a workplace incentive system for increasing the level of employee exercise activity is offered as an example. An eleven-step process is outlined below in Exhibit 8–2. However, the number of actual steps may vary according to the specific characteristics of the type of program involved.

OPPORTUNITIES FOR THE USE OF INCENTIVES

When considering where incentives can be used in health promotion programs, it is useful to categorize their potential uses. One conceptual framework for organizing both community and workplace health promotion programs is portrayed in Exhibit 8–3. The framework includes four major program components and a brief description of each component. Potential incentive opportunities are then identified.

STRENGTH OF INCENTIVES

The extent to which an incentive system will contribute to behavior change is directly related to a number of aspects of the design and implementation of the incentive system. However, the ultimate behavioral effects of the incentive system are also affected by a large number of other extraneous variables that generally influence our behavioral choices. Despite the role these extraneous variables play, it is important to design and implement incentive systems that have maximum potential to help people change their health behavior. The following features of a formal incentive system are important in maximizing its behavior change effects:

- The degree of congruence between the pay value of the incentive system and the pay values that are important to the target group affected by the incentive
- The participant's perception of the probability of successfully accomplishing the required actions/behavior
- The participant's perception of the probability of actually receiving the pay value as a result of successfully accomplishing the required actions/behavior
- The clarity of the rules governing the incentive system
- The extent to which the incentive rules are communicated to the target group

Exhibit 8-2 Design Process for Incentive Systems

Step	*Example*
Step 1: Determine what actions or behaviors you want to increase (or decrease) with the incentive.	For a specific workplace population at a local business you determine that about one-third of the employees exercise vigorously three or more times a week. A national survey shows that normally 54 percent of a workforce is involved in regular vigorous exercise three or more times a week. Therefore, a program objective is established in order to increase those reporting regular vigorous exercise to 50 percent of the workforce by the time of next annual survey. The behavior that is to be the focus of the incentive system is regular vigorous exercise. The current nonexercisers constitute the primary target population for the incentive.
Comment: By identifying the desired action/s or behavior/s early you increase the chances that the rest of the incentive system will in fact accomplish what it is intended to accomplish. This process should also result in an identification of the target population as well as the target behaviors.	
Step 2: Research the values that hinder or would catalyze adoption of the desired behavior/s.	In the survey, inquiry is made into why people don't exercise; 22 percent say that if it were possible to exercise at lunchtime they would. Another 13 percent say they lack motivation. An additional 8 percent say that it's too boring.
Comment: This step should identify the major types of pay values that would help nonexercisers adopt and maintain a new exercise behavior. The primary focus of this step is to determine what types of pay values would have the greatest potential effect on the exercise behavior of the target population. Basic market research techniques can be used to help accomplish this step.	
Step 3: Select the formal and informal pay values that are feasible for inclusion in the incentive design that will produce the strongest behavior change effect.	Recognizing that development of a fitness center is too expensive, a decision is made to conduct an eight-week fitness contest combined with on-site lunchtime aerobic exercise sessions based on the survey results. This approach includes the pay values of access improvement, group and individual challenge, and belonging. The fitness contest will include departmental competition with an additional day off for the department with the highest participation rates. A policy of flextime for participation is approved by management. Another incentive pay value is incorporated
Comment: From the list of types of possible incentives presented above, it is important to select those that are feasible to implement and those that will have the strongest incentive effect related to the resources required to implement the incentive. An effort should be made to include program design modifications that build in as many additional incentive dimensions as	

Exhibit 8–2 continued

Step	*Example*
possible. For example, by consistently writing up in an employee newsletter those people who have made a significant change in lifestyle, you incorporate recognition, approval, self-mastery, personal challenge, good exemplars, and high visibility types of incentives in one program component. Estimates of what resources will be required to implement the incentive should also be developed.	by offering points for individuals that will be totaled for receipt of material goods. The aerobic exercise session at lunch is designed so that it provides double the aerobic points of other exercise options. The cost of the material goods to be given to participants is $300 with a $3 entrance fee to cover all other costs. Existing shower facilities will be used. The final incentive system includes the pay values of ease of access, group and individual challenge, belonging, time off, and material goods.
Step 4: Develop incentive system rules.	Rules are developed for the fitness contest and for the aerobics class. A draft employee newsletter article is prepared in order to market the fitness contest to non-exercising employees. The incentive pay values are written into the rules.
Comment: It is necessary to determine basic rules as to who is eligible, what the reward (or penalty) is, what separates "winners" from "losers," and the timing and requirements for operating the incentive system. Customarily, a series of documents are necessary to implement the incentive system.	
Step 5: Examine the draft incentive rules for unintended artifacts.	The draft rules are analyzed for their effect on existing exercisers and nonexercisers.
Comment: Sometimes the best approach for determining unintended artifacts is to ask yourself (and others) how you (and they) would react to the proposed incentive. The opportunity for people to circumvent the rules for the incentive system should also be examined.	
Step 6: Use a focus group or groups of employees picked at random or an existing group and elicit their response to the incentive system.	The draft rules and draft newsletter article are then given to an employee advisory group for specific feedback on the incentive system design.
Comment: Use the draft materials with little verbal explanation, then ask the group questions about their perceptions of how the incentive system will operate, how it can be outwitted, anticipated employee reaction, possible problems, etc.	
Step 7: Develop and refine a communications plan for the incentive system.	Some changes are made in the rules resulting in the addition of points for weight loss, smokeless days, and low absenteeism.

Exhibit 8–2 continued

Step	Example
Comment: Based on the feedback from the focus groups, refine the incentive system materials and develop a communications plan including message content, timing, and types of communication vehicles. It is important to communicate using several vehicles and to provide frequent reminders.	The employee newsletter article and the rules are finalized. A reminder memo is also developed.
Step 8: Field test the incentive system with a pilot group.	A presentation is made to the staff of a small department and feedback is received. Those responding recommend that the entire program be repeated in the fall each year. A true pilot is perceived to be not feasible to carry out.
Comment: If it is possible to carry out a pilot test with a subsidiary, division, or plant, it may help determine if there are any features of the incentive design that should be modified prior to full-scale implementation.	
Step 9: Evaluate the field test, modify the design, and implement organizationwide.	Final changes are few. The program is kicked off in the month of May for an eight-week period.
Comment: Once the incentive system has been piloted and results are identified, full-scale implementation should be carried out.	
Step 10: Provide ongoing maintenance for incentive system.	A reminder message is issued in early May to all employees and a write-up in the employee newsletter is provided in June. Numbers of participants are identified. The program is repeated again in the fall.
Comment: The strength of the incentive's effect is directly proportional to the extent to which incentive rules are communicated to the primary target group. This also includes reminders and feedback on group performance.	
Step 11: Periodically (i.e., at least annually) evaluate the effects of the incentive system.	The employee survey is repeated one year later and 52 percent of respondents indicate that they engage in regular vigorous exercise. The fitness contest is identified as a primary factor in helping the nonexercisers to become exercisers.
Comment: Identifying the target actions or behaviors at the beginning of the design process significantly simplifies the evaluation process because it provides a clear opportunity to monitor the desired results of the incentive effort. The direct and indirect costs associated with the operation of the incentive system should ultimately be compared with the organizational gains from the changes in employee behavior.	

Exhibit 8–3 Opportunities for Incentive Use

Program Component	Brief Description	Use of Incentives
Awareness/ Communications	This component generally deals with communication of health information and program information.	• To promote learning • To promote awareness of program activities for internal marketing purposes
Health Management Process	This component generally involves individual fitness and health testing, use of a health risk appraisal, counseling, development of a wellness prescription and a follow-up protocol.	• To participate in the process • To meet personal wellness objectives • To improve test scores
Group Interventions	This component generally deals with group activities covering the full spectrum of health promotion topics, including health fairs, workshops, support groups, runs, walks, par courses, fitness contests, etc.	• To encourage participation • To encourage completion of activities • To encourage behavior change • To encourage health service use changes
Supportive Environment	This program component generally deals with the introduction of changes in workplace policies, formal incentive systems, changes in the type of food available to employees, seatbelt laws, etc.	• To encourage behavior change • To encourage health service use changes

- The extent to which reminders about the incentive are periodically given to the target group
- The absence (or presence) of any extraneous factor that would affect the desired behavior

Additional examples of incentive systems are contained in Appendix 8–A.

SUMMARY

Formal as well as informal incentive systems should be an important feature in the design of community and workplace-based health promotion programs. The difficulty of initiating and maintaining long-term health behavior change requires us to consider the use of a variety of types of incentive systems. The effective design of incentive systems calls for a rational stepwise approach that considers target behaviors, pay values necessary to help people initiate and maintain the target behaviors, incentive rules, feasibility, unintended artifacts, communication plan, and evaluation steps. Multiple types of pay values can be combined into a formal incentive program in order to enhance the incentive effect. Many potential modifications are possible, limited only by our ingenuity in designing and implementing formal and informal incentives for health behavior change.

NOTES

1. Robert M. Goldenson, ed., *Longmans' Dictionary of Psychology and Psychiatry* (New York: Longmans, 1984), 371.

2. Ibid., 371.

3. Larry Chapman, "Creative Incentives for Health Behavior Change" (Paper presented at the Wellness in the Workplace Conference, Norfolk, Virginia, May 1985).

4. Goldenson, *Longmans' Dictionary*, 232.

SUGGESTED READINGS

Alderman, M. "Hypertension Control Programs in Occupational Settings." *Public Health Reports* 95 (1980): 158–163.

Arnold, D.D. "The 'Ceiling Effect' or Traditional Incentive Plans: How to Encourage Low Worker Performance." *Industrial Management (US)* 25 (Nov.–Dec. 1983): 7–13.

Bainum, R. "Bonus Incentives Can Promote Image and Care." *Journal of the American Health Care Association*, May 1985, 50.

Bernacki, E.J., and W.B. Baun. "The Relationship of Job Performance to the Exercise Adherence in a Corporate Fitness Program." *Journal of Occupational Medicine*, July 1985, 529.

Browne, D.W., et al. "Reduced Disability and Health Care Costs in an Industrial Fitness Program." *Journal of Occupational Medicine*, November 1984, 809.

Brownell, K.D., et al. "Weight Loss Competitions at the Work Site: Impact on Weight, Morale and Cost-Effectiveness." *American Journal of Public Health* 4 (1984): 1283.

Colodin, Juana. "Employee Incentive Plans in Greensboro." *MIS Report*, 16 (September 1984): 12–13.

Elder, J.P., et al. "Applications of Behavior Modification to Community Health Education: The Case of Heart Disease Prevention." *Health Education Quarterly* 12 (Summer 1984): 1251–1258.

Elling, Bruce. "Incentive Plans: Short Term Design Issues." *Compensation Review* 13 (Third Quarter 1984): 26–36.

Fein, Mitchell. "The Case for Rewarding Employee Involvement in Productivity Improvement Programs." *Quality Circles Journal* 7 (September 1984): 20–23.

Forster, J.L., et al. "A Work-Site Weight Control Program Using Financial Incentives Collected Through Payroll Deduction." *Journal of Occupational Medicine* 27 (1985): 804–808.

Frederiksen, L. "Using Incentives in Worksite Wellness." *Corporate Commentary,* November 1984, 51–57.

Gray, F. "Health Promotion: Accentuate the Positive." *Health Social Service Journal,* March 1984, 380+.

Guy, J. "Incentive Bonus Schemes: Tackling the Bonus Bogeyman." *Health and Social Service Journal,* March 22, 1984, 348+.

Harden, David. "Using Employee Incentives as a Motivational Tool." *MIS Report* 16 (September 1984): 8–11.

Jeffery, Robert W., et al. "Promoting Weight Control at the Worksite: A Pilot Program of Self-Motivation Using Payroll-Based Incentives." *Preventive Medicine* 14 (January 1985): 187–194.

Johnson, F. "Bonus Incentive Schemes: Face-Saving Schemes." *Health and Social Service Journal,* June 21, 1984, 730–731.

Kendall, R. "Rewarding Safety Excellence." *Occupational Hazards* 46 (March 1984): 45–50.

Kopelman, R.E. "Using Incentives to Increase Absenteeism: A Plan That Backfired." *Compensation Review* 15 (February 1983): 40–45.

Kurt, T.L. "Savings Possible with Reimbursement Accounts." *Occupational Health & Safety* 52 (November 1983): 18–19.

Renken, H.J. "An Employee Incentive Program Can Be the Answer to Increased Productivity." *S.A.M. Advanced Management Journal* 49 (February 1984): 8–12.

Robins, J., and M. Lloyd, "A Case Study Examining the Effectiveness and Cost of Incentive Programs to Reduce Staff Absenteeism in a Preschool." *Journal of Organizational Behavior Management* 5 (March-April, 1983): 175–189.

Scarpello, Vida, and John P. Campbell. "Job Satisfaction and the Fit between Individual Needs and Organizational Rewards." *Journal of Occupational Psychology,* 56, no. 4 (1983): 131–134.

Shepard, D.S., et al. "Cost-Effectiveness of Interventions to Improve Compliance with Anti-Hypertensive Therapy." *National Conference on High Blood Pressure Control.* Washington, D.C., Government Printing Office, 1979.

Sider, H. "Economic Incentives and Safety Regulations: An Analytical Framework." *American Economist* 28 (January 1984): 18–24.

Smith, I. "Matching the Incentive to the Performer." *Personnel Management,* January 1984, 27–30.

Sullivan, Timothy. "Underrated Incentives." *Management* 4, no. 4 (1984): 23–25.

"Tax Ruling Upcoming on Awards and Incentives." *Occupational Hazards* 46 (March 1984): 51.

Warner, K.E. "Economic Incentives for Health." *Annual Review of Public Health,* 1984, 107–133.

Yenney, Sharon L. "Using Incentives to Promote Employee Health." Background paper prepared for the Washington Business Group on Health under a Cooperative Agreement from the Office of Disease Prevention and Health Promotion, U.S. Department of Health and Human Services, 1985.

Appendix 8–A*

Examples of Incentive Systems

A. *Company:* Bankers First, Augusta, GA
Contact: Jim Gray or Sally Rumor
Phone: (404) 823-3200

Incentives combined with some form of competition seemed to be particularly effective at Bankers First. Employees interested in a weight-loss program formed teams to compete among branch offices to see which teams could lose the most weight. Each team member paid $5 for a ten-week course in safe and permanent weight loss and nutrition. For each pound lost during that time (up to 24 pounds), the employee received $1. Members of winning teams received jogging suits, new clothing, and T-shirts. Any employee who met his/her goal received a three-month membership in a local health club. The individual who lost the most weight received a gift certificate and all "graduates" received coffee mugs and T-shirts. The friendly spirit of competition helped many of the participants to stay on the program when they were tempted to overeat.

B. *Company:* Bonne Bell, Lakewood, OH
Contact: Connie Schafer
Phone: (216) 221-0800

Bonne Bell promotes good health among its employees and makes a major commitment to consumer health awareness as well. The company has some unusual and effective incentives for its employees. Employees may

---

* Reprinted with permission from "Using Incentives to Promote Employee Health," a paper prepared by Sharon L. Yenney for the Washington Business Group on Health under a Cooperative Agreement with the Office of Disease Prevention and Health Promotion, U.S. Department of Health and Human Services, 1985.

The "Summary of Pay Values" was prepared by Larry Chapman.

take an extra 30 minutes at lunch time if they wish to exercise. Discounts are provided for sports equipment such as running suits, shoes, and bicycles. And employees have permission to wear exercise clothes at work following an afternoon workout.

To encourage physical exercise during inclement winter weather, runners are paid $.50 per mile during January, February, and March; walkers are paid $.25 per mile. Runners must complete 10 miles each week to qualify.

Other incentives are offered for those who are trying to drop some bad habits. If smokers quit for six months, there is a $250 bounty. If they begin again, they are asked to give $500 to the corporate charitable foundation, which donates it to a community group supporting nonsmoking efforts.

If an overweight employee loses at least 10 pounds, he/she will receive $5 per pound over a six-month period. To discourage too great a weight loss, rewards are not offered for more than 50 pounds. For every pound gained back, the employee is asked to pay $10 to the corporate charitable foundation.

C. *Company:* DuPont, Waynesboro, VA
Contact: James W. Pruett, Safety Director
Phone: (703) 949-2000 Ext. 2351

Efforts to reduce the number of lost work days due to nonwork automobile accidents resulted in a seatbelt safety program at this DuPont plant. A committee of hourly workers who were asked to study the problem recommended an audit of incoming traffic two days each week to determine the percent of workers using seatbelts. To make the effort visible to employees, every tenth car in which passengers were wearing seatbelts received a "reward"—cheese and crackers and other snacks. At the time of the first audit, 25 percent of the employees wore seatbelts regularly.

The incentive that was established to improve seatbelt usage was tied to the performance of the total plant. If no employee was involved in a nonwork automobile accident that resulted in lost work time for two months, each employee received a Board of Directors Award—a catalogue of gifts with an average value of $16. Included in the catalogue were household items, garden supplies, tools, personal items such as hairdryers. During the period studied, all employees won a gift because seatbelt usage rose to 90 percent.

Later, the employee committee recommended more difficult rules: the audit was conducted three times each week on both incoming and outgoing traffic and three months of over 90 percent seatbelt usage was required. The employees won again.

Now the plant is auditing traffic (and providing the food prizes to every tenth car), but no longer needs to provide the incentive gifts. The average seatbelt usage in 1985 remained at 88 percent. The traffic audit and snack prizes demonstrate the continued concern of management and help to reinforce the employees' new seatbelt habits.

Results:
Three-year period before seatbelt campaign:
25 percent of the employees used seatbelts regularly
14 non-work injuries due to auto accidents
394 work days lost
Three-year period after the start of the campaign:
88 percent wear seatbelts without incentive program
90 percent wore seatbelts during incentive program
7 non-work injuries due to auto accidents
51 work days lost
In 1984—just one accident and one day lost.

D. *Company:* Flexcon Company, Spencer, MA
Contact: Bob Quentin, Data Processing Manager
Phone: (617) 885-3973

Flexcon uses gifts to encourage their employees to reduce or quit smoking. Every third Thursday, quitters and nonsmokers receive a gift certificate. A similar gift certificate also goes to those who reduce smoking. An important aspect of this program is that those with good health habits (the nonsmokers) are rewarded at the same time that smokers are being encouraged to adopt healthier behaviors.

Flexcon has 398 employees—214 nonsmokers and 184 smokers. In a six-month period in 1984, 42 employees quit smoking and 17 cut down. The company has given out $24,000 in gift certificates.

E. *Company:* Intermatic, Inc., Spring Grove, IL
Contact: Mary Kay Rundblad, RN
Phone: (815) 675-2321

For the past three years, Intermatic has run a fitness program with incentives. Aerobic points are earned and accumulated for six months. In the first year, points could be used for T-shirts, sports jackets, exercise shoes. In the second year, they received T-shirts and golf caps.

The Chairman of Intermatic asked employees who smoked to "bet our money—not your life." Those who gave up smoking for one year were eligible for a lottery. The grand prize was a trip for two to Las Vegas, with two nights lodging and $200 expense money. Others who quit but didn't win the Las Vegas trip got a day at the local horse races—admission tickets for two and a free $2 betting ticket. In addition, employees could bet up to

$100 on themselves at the beginning of the program. If they were able to quit smoking, they got money back. If they didn't succeed, the money was donated to the American Cancer Society or the Heart Association. Anyone who had not smoked in one year was eligible for the lottery, so nonsmokers could participate, too.

Intermatic also has "birthday fitness awards." A $25 check is available on the employee's birthday. When picking up the check in the medical department, employees get their blood pressures checked, glucose levels screened, weight, hearing, and vision tested—and a friendly reminder to get a regular checkup for good health.

F. *Company:* L.L. Bean, Freeport, ME
Contact: Nonie Bullock
Phone: (207) 865-4761

Recreation is a way of life for Bean employees and the company has geared its incentives for good health to that life. A 90-acre tract provides an inducement for employees to exercise regularly. Trained personnel offer a wide range of lifestyle programs and clinics.

The most innovative incentives for good health are through the recreational program. Canoes, tents, sleeping bags, and camping and recreational gear for outdoor sports are loaned free of charge to employees and their families. The company owns five cabins on a lake which are available year round to employees on a lottery basis (and small weekly fee). The company also subsidizes travel and lodging expenses for groups interested in entering marathons, ski races, and other competitive activities.

Bean employees who wish to lose weight receive a subsidy for fees in a local program. Members of the runners club who log 200 miles receive T-shirts (long-sleeved, because it is in Maine!), and those logging 500 miles receive a pair of running shorts.

If employees attend 90 percent of the 10-week aerobics classes, they receive a 50 percent rebate of the $24 fee and an award certificate. Smokers who want to quit pay $26 to enroll in a cessation program and get $13 back after three months of being smoke-free.

G. *Company:* Scherer Brothers Lumber Company, Minneapolis, MN
Contact: Bob Peters
Phone: (612) 379-9633

Scherer Brothers was one of the pioneers of "well pay"—rewarding employees for staying well and coming to work daily. Any union employee not absent or late for work for one month receives two hours' extra pay.

Office workers who do not use any sick leave during the year get a $250 bonus.

Another creative incentive was established to promote awareness of personal safety. Each employee in the shop (not office) can receive three $100 bonuses each year: $100 if no time has been lost from the job due to a work-related injury, $100 if no injury required more than first aid, and $100 if the company has a better safety record during the year than the previous year.

Noontime meals are complimentary for the office staff of about 50 people. The cafeteria has installed a salad bar along with nutritious hot lunches and has removed salt, butter, sugar, processed luncheon meats, high-fat foods, and caffeinated coffee.

H. *Company:* Westlake Community Hospital, Midwest Center for Health Promotion, Melrose Park, IL
Contact: Betsy K. Adrian
Phone: (312) 681-3000 Ext. 3300

Westlake operates a Good Health Plan for employees with five incentive plans that can mean money in the pockets of employees, as well as support for their good health.

Westlake conducts an annual health appraisal (computerized risk appraisal, height, weight, blood pressure and blood tests) for all employees. Employees receive a bonus of $50 for participation. At the time of the appraisal, employees can qualify for additional bonuses. If blood pressure is within normal limits, the bonus is $25; weight within normal limits, $25; nonsmoker, $25; seatbelt user, $25; annual dental checkup, $25. Guides to determine "normal limits" are provided to all employees.

The Westlake medical insurance plan for employees establishes a $150 deductible for a low-option program and $250 deductible for high option. If an employee has blood pressure and weight within normal limits and does not smoke, $150 of the deductible is waived if the employee files an insurance claim.

If an employee is injured in an automobile accident and is using a seatbelt at the time of the accident, 100 percent of any emergency care is paid (no deductible, no co-payment).

I. *Company:* Xerox, Webster, NY
Contact: Richard E. Miller
Phone: (716) 422-9051

The Xerox Health Management Program—called Take Charge—conducts quarterly activities with new incentives established for each quarter. For example, a weight control program—The Great Weight Race—uses five-person teams of employees and spouses who compete for trophies, merchandise, and health information packets. Each team sets a weight-loss goal of six to 20 pounds for each member to be lost over a 10-week period. Guidelines for safe weight loss are provided. Each person must lose at least seven pounds to be eligible for the prizes. Scoring is based on the percentage of weight lost toward the goal. The winning team gets a National Champion's trophy and the second through fifth place teams receive smaller trophies. Individual members of the winning teams choose a prize (scales, nutrition and cook books, jump ropes, golf shirts, sports bags, etc.). All participants receive a copy of a self-help guide to nutrition and healthy eating. In 1984, 196 teams completed the program. Anyone who loses at least 50 percent of the target weight loss gets a T-shirt.

The following is a summary of the various pay values used in the incentive systems examples:

Summary of Pay Values

Example	Name	Pay Values
A	Bankers First	Group and individual challenge, financial reward, material goods, belonging
B	Bonne Bell	Time reward, financial reward, special privilege, financial penalty
C	DuPont	Material goods
D	Flexcon Company	Material goods
E	Intermatic, Inc.	Material goods, gambling urge, financial reward
F	L.L. Bean	Material goods, financial reward
G	Scherer Brothers Lumber Company	Financial reward, material goods
H	Westlake Community Hospital	Financial reward
I	Xerox	Belonging, group and individual challenge, material goods, recognition

Chapter 9

Creating the Healing Connection

John L. Coulehan, MD, FACP, and Marian R. Block, MD

This chapter deals with how practitioners can use themselves most effectively to promote patient involvement in health care. Our perspective is that of primary care physicians. The authors will show how the practitioner-patient interaction is a learning experience, one that can be used to encourage personal responsibility and behavioral change. The interaction can also be used to teach passivity and "medicalization"; it can teach that medicine has all of the answers and does the healing. Or it can give contradictory messages. For example, some physicians and other practitioners recommend treatment but do not offer explicit instructions or determine whether the patient understands the illness and treatment. In order to make these messages clear, the practitioner must know how to promote active patient involvement and then set about creating a "healing connection" in which the patient learns such involvement. In this chapter we will use excerpts from interviews with patients in our own practice to illustrate how a practitioner can influence patient involvement.

From the moment ill persons become clients or patients, they begin to look at their world differently and to revise beliefs about the nature of their problem, its meaning, and what should be done about it. Patients already have some understanding of the nature of illness in general and their problem in particular, but now have decided to seek help from a professional. They know their disability and suffering to some extent, and practitioners should be prepared to help them understand and organize that knowledge further.[1] The practitioner might give the illness a name, provide an explanation, detail what must be done and what role the patient must play in the healing.

Talking with patients inevitably modifies a patient's knowledge about a problem. How practitioners ask a question, how they listen, and how much information is needed all contribute to the educational potential of the healer-patient relationship. Different case histories from the same patient may be obtained because of different communication styles and educational techniques; these various styles indicate to the patient which symptoms matter and which do not. Unfortunately, practitioners don't always see themselves as teachers. They may be more aware of their other roles, such as healer, scientist, or technician.

The degree of teaching and patient involvement depends upon the nature of the condition. In acute and overwhelming illness, it is true that patient involvement may wait while the practitioner takes quick, aggressive action on behalf of the patient. For moderate, chronic, or self-limited illnesses, patient involvement is critical and different types of teaching may be necessary.

If practitioners never think of themselves as teachers, the quality of education and patient involvement may be poor. Commonly, practitioners do not consider health education as an integral part of clinical care. Therefore, the patient may receive mixed messages and the teaching may be vague or nondirected. The doctor might suggest "stop smoking" but not put the message in context, or consider the patient's specific needs or beliefs. The practitioner may share the widespread belief that most people don't have enough "will power" to change their health habits, so why attempt to help them to change? The practitioner with these beliefs teaches defeatism and rationalization.

PATIENT-CENTERED HEALTH CARE

A "healing connection" is a relationship between practitioner and patient based upon the mutual participation model: both practitioner and patient work actively together to promote healing.[2] The "connection" requires active patient involvement for medical, psychological, and ethical reasons.

Engagement in Therapy

Practitioners ask patients to change their habits, to stop smoking or drinking, to embark upon cardiovascular conditioning exercises, to identify stress management techniques, and to articulate their health care needs. Such life changes cannot be undertaken in a passive, unthinking manner. These behavioral changes are crucial in preventing or treating major chronic disease, and they require a practitioner and patient to form an *alliance* based on mutual participation that leads to patient engagement. In contrast to compliance, patient engagement means the patient must participate in the decision-making process for a successful therapeutic regimen. Compliance indicates passivity—engagement indicates activity.

Empirical research demonstrates that patient cooperation in taking medications is on average 50 percent.[3] In some acute illness situations, cooperation may reach 80 percent. A variety of patterns explain this compliance rate. While some patients fail to take any prescribed medications, others take more than is prescribed. Of those who do cooperate, some will take too much and others only partial amounts at sporadic times. What factors account for differences in patient cooperation? Personal characteristics such as age, sex, socioeconomic group, educational level, and personality do not necessarily influence how well people follow medical regimens. Many other factors, such as physical disabilities, environmental conditions, family and physician support have a more direct bearing upon compliance.

Table 9-1 presents cognitive, affective, and physical factors that directly influence patient cooperation.[4] For factors listed in Table 9-1,[5] a practitioner can initiate a process of communication that modifies each and potentially promotes a high level of cooperation. A practitioner needs to transfer information by attending to cognitive, affective, and physical factors. Listening to what a patient believes and expects forms a basis for cooperation. Active listening must take place on the part of both practitioner and patient.

Here is an example of a physician directly addressing the issue of a patient's cooperation. A sample conversation might sound like this:

> Dr: Well, what I'd like to do is to have you start taking the Motrin. And I'd like you to *try* to take it three or four times a day.
>
> Pt: Okay.
>
> Dr: And let's *try* that for about a week. (Doctor waves hand to emphasize the point, leaning forward.)

Table 9-1 Factors That Influence Patient Cooperation with Medical Regimens

Cognitive
- Belief that the illness is significant and medical treatment can help one get better
- Degree to which patient expectations are fulfilled during the encounter
- Degree to which patient recalls and understands instructions

Affective
- Trust in what doctor is saying
- Satisfaction with the doctor and other aspects of the care setting
- Confidence and trust that medicine or treatment will not be harmful
- Feeling that the doctor is working in patient's best interest

Physical
- Capability to participate in treatment
- Treatment that involves minimal pain or discomfort

Pt: Mm. Ah hah.

Dr: I'd like to see you back, either later this week, like Friday, or early next week, whenever you can make it back.

Pt: All right.

Dr: Okay, is that going to be a problem for you?

Pt: No. I can get back.

Dr: And I'd also like to talk some more about some of these things that worry you. To see whether I can be of any help *that* way.

Pt: All right.

Dr: Does that sound fair?

Pt: Okay, Yes, ah hah.

Dr: Okay. I'm going to write your prescription.

Pt: I'm going to get myself together. My doctor, my family doctor, he was treating me for anxiety. And I was taking a nerve pill but I don't want to lean on a nerve pill.

Dr: Mm hm, I know.

Pt: First, he was giving me tranquilizers, and the price of it. . . . But I said I have to get myself together. I can't stay on these things.

Dr: Well, I understand your desire to help yourself and that's how people get over this.

Pt: Ah hah. Ah hah.

Dr: And you're the one who is going to do it. But I'd like to see if I can be of any assistance to you. Okay? Just kind of a person for you to talk to.

In this illustration the authors note the fine line the doctor and patient walk between patient responsibility ("I have to get myself together") and medical intervention ("You're the one who is going to do it, but I'd like to see if I can be of any assistance to you") that ultimately results in patient engagement. In summary, patient engagement occurs when patients feel a sense of control over their recovery as well as support from their environment and significant others.

Engagement and Loss of Control

There are several reasons why active participation is critical in creating a healing connection. Active patient involvement addresses illness beliefs, patient anxiety, and the individual's loss of control, which commonly occurs in an illness situation. In addition, effective activities require the patient's participation for success. The following summarizes the reasons why active patient involvement is essential for optimal health care:

- The therapeutic reason: Need for patient engagement in treatment
- The psychological reason: Need for patient to regain control to become well
- The illness beliefs: Need for judgments to be based upon patient beliefs and values

Illness signifies loss: the threat of death, the loss of control over our own lives and destiny.[6] Illness has historically required that we be passive in the healing process and withdraw from our normal activities. The anxiety and suffering associated with illness have arisen out of loss of control. The future may seem meaningless, and a feeling of being pawns moved by inexplicable forces out of one's control is generated. This patient was reflecting upon the moment his doctor told him he had cancer:

> Pt: One of the things that happens to you is that your status change is just dramatic. You go from being someone who does things to someone everything is done to. . . . For me the uncertainty was much worse than finally knowing exactly where I stood. The uncertainty created a tremendous anxiety . . . and I think it's clear that once you found out what you're up against, it's not easy but it's somehow relaxed and it takes out the anxiety . . . getting rid of the anxiety is tremendously important.

When he knew what he was up against, he was ready to fight the illness. The healing process is facilitated as control is regained. From a practitioner perspective this presents a classic quandary: which comes first, the healing or the regaining of control? In chronic illness the practitioner has to pay attention to both. Health care providers who ignore the issue of control nonverbally imply that their patients should be passive participants in their care. A doctor, for example, might feel that he or she is an expert on diabetes and will tell the patient what dose of insulin to take, what to eat, and be available to help if the patient gets into trouble. These attitudes would result in a passive patient who lets the doctor control the patient's diabetes. Another doctor, however, who stresses patient independence might find that his or her patients adjust their own insulin doses, change their diets to reflect daily activities, and may even miss follow-up appointments because they are too busy doing other things. These patients are engaged in therapy because they have taken charge and are active participants in their own health care.

Engagement and Human Values

The final reason for patient involvement in the healing connection relates to values. The most fundamental value of health practitioners is to help sick people get well and function better. Usually, the patient and practitioner share this general value, but in specific situations conflicts can occur. For example, one patient's religious beliefs may preclude certain kinds of medical treatment goals. Another patient's love of travel and eating in restaurants may interfere with a strict adherence to a low-salt diet. A third patient's desire to have children may be more important than the added risk of pregnancy imposed by her lupus.

Medical decisions should be made by the patient, not the practitioner. Thus, at the most basic ethical level patient involvement in decision making is crucial. It requires that the patient be encouraged to actively express his or her values, goals, and life style preferences. Textbook treatment is abstract; it must be individualized for each patient. A paternalistic approach to health care, no matter how subtle, ignores the patient's values and attempts to impose the practitioner's own values on the situation. Recognition of patient autonomy and engagement demands that practitioners foster active decision making on the part of their patients.

Practitioners As Educators

Patients learn active involvement from their interactions with practitioners. But how does the practitioner convey this attitude? How does the practitioner foster patient involvement in health care? Is it a question of tagging something on to each office visit, such as little talks on influenza or diabetes? Does it require handing out pamphlets or perhaps showing videotapes in the waiting room? Videotapes, educational materials, and discussions may be useful, but they are not central to the practitioner's role as an educator.

A practitioner-patient interaction is potentially educational. The practitioner, aware of it or not, is teaching. Of course, the converse is also true; the patient should be teaching the doctor as well. Sensitive and astute practitioners can learn a great deal from their patients using active listening and empathy skills.

THE PROCESS OF CREATING PATIENT INVOLVEMENT

The practitioner begins to establish a healing connection by careful attention to process. First, the practitioner involves the patient in the process of data collection and analysis. This requires that the practitioner demonstrate respect for the patient as a person and as a historian, and it involves the skills of active listening, accurate responding, clarifying the real problem, and learning how the problem impacts on the person.

The second step is to engage the patient in decisions about what to do and how to do it. This calls upon the skills of negotiation. The third step is to extend the practitioner's influence beyond the office and into the future, in other words, influencing the patient to *change*. These activities engage the person as an educated consumer, client, and patient. Each of these will be discussed in more detail in the following sections.

Setting

The setting for data collection is the clinical interview and examination. The patient is the best source of data about the disease from which he or she suffers. Practitioners cannot observe diseases directly but only assess them indirectly through conversation with the patient, observation, physical examination, and laboratory studies. Experienced clinicians know that, despite all our technology, perhaps 70 percent of useful clinical information comes from the medical history.[7]

Unfortunately, it isn't possible to simply let patients tell their own story because, though they have expert knowledge about their experiences, they do not have expert knowledge about the disease. They do not read health care textbooks. They may not know what particular symptoms or characteristics of the symptoms are important for the practitioner to know in making a diagnosis. Consequently, patients must be guided or encouraged to provide accurate and precise data. This means the clinician must be neither a passive figure who asks only general, open-ended questions nor a paternalistic figure who assumes a controlling style and dominates the conversation. Good health care should nourish patient autonomy and decision making. This begins with sensitive and careful medical interviewing that nourishes the patient's active—albeit guided—involvement in data collection.

Demonstrating Respect

How do clinicians help their patients to become more active in the interview process? There are three major steps. First, physicians must communicate *respect* for their patients. Sick persons who experience respect will be more likely to use their limited energy as active participants, to ask questions, and to reveal deeper feelings and concerns. The term "respect" refers to a basic attitude and specific behaviors of the practitioner that convey "positive regard" for the patient.[8]

Practitioners may communicate lack of respect through thoughtless behaviors, such as failing to knock at the door of the examining room, introducing themselves in a hasty mumble, mispronouncing the patient's name, or conducting the interview while standing and looking down at the patient who is undressed and wearing a hospital gown. Practitioners demonstrate a controlling style that communicates that the patient should be passive each time they ignore the emotional content of the patient's statements. Often, practitioners fail to comment on their findings or plans, and leave the room before the patient has an opportunity to ask questions.

Whatever a practitioner's attitude toward the patient, he or she must demonstrate respect by consciously attending to certain actions. Respectful behaviors include:

- Introducing oneself clearly
- Maintaining good eye contact
- Not using the patient's first name during an initial interview. Demonstrating that the patient is your equal sets the stage for mutual participation.
- Inquiring about and arranging for the patient's comfort and continuing to consider it during the course of the evaluation. The patient is sick or in need of help.
- Conducting the interview while sitting at the patient's level in a position where one can be easily seen and heard
- Warning the patient when one intends to do something unexpected or painful, particularly in the physical examination
- Encouraging the patient to ask questions and building in opportunities for the patient to do so
- Maintaining general sensitivity to the individual and situation

Active Listening

The second step is to listen and respond accurately not only to cognitive but also to affective components of the patient's communication. This active listening and responding is sometimes called *empathy*.[9] Empathy is not an emotional state of sympathy or feeling sorry for someone; in a medical interview, being empathic means being aware of the total communication—words, feelings, gestures—and letting the patient know that he or she has been understood. By doing this the clinician completes a feedback loop and gives positive reinforcement. Behaviors that demonstrate that the clinician is both listening and understanding encourage patients to continue to tell their story.

A busy practitioner can easily fail to do this. Some clinicians some of the time simply *ignore* what the patient has said and act as if they did not hear it. For example:

> Pt: Most days my arthritis is so bad the swelling and pain are just too much.
>
> Dr: And have you ever had operations?

Often practitioners respond to symptoms, and particularly feelings about symptoms, in a way that *minimizes* them. For example:

> Pt: I was in agony with the pain and terribly frightened.
>
> Dr: So you had a little pain and anxiety. Well, everything's going to be okay.

Neither of these types of response is effective and, therefore, will not foster a healing connection. An accurate response indicates that practitioner is comprehending exactly what the patient has said and felt. For example:

> Pt: Most days the arthritis is so bad the swelling and pain just get too much. I can't seem to do anything at all anymore and nothing seems to help.
>
> Dr: It seems as though the pain and disability are really getting to you.

When the practitioner learns to engage in reflective listening, he is likely to find that this has a positive effect on the patient's ability to be active in giving an accurate history and in talking about what he or she is feeling. By optimizing this opportunity, the practitioner may more easily facilitate behavior change.

Skillful Interviewing

The third step in encouraging patients to become more involved in the process of data gathering has to do with the style of the conversation itself. Respect and accurate responding encourage the patient to be more involved and active, but the practitioner must then guide the conversation by using specific interview skills to yield accurate and precise data. We cannot review all of these skills in this chapter, but three points deserve explicit emphasis.[10]

First, the clinician should use language the patient understands. A physician, for example, may talk about hematemesis rather than vomiting up blood or about paresthesias rather than pins-and-needles sensations in the fingers. Both hematemesis and paresthesias are quite precise and useful words, but they are not conversational English. Many times patients do not let on that they have failed to understand the practitioner's statement. They do not feel comfortable asking "What do you mean?" This becomes a particular problem with closed-ended or yes/no types of questions where minimal patient response is requested or with explanations and instructions where no response is sought.

The second skill is to indicate where you are and where you are going in the interview. Much of this can take place at various transitional points during the interactions as the practitioner *summarizes* what the patient has said, *asks* if there are any questions or remaining concerns, and then *states* what is coming up next and why. For example: "Anything else? Okay, now I'd like to get a better idea about how this illness has influenced you at work. Let's talk about your daily activities."

The third skill is using the physical examination to provide information to the patient, while at the same time obtaining the information that is needed. This is particularly important in terms of specific activities relating to sexual matters. The following dialogue between a doctor and his new patient demonstrates this process. The patient requested a diaphragm for birth control but knew little about contraceptives or about the relevant anatomy and physiology.

Dr: What do you know about the diaphragm?
Pt: Well, I have just read about it in this book (patient indicates pamphlet on different contraceptive methods the nurse gave her to read while she was waiting).
Dr: Okay. Have you ever had a pelvic exam before?
Pt: No.
Dr: The diaphragm is a good method of birth control, but it takes some time and patience to learn how to use it. Okay? And you do have to be comfortable with your own insides, with your vagina, with touching it and putting something inside when you have intercourse and then taking it out.
Pt: Um hum.
Dr: What I would like to do is to just go through an exam with you, and I will explain things to you as I go along. Okay? And then we will go through fitting you with the diaphragm and talking about what it is like to use it and then you can decide whether that's something you would like to try. (Patient nods.) Do you have any questions before we do your exam?
Pt: No, uh uh.
Dr: And as I do things I will tell you what I am doing. All right. What I am going to do first is look at the outside of you. I am checking the labia or lips. That's good, you are doing fine, and now you are feeling my finger at the edge of the vagina,

and now inside, feeling where your cervix is. Do you know what your cervix is?

Pt: No.

Dr: Okay. It is the opening to your womb or uterus. I am just locating it first, okay, and now you're going to feel the metal thing I showed you before and I'm inserting it very gently, this muscle here stretches real easily, and now I can see your cervix very clearly and . . .

Pt: Is that where I put the diaphragm?

Dr: Exactly. That is exactly where you put the diaphragm. Okay. Now I am just using one of these Q-tips to do the Pap test . . . and now I'm taking the speculum out. Okay, are you still with me?

Pt: Yeah.

Dr: Okay. Now I'm checking back inside your vagina, and where my fingers are is where you put the diaphragm. Okay? I am touching your cervix right now and on you it is a little bit off to your left side and it feels like the end of your nose when you touch it. Now when I put one hand here (Doctor places hand on lower abdomen), between the two hands I can feel your womb or uterus. I am touching it now and it feels completely normal. And I am checking on each side for your ovaries . . .

Pt: You can feel all that?

Dr: You can feel all that, especially in someone like you because you are very relaxed and I can feel everything.

The practitioner set the stage for patient involvement—obviously crucial for the success of this birth control method—by using the history and physical examination to educate, instead of allowing the patient to feel passive and exposed. This kind of informative interaction should take place routinely. Note, too, how the physician checked back frequently and used both medical and lay terms (labia/lips, uterus/womb). The physician went on to fit the diaphragm and allowed the patient to practice inserting it, thereby employing repetition of the information and reinforcement of the patient's understanding and ability.

Below is a list of the deterrents discussed in this section. These are practitioner attitudes or practices that promote passivity, misunderstanding, and lack of patient involvement.

- Negative assumptions about the patient's competence or ability to change

- Disrespectful behavior
- Failure to listen and respond to both cognitive and affective communication
- Overuse of medical terminology
- Disorganized interview
- Failure to use clinical procedures as teaching opportunities

INTERACTIVE DECISION MAKING: NEGOTIATION

Negotiation is the process by which we use discussion and compromise to arrive at the settlement of some issue. It is that component of the clinical transaction in which we actively engage patients in decisions about their own health care.[11] When the stage is set for patient engagement, the practitioner can then encourage the patient to be more active in making those decisions that affect health and medical care (Figure 9-1).

Clinical judgments are always made in the context of information scarcity; we never deal with disease in the abstract where everything can be known, but only as it manifests itself in individual illness of real people. The individual's own genetic makeup, immunological resistance, life stresses, and personality may all modify the nature of his or her particular illness. Likewise, his or her activities, beliefs, values, and goals may all modify how the illness should be treated. Important medical decisions must take all of these factors into account. This means that the decisions cannot be made solely by a clinician who then imposes a course of action; nor should the clinician fail to accept responsibility for decisions by merely presenting alternatives for patients to accept or reject. The practitioner

---

Figure 9–1 Promoting Patient Involvement in Health Care

Process	DATA	Outcome
• Respect • Accurate Listening • Interview Skills	**DATA** ⬇	• Cognitive and Affective Understanding
• Negotiation • Cost/Benefits • Health Beliefs	**DECISIONS** ⬇	• Plan of Action
• Clear Communication • Explicit Goals • Reinforcement	**GOALS**	• Healthy/Functional Outcome

should neither act paternalistically nor like a neutral consultant; rather, the practitioner should encourage the process of negotiation.

Negotiation is an interactive process; we use the word to express both the "maneuver to find a path" and "give-and-take bargaining." (You give a little, I'll give a little, let's both try to find a way out of this mess.) Negotiation requires a number of features we have already discussed, such as conducive atmosphere and putting the patient at ease. It also requires dialogue; practitioner and patient participate together as new data are sequentially added. The patient is himself or herself a resource in solving the problem.

Consider this example of a 25-year-old woman with persistent and severe vaginal itching. The physician performed an examination, and, after looking at a specimen under the microscope, returned with the news that the infection was caused by trichomonas and could be treated with a single dose of medication. But seeing the name of the drug as the physician wrote it on the prescription pad, the patient unexpectedly hedged:

> Pt: Isn't there anything else I could take besides Flagyl?
> Dr: (functioning in the context of certainty) It's the best for it.
> Pt: (commenting) Okay, but I might . . . I'll try it.

Several scenarios could be imagined here with the clinician simply saying "fine" and the patient being left to her own doubts about the drug, perhaps taking it, perhaps not. Instead, the clinician, hearing the patient's hesitation ("but I might"), uses the patient as a resource to solve the problem:

> Dr: What's the problem?
> Pt: But I think I was allergic to that.
> Dr: Why do you think that?

Negotiation is particularly necessary when any uncertainty arises in the course of the interaction. As the dialogue unfolds, it becomes clear that in this case the uncertainty is whether the patient is allergic to the drug and, more important, whether or not it is safe for her to take it. So the context has suddenly changed from one of certainty to one of doubt. The elements of negotiation that this case illustrate include:

- presentation of information or data
- verification of the data
- interpretation of the data
- weighting of risks and benefits
- formulation of a plan of action

The physician has now asked the patient for information (why do you think that?) and she replies:

> Pt: Because I remember taking Flagyl before, and it did something . . . I think I broke out in hives.

Next the clinician tries to verify the data, at first expressing, perhaps, some disbelief:

> Dr: Really?
> Pt: But I'll try it and if I break out, I'll let you know . . .
> Dr: That's a worry. Let me check your record (flipping through old chart). What it says is that you were sensitive to Ampicillin and Sulfa and . . . . Yes, it also says Flagyl.

Physician and patient now seem to agree on the information; but they have some difficulty agreeing on the interpretation of that information: is hives a serious side effect to consider or not? In order to mobilize cooperation, the clinician must understand the patient's health beliefs. The components of a patient's beliefs required for cooperation in health care are:

- Personal susceptibility
- Illness seriousness
- Treatment efficacy
- Ability of one's own actions to influence outcome

In this instance, the patient seems to believe that a possible allergic reaction is trivial, at least compared with the intractable itch. She may also believe that she is no longer susceptible to a reaction:

> Pt: I think it was just hives. Maybe I've outgrown it.
> Dr: I don't want you to take it if you had hives from it.
> Pt: Well, maybe I've outgrown it 'cause I think, it's been a while back. It can only break, break me out in hives a day and like it will probably go away in the morning.
> Dr: I would be kind of worried about that, before prescribing it to you, because you could get an even more serious reaction to it.

Explanations and "teaching" may be futile unless the patient believes she is susceptible, the treatment effective, and her own actions important.[12] In this instance, the clinician (who has already described Flagyl as "the best") seems about to propose an "alternative" therapy to a patient who believes she is not susceptible to any serious consequences of the *best* therapy.

Listed below are additional questions that are helpful in eliciting the patient's beliefs about a particular illness or therapy.[13] These questions may not always be appropriate to a patient with mild illness. However, they may be crucial to the negotiation of decisions about severe or chronic illness, particularly for cases in which the patient seems to be getting worse despite "good" medical care.

1. How would you describe the problem that concerns you most?
2. What are the main difficulties this problem (sickness, illness, disease, misfortune) has caused you?
3. What do you think is wrong, out of balance, or causing your problem?
4. What does it do to you? How does it work?
5. Why did it start when it did?
6. What kind of treatment do you think you should receive?
7. What are the results you hope for with treatment? Without treatment?
8. Apart from me, who else can help you get better? What else can you do?
9. Why did you, as opposed to somebody else, get sick? And get sick now?
10. What do you fear most about your sickness?*

In our example, the practitioner now has an understanding of the patient's particular beliefs about this problem, and this facilitates her role of negotiator. Patient and clinician must next discuss alternative therapy and must weight the risks and benefits of any course of action. These features of the negotiation process are critical to patient autonomy and informed consent. The point negotiated in this continuing dialogue is how the patient can safely take the best medication available for her problem:

Pt: But they. . . . It was a while ago.
Dr: But it does say you're allergic to it.
Pt: That's because I told them that.
Dr: I'll tell you what I want you to do . . .
Pt: I'd rather take the Flagyl, it won't be your fault.
Dr: Well, let's, just to be on the safe side, let's use a test dose . . .
Pt: Okay.

Source: Adapted from *Annals of Internal Medicine,* Vol. 88, pp. 251–258, with permission of American College of Physicians, © 1978.

Dr: Because trichomonas, while it's uncomfortable, it can't kill you.

Pt: Yes, but it can drive you mad.

Dr: I know, but the point is, we don't want to do anything that would be harmful to your health.

People usually trust health professionals and do not prefer a tedious rundown of all possible risks and side effects.[14] Indeed, this patient never asks what the clinician means by "an even more serious reaction." A sick person may have little interest in discussing alternative therapies unless, as in this example, the practitioner proposes a therapy inconsistent with his or her beliefs. This patient believes that she would not suffer serious reaction to the best therapy and that the physician was about to propose a less effective alternative. She even tried to turn the clinician into a neutral consultant ("It won't be your fault"). She clearly expressed her willingness to risk possible hives for the undisputed benefit of eliminating the itch. The physician, on the other hand, was much more concerned about a possible allergic reaction. They assigned different weights to the risks and benefits of therapy. However, they were still able to formulate a plan by negotiating a compromise utilizing a test dose of medication.

PERSONAL CHANGE

Although the clinician may have gathered all appropriate data and arrived with the patient at mutually acceptable decisions, the patient himself or herself must then take the medication or carry out the recommendations. In other words, the patient must in some way "change" and the practitioner's role is to influence the patient or help that change occur. Some practitioners are sanguine or pessimistic about persons being able to stop smoking, significantly alter their diet, or engage in cardiovascular exercises. This elite, authoritarian attitude on the part of health care providers restricts the patient's acceptance of treatment by focusing entirely on what the practitioner can do to the patient as opposed to what the patient can do to help himself or herself. Thus, practitioners should attempt to encourage their patients toward change, toward a healthier lifestyle in which they are more in control of factors that influence illness. There is no essential difference between influencing the patient to maintain health and in influencing the patient to follow a medical regimen. The five components are shown below:

1. Practitioner's belief in the potential for change
2. Selecting treatment options with the involvement of the patient

3. Communicating information needed to make a decision in such a way that the patient will be able to understand it and use it
4. Stating explicit goals and detailed ways for achieving them
5. Providing reinforcement at periodic intervals

Recall of Medical Information

Investigators who have studied the recall of medical information agree that patients on the average remember 50 to 60 percent of the data immediately after it is given, and remember 45 to 55 percent of it several weeks later.[15] Interestingly, neither the patient's intelligence nor his or her age seem to be important factors determining how much is remembered. There are factors, however, that do influence how much information is remembered. They are listed below and relate to the manner in which the practitioner presents the information. Health educators will recognize these factors as basic tenets of adult education.

- Presentation in words and phrases likely to be understood
- Statement in concrete and specific terms, rather than abstract and general terms
- Statement of the most important data first
- Repetition to bring home salient points
- Specific inquiry by the practitioner about what the patient understands
- Written description to supplement and reinforce the discussion

Explicit Goals and Protocols

The next step requires presenting explicit goals and protocols for achieving the desired outcomes and methods to evaluate these outcomes. Some practitioners, more comfortable with diagnostic tests and medications, may give very explicit and concrete descriptions of these but make global statements about diet or exercise. Statements like "You have to watch your cholesterol" or "You should cut down on salt" do not give the patient enough information with which to proceed. They are simply slogans or admonitions rather than specific treatments. The results of this type of "patient involvement" are less than satisfactory. If lowering cholesterol is the issue, and the patient agrees it is a desirable goal (engagement begins), then the patient must be given specific information about what foods to eat and to avoid, how this will change his or her usual eating habits, and what amount of cholesterol lowering to expect. Such an approach requires that the practitioner learn something about diet, exercise, and behavioral change techniques so that they can be presented knowledgeably and explicitly to the patient. It does not require that the practitioner become an expert, but only that he or she is able to help patients with a step-by-step approach rather than by making vague references to "watch your diet" or "reduce stress."

The patient and clinician must then design a treatment plan with specific objectives and short-term goals and strategies for change. A very useful behavioral technique to facilitate behavioral change is that of self-monitoring or the use of patient log books. These can be used by the patient to monitor the presence and severity of symptoms on a day-to-day basis and to ascertain their relationship to other factors in the patient's life. They may also be used to monitor behavioral goals such as a modification of diet, an exercise program, or reduction in coffee drinking or cigarette smoking. In this way the patient not only has a record to provide needed information, but the process of making the record and his or her reflection upon it can, in itself, assist the behavioral change.

Reinforcement

The final component of encouraging change is a provision for reinforcement or "booster doses" at periodic intervals. This notion is analogous to that of vaccination, in which the initial antibody response might be large and effective, but antibody levels will gradually decline unless booster doses are given. Because of immunological receptivity induced by the first vaccination, the small boosters may produce very large (anamnestic) antibody responses. Similarly, patients who are engaged in an active health-promoting program should have periodic access to their practitioner, not because they are "sick" again but because they need reinforcement and feedback. If the clinician is not available to do this or it is too costly, a "booster person" should be assigned who is more accessible (i.e., a family member, friend, colleague, or possibly a "buddy" attempting similar behavior changes).

Follow-up can take the form of periodic visits to the clinician, group meetings of persons who have similar problems and objectives, or occasional telephone calls to "report in." Both clinician and patient should examine a flow sheet, a more condensed and much less detailed version of the patient log book, which can demonstrate progress (for example, in weight reduction) over longer periods of time. A flow sheet allows a more global perspective, shorn of the daily vicissitudes that are inevitable in attempting to change.

Each of these methods can provide the opportunity for clarification, reinforcement, and support. One of the most attractive features of a long-term practitioner-patient relationship is the accessibility of the clinician to answer questions and to provide information as a method of promoting continued good health.

SUMMARY

Understanding the educational process is a major activity in effective practitioner-patient interactions. Practitioners cannot avoid educating their patients *in some way* but, unless they attend consciously to their educational role, they may encourage the patients' passivity or may give contradictory, negative messages. Effective health care, however, requires active patient participation for important medical, psychological, and ethical reasons. Realizing this, clinicians should use their skills to provide patients with needed information to enable them to gain more control over their illness process and to maintain a healthier life. The main obstacles to achieving such patient involvement are the practitioner's negative assumptions, disrespectful behavior, failure to listen, use of jargon, poor understanding of the patient's health beliefs, failure to negotiate, lack of explicit goals and reinforcement, and a personal attitude of omnipotence.

The practitioner can initiate patient involvement in the process of data gathering and diagnosis. This requires behaviors that demonstrate respect for and accurate understanding of the patient and interview skills with which both engage and educate. These lead to the next steps of patient involvement in making medical decisions, an objective promoted by the clinician's explicit attention to patient beliefs, values, and expectations in the process of negotiation.

Finally, the practitioner's teaching role extends beyond the immediate situation when he or she influences the patient to seize control and change behavior in a healthful manner. The practitioner accomplishes this through a belief in the potential for change, clear communication of information, selection of an engagement-oriented treatment plan, setting of realistic and explicit goals with the client, and regular reinforcement in a sustained clinician-patient relationship.

NOTES

1. Michael Balint, *The Doctor, His Patient and the Illness* (New York: International University Press, 1957).

2. Eric J. Cassell, *The Healer's Art* (Philadelphia: J.B. Lippincott, 1976); and Thomas S. Szasz and Marc H. Hollender, "A Contribution to the Philosophy of Medicine: The Basic Models of the Doctor-Patient Relationship," *Archives of Internal Medicine* 97 (1956): 585–592.

3. David L. Sackett and R. Brian Haynes, *Compliance with Therapeutic Regimens* (Baltimore: Johns Hopkins University Press, 1976).

4. Philip Ley, "Satisfaction and Communication," *British Journal of Clinical Psychology* 21 (1982): 241–254; Vida Francis, Barbara M. Korsch, and Morie J. Morris, "Gaps in Doctor-Patient Communication," *New England Journal of Medicine* 280 (1969): 535–540; Philip Ley, "Patients' Understanding and Recall in Clinical Communication Failure," in *Doctor-Patient Communication,* eds. D. Pendelton and J. Haser (London: Academic Press, 1983), 89–107; and Marshall H. Becker and Lois A. Maiman, "Sociobehavioral Determinants of Compliance with Health and Medical Care," *Medical Care* 13 (1975): 10–24.

5. Szasz and Hollender, "A Contribution to the Philosophy of Medicine," 585–592; Sackett and Haynes, *Compliance;* Ley, "Satisfaction and Communication," 241–254; and Francis, Korsch, and Morris, "Gaps," 535–540.

6. Cassell, *The Healer's Art.*

7. Paul Cutler, *Problem Solving in Clinical Medicine* (Baltimore: Williams & Wilkins, 1979).

8. Carl R. Rogers, "The Interpersonal Relationship: The Core of Guidance," *Harvard Educational Review* 32 (1962): 416–529; and Allen E. Ivey and Jerry Authier, *Microcounseling* (Springfield, Ill.: Charles C Thomas, 1978).

9. Ibid.

10. Eric J. Cassell, *Talking With Patients,* Vol. 2, *Clinical Technique* (Cambridge: MIT Press, 1985); and John L. Coulehan and Marian H. Block, *The Medical Interview: A Primer for Students of the Art* (Philadelphia: F.A. Davis, 1986).

11. Stephen A. Eraker and Peter Politser, "How Decisions Are Reached: Physician and Patient," *Annals of Internal Medicine* 97 (1982): 262–268; Mark Siegler, "The Physician-Patient Accommodation. A Central Event in Clinical Medicine," *Archives of Internal Medicine* 142 (1982): 1899–1902; David S. Brody, "The Patient's Role in Clinical Decision-Making," *Annals of Internal Medicine* 93 (1980): 718–722; and Wayne Katon and Arthur Kleinman, "Doctor-Patient Negotiation and Other Social Science Strategies in Patient Care," in *The Relevance of Social Science for Medicine,* eds. L. Eisenberg and A. Kleinman (Dordrecht: D. Reidel, 1981), 253–279.

12. Becker and Maiman, "Sociobehavioral Determinants," 10–24; and Albert R. Martin, "Exploring Health Beliefs. Steps to Enhancing Physician-Patient Interaction," *Archives of Internal Medicine* 143 (1982): 1773–1775.

13. Arthur Kleinman, Leon Eisenberg, and Byron Good, "Culture, Illness and Care. Clinical Lessons from Anthropologic and Cross-Cultural Research," *Annals of Internal Medicine* 88 (1978): 251–258. Adapted with permission of American College of Physicians, 1978.

14. Charles W. Lidz, Loren H. Roth, E. Zerubavel, et al., *Informed Consent: A Study of Psychiatric Decision-Making* (New York: Guilford Press, 1983).

15. Ley, "Patients' Understanding and Recall," 89–107.

SUGGESTED READINGS

Cassell, E.J. *Talking with Patients. Volume 1, The Theory of Patient Communication.* Cambridge: MIT Press, 1985.

Hulks, B.S., J.C. Cassell, L.L. Kupper, and J.A. Burdette. "Communication Compliance and Concordance between Physicians and Patients with Prescribed Medications." *American Journal of Public Health* 66 (1976): 847–853.

Melamed, B.G., and L.L. Siegel. *Behavioral Medicine: Practical Applications to Health Care.* New York: Springer, 1980.

Part III

Strategies for Participation

Chapter 10

Self-Care Education

Barbara Caporael-Katz, RN, MSN, and Lowell S. Levin, EdD, MPH

This chapter defines self-care and its basic assumptions. We will outline why self-care is important and provide examples of successful self-care demonstration programs. Self-care teaching methods will be described and illustrated with educational tools used in actual practice. The issues of client empowerment and professional participation in self-care education and potential problems and obstacles will be discussed.

SOME DEFINITIONS

"Every man his own doctor" was the rallying cry of a nineteenth-century self-care movement that arose in reaction to the invasive and ineffective medical care of the day.[1] In the latter days of the twentieth century, lay people are again attempting to gain control of their own health in the face of an impersonal, technological, and very costly health care system.

The modern form of self-care consists of activities that an individual or family undertakes to regain or maintain his or her own health. Treating minor illness at home, instituting an exercise, stress management, or dietary program, or weighing the pros and cons of recommended diagnostic testing and prescribed medication are all examples of self-care activities.

Self-management of a chronic disease such as arthritis, asthma, or diabetes through monitoring of symptoms, regulation of medication doses, and alteration of diet and activity regimens is another facet of self-care.

Preventive self-care focuses on lifestyle modification to reduce the risk of heart disease, cancer, and other chronic ailments. Smoking cessation, weight control, stress management, fitness, and adoption of a diet high in nutrients are specific self-care techniques used to attain an optimal state of health.

While self-care is not a well-defined political movement, some advocacy organizations such as the Peoples Medical Society, a lay version of the American Medical Association,[2] have developed lobbying efforts, newsletters, and resource materials. Such organizations are designed to implement large-scale self-care activities such as:

- Provision of data on the quality of medical care services
- Investigation of potentially harmful or ineffective drugs, treatment modalities, and medical devices
- Development of codes of practice and patient rights statements for voluntary use in health facilities

A common theme runs through all of these self-care activities. It is the idea that the average person, given sufficient information, a bent towards self-responsibility, and some consultation from health professionals, can make intelligent decisions about health practices that are in his or her best interests.

THE EMERGENCE OF SELF-CARE

Self-care is a very ancient and pervasive social practice. While all societies have professional healers, the individual and family have always been the primary unit of health when it comes to health promotion, prevention, care for minor illnesses and injuries, daily care for chronic conditions, and efforts to restore health. Studies in this country and in Europe support the idea that, conservatively, 85 percent of all health care is provided by lay people to themselves and each other.[3]

The borderline between self-care and professional care has been fluid through history, with one or the other segment dominating as diseases, treatment concepts, and technology changed. In the United States, self-care is currently on the ascendancy for a variety of reasons:

- Chronic diseases, which respond more to lifestyle modification than medical treatment, have become the major source of morbidity and mortality in the United States.[4]
- Mass media exposure has greatly increased public sophistication about health matters and created more demanding consumers.
- Nonprescription drugs and home medical technologies such as home glucose monitoring have eliminated many visits to physicians and medical laboratories for such purposes.[5]

- The limits and hazards of curative, technological medical treatments such as coronary bypass surgery are becoming widely publicized.[6]
- As industry and government institute health care cost-containment measures, access to professional care becomes limited by financial constraints.[7]

The womens' movement must be given credit for the current surge of self-care interest. With the publication of the first edition of the book *Our Bodies, Ourselves* in 1969, women gave credence to the notion that lay persons could provide prudent health advice and intelligently critique the medical care system.[8]

In the years since this initial effort, parents' groups advocating for more humane childbirth practices, health promotion programs emphasizing personal self-responsibility, and medical self-care courses that transfer medical skills to the public have further blurred the boundaries between professional and lay care.

WHAT IS A SELF-CARE PROGRAM?

There is no such thing as a "typical" self-care program. Formats range from the interactive self-care displays in the Cold Self Care Center at the University of Massachusetts student health center to the Cooperative Care Center, a full-fledged inpatient unit based on self-care principles at the New York University Medical Center.[9]

Resource centers like the Center for Medical Consumers in New York City and Planetree in San Francisco provide lay people with free access to medical books, magazines, and pamphlets.[10]

Self-care skills training is the focus of medical self-care programs such as Healthwise of Boise, Idaho, which, through classes and videotapes, teaches participants the principles of home diagnosis and treatment of minor illness.[11]

Industries have even entered the self-care arena by offering employee courses on health consumerism in conjunction with health care cost-containment efforts. The Consumer Health Skills program at Southern New England Telephone Co. was developed to enable participants to make informed health decisions and help them reduce their health care costs. For example, a chapter entitled "Medical Decisions—Chances to Choices" introduces participants to the concepts of informed consent, second opinions, and cost-benefit health decision making.[12]

As the self-care philosophy becomes more prevalent, even traditionally oriented chronic disease programs have begun to emphasize self-management skills. In programs like the American Red Cross Lowdown on High Blood Pressure, lectures on the nature of the disease process are being supplemented by demonstration and practice sessions in home blood pressure monitoring.[13]

Holistic health programs such as those offered at the Omega Institute in Rhinebeck, New York, provide some of the most extreme forms of self-care instruction.[14] Participants who opt for self-healing outside the boundaries of the traditional medical care system are offered courses in acupressure, therapeutic touch, macrobiotics, and a variety of other alternative therapies.

Self-care in the form of mutual aid and self-help groups such as Overeaters Anonymous involve an estimated 15 million people in 500,000–700,000 separate groups. Lay voluntary organizations such as hotlines, peer counseling services, and crisis centers have also become widespread self-care resources.[15]

THE OUTCOMES OF SELF-CARE

Self-care often takes place outside the boundaries of the formal medical care system such as within families, between friends, colleagues, or neighbors. Because these activities are rarely managed by health professionals and have generally not been subjected to controlled, scientific study, their importance is underrated by the medical establishment and health policymakers.

An examination of current social, epidemiologic, and economic trends suggests that self-care may have a significant impact on both the lay public and the health care system. Some of the outcomes of a widespread self-care movement might include:

1. A significant reduction in health care costs—As industrial and governmental health care cost-containment efforts raise barriers to the utilization of expensive diagnostic and inpatient services and encourage early hospital discharges, self-care will, of necessity, become more prevalent. A self-care program entitled "I'm in Charge" developed by a benefits consulting firm is an example of self-care instruction specifically designed to lower health care costs by encouraging consumers to make effective cost/benefit decisions about medical tests and treatment.[16]

2. Protection from iatrogenic illness and injury—Self-care programs and materials such as the Peoples' Medical Society book *Take This Book to the Hospital* teach clients to question the necessity and purpose of medical tests, hospitalization, and surgery.[17] Such assertiveness could

potentially reduce the incidence of excess x-ray radiation, medication errors, and unnecessary surgery.
3. Reduction in the number of medical lawsuits—Lawsuits against hospitals and medical personnel are often initiated by patients who have received inadequate information about the potential risks and benefits of proposed surgery or diagnostic testing.[18] Patients who have completed a self-care program are prepared to participate fully in the informed consent process. Armed with a set of questions for the physician prior to hospital admission, such patients will be more realistic about the outcomes of medical procedures and less likely to sue unnecessarily.
4. Improved health status of the population—Experts estimate that a significant number of deaths from cancer and heart disease could be prevented by adoption of healthier lifestyles.[19] With its emphasis on personal responsibility for health practices, self-care encourages people to consider the implications of unhealthy behavior and to make positive changes that will ultimately result in a reduced risk of premature death. Effective self-management of chronic diseases such as hypertension, arthritis, and diabetes has been shown to have a positive impact on unnecessary hospitalizations and development of complications.[20] The hypertensive patient who has completed an educational program and undertakes a self-care regimen of salt restriction, stress reduction, exercise, and home blood pressure measurement is far less likely to end up in an emergency room suffering from severe chest pain than one who avoids self-care.

SELF-CARE VS. TRADITIONAL HEALTH EDUCATION

The assumptions underlying self-care learning are profoundly different from those of traditional health education. The guiding principle of self-care is that the lay person is the primary health decision maker while the health professional acts as a consultant and resource person. Such a relationship requires the health educator to abandon the role of informational expert, to deemphasize compliance in favor of cooperation, and to become a facilitator as opposed to a provider of learning experiences.

In Table 10-1 the assumptions and methods of traditional health education are contrasted with those of self-care learning.

A thoughtful reading of these contrasting approaches indicates that self-care learning requires far more involvement, risk taking, and commitment from educators, participants, and sponsoring institutions than traditional health education.

Table 10–1 Comparison of Traditional Health Education and Self-Care Learning

Traditional Health Education	Self-Care Learning
1. Educational objectives defined by the instructor.	1. Educational objectives defined by the learner.
2. Learner's existing health values, beliefs, and knowledge are often considered irrelevant.	2. The learner's existing health knowledge and beliefs are considered a baseline for further self-care learning.
3. Emphasis on compliance with prescribed medical regimens.	3. Emphasis on careful weighing of treatment options.
4. Only the theories of allopathic medicine (the traditional system of medicine and surgery) represented.	4. Theories of allopathic and "alternative" medicine (chiropractic, homeopathy, etc.) are presented and considered as options.
5. Passive learning methods such as lectures favored.	5. Participative learning methods such as simulations and role plays favored.
6. Instructors act as informational experts.	6. Instructors act as resource persons and learning facilitators.

The learner in self-care must be willing to forsake the safer role of the dependent, passive patient for one of a more active responsible, decision maker. The educator must be willing to drop the mask of an impersonal expert and become personally involved in the learning process. A health care institution that sponsors self-care programs takes a radical step for a bureaucracy: that of sharing information and power with its clients, and exposing itself to criticism.

The rewards for all parties involved in self-care activities are proportionate to the risks: the learner feels more satisfied with his or her health care, the educator achieves his/her learning objectives and develops a sense of personal effectiveness, the sponsoring facility gains positive public relations, and more cost-effective patterns of health services utilization.

SELF-CARE EDUCATION—A CASE STUDY

The Yale University/Kellogg Foundation Self Care project explored techniques for development, implementation, and evaluation of self-care education in four diverse communities in the New Haven, Connecticut, area. Over a three-year period (1979–82), project staff worked within a university HMO, The Yale Health Plan, two community health centers, The Hill Health Center and the Fairhaven Clinic in the inner city, and a small hospital, Griffin Hospital, in an industrialized community to determine the self-care interests of clients and the most effective techniques for fostering health empowerment.

The project sought to answer questions such as:

- What motivates clients to participate in self care?
- Is it possible to implement self-care programs with minority populations in lower-income communities?
- What educational techniques work best for self-care learning?
- How can health professionals become appropriately involved in self-care learning?

In the course of its life, the project explored a variety of approaches to self-care program development and promotion.[21] The stages in this process and the techniques used at each stage are described in Table 10-2.

TAILORING PROGRAMS TO CLIENT NEEDS

Needs assessment procedures in self-care are similar to those used in traditional health education programs. However, they are used more frequently and more intensely to ensure client involvement in program development. Effective self-care programs can be compared to customer service-oriented corporations. They constantly solicit clients' opinions and perceived needs and continually adjust their programs to meet these needs.

Interviews with church, civic leaders, and directors of local health and counseling agencies were used in the initial stages of all the Yale/Kellogg Self Care Program sites to identify broad categories of need, potential groups for program co-sponsorship, and sources of opposition. Questionnaires distributed through physicians' offices, health fairs, screening programs, and senior centers were another method used to investigate self-care interest areas.

Advisory groups were developed at all sites and were taken very seriously. Members were recruited from the ranks of early program participants, community leaders, and employees of sponsoring organizations. Group members suggested program ideas and promotional methods, and reviewed curricula and program materials. They personally "sold" self-care to friends, neighbors, and colleagues. In many cases, advisory group members went through leadership training and functioned as program assistants.

Custom-designed programs co-sponsored with community groups were found to be the most truly client oriented. In the Griffin Hospital Self Care Program, some of the groups that approached program staff to co-sponsor programs included a tenants association in an apartment complex, a senior

Table 10–2 Program Development Steps and Techniques for Self-Care Learning

Program Development Step	Techniques
1. Tailor programs to meet clients' expressed needs.	• Surveys • Interviews • Co-sponsorship with existing organizations • Advisory groups
2. Integrate the self-care program into the structure of the sponsoring organization.	• Organizational analysis and problem solving • Program mentor • Self-care programs for employees
3. Reinforce clients current self-care knowledge and skills.	• Oral history • Values clarification • Ethnic sharing
4. Provide open access to a wide range of medical information sources.	• Newsletters • Resource centers • Annotated bibliographies • Medical terminology instruction • Audiovisual programs
5. Utilize participative learning techniques to foster clients empowerment.	• Demonstration/practice • Simulations • Role plays • Self-care "tools" • Case studies • Panel discussions
6. Involve clients in program development, implementation and evaluation.	• Leadership training • Peer teaching • Client written materials
7. Evaluate the self-care program based on criteria developed by clients and sponsoring institutions.	• Questionnaires • Utilization reviews • Cost/benefit analysis • Funding assessment

citizen center, a teen job training program, a women's club in an affluent suburb, and an English language program for recent immigrants. In each of these cases, project staff designed programs with group leaders and conducted classes at a location chosen by participants. The "Healthstyles" class held in the basement of an apartment complex offered practical instruction in the use of home medical tools. It also featured an energetic toddler riding his tricycle in the background. Such a class was sorely lacking in the amenities of a classroom but provided a convenient and familiar environment for a dozen women to discuss health, family relationship, and assertiveness issues.

The willingness of self-care staff to provide programs at client-selected locations and on their terms was an important psychological gesture that indicated that clients were truly in control.

ORGANIZATIONAL INTEGRATION AND SELF-CARE

Until recently, health care institutions have been rigidly hierarchical, with physicians and administrators on the top and nurses, technical staff, and patients on the bottom of the power structure. Self-care programs, with their emphasis on open information sharing and patient empowerment, must be gingerly integrated into the organizational fabric of those hierarchies to ensure ongoing program viability.

The comment of one financial officer in a sponsoring facility illustrates the type of organizational obstacles faced by self-care programs. He was overheard to say "Why are we running programs that keep people healthy? We make money by getting them to use more of our services."

Good public relations through programs like an "I Can Cope" series for cancer patients that won public recognition and positive editorial comment in the local paper have gone a long way towards overcoming this type of hostility by presenting the hospital as a community-oriented organization.

Sponsorship of programs for facility employees has also been helpful in integrating self-care into the organizational fabric. Stress management sessions for employees at one community health center site helped alleviate a serious morale problem. Nursing staff at another site attended seminars on patient communication and personal self-care.

The use of facility staff as teachers of community self-care programs and members of advisory committees has also contributed to developing grass roots support in various levels of the organization.

At one hospital self-care program site, an influential physician with an interest in preventive medicine was enlisted as program "medical advisor." He briefly reviewed curricula and newsletters and fielded questions and objections about self-care from other hospital medical staff. Such attempts at organizational integration do not guarantee continued program sponsorship, but they do help to build a sense of ownership for the self-care program.

REINFORCING CLIENTS' SELF-CARE KNOWLEDGE

Clients came to self-care programs with extensive knowledge about health derived from the media, from family traditions, encounters with doctors, and hospitalizations. An excessive reliance on the medical care system for treatment of every symptom teaches many people to distrust their own health expertise. As one client noted, "Until I took a self-care course, I didn't know that my common sense was hidden medical knowledge."

The Kellogg Self Care Program sites built on the base of a client's previous knowledge by searching out home remedy recipes, featuring stories of personal triumphs over health problems, and encouraging program participants to share their unique methods of health promotion. Ethnic sharing, oral history, and values clarification were used to help clients explore their personal and family health cultures.

In ethnic sharing, clients and facilitators describe their ethnic heritage and its influence on their health beliefs: "I come from an Irish family, and we never discussed illness or gave in to it." A discussion of the implications of family traditions and current health behavior follows the exercise.

"Health Story," an oral history of local health practices in a community of five industrial towns, probed indigenous diet, stress management, home remedy and illness care practices. Participants were a diverse group including physicians, a mother of 12 children, a diabetic, members of a weight reduction self-help group, and an herbal healer. The interviews were tape recorded, edited, and published in the program newsletter.

The oral history uncovered fascinating stories of self-care practices such as that of the executive who took garlic pills to supplement his regular medication for hypertension or the surgeon whose mother saved his life by diagnosing an almost fatal case of septicemia from abscessed teeth that had eluded the expertise of his medical school professors.

The oral history legitimized some of the common-sense health promotion techniques being used in the community. It uncovered a variety of dietary, self-medication and exercise techniques that are being practiced completely outside the realm of organized medical practice and generated a new respect for the ability of people to care for themselves.

Values clarification in the form of sentence completion exercises such as "My doctor makes me feel . . . " were used to explore attitudes related to health. Positive and negative attitudes toward gynecologic exams, breast cancer treatment, aging and exercise came to light during a values clarification exercise with a group of older women. Such exercises help clients and program facilitators recognize the part that attitudes and feelings play in health decision making.

ACCESS TO HEALTH INFORMATION

The provision of accurate health information has always been the heart of health education practice. However, many health professionals believe that too much unadulterated medical information can be dangerous. This belief has led to the practice of editing and laundering the medical information that is passed along to clients. Information about iatrogenic disease (illnesses and injuries caused by medical treatment), the waxing and waning of fashions in medicine, and power struggles over therapeutic approaches are carefully hidden from clients. Many of these editorial efforts produce the illusion that there is only one authoritative view on a specific medical issue.

In self care, the key word is *options*. Every effort is made to present currently accepted medical theories while helping clients develop the capacity to critically evaluate them. For example, clients in self-care programs learned about the popularity of coronary bypass surgery and the controversy about its long-term effectiveness.

In the Kellogg self-care project, medical books and magazines were used in class and made readily available to clients. Proper medical terminology was always used and accompanied by an appropriate explanation. Clients were taught to understand the difference between anecdotal and scientific evidence and to recognize the shortcomings of medical research methods. Samples of medical product advertising were brought to class and critically analyzed for message, visual impact, bias, and content. Alternative healing practices were subjected to the same scrutiny as those of mainstream medicine.

Each site in the self-care project maintained a resource center of books, magazines, and audiovisuals for client and staff use. Newsletters containing project information, staff- and client-written articles, and community resources were published by each of the self-care projects. Annotated bibliographies of health-related books were developed by project staff to help clients sort out useful information from the myriad of unsubstantiated and commercially biased materials on the market.

Traditional instructional techniques such as lectures and audiovisual presentations were all used extensively in the self-care project to provide information. However, the principles of critical analysis and examination of options and alternatives were always emphasized.

Guest speakers were invited to address self-care sessions, but care was taken to dilute the authoritative aspect of presenting one particular viewpoint. For example, in one session of a Griffin Hospital program entitled "Kids, Parents and Health," a panel discussion on family nutrition featured a conservative nutritionist, a physician advocate of moderate preventive nutrition practices, and a lay vegetarian and vitamin user. In the subsequent question-and-answer period, each panelist was challenged on his or her presentation by provocative questions from the audience.

PARTICIPATIVE LEARNING IN SELF-CARE EDUCATION

Self-care education emphasizes practical skills that can be applied in real-life situations. Simulations, demonstration and practice sessions, role plays, and case studies are experiential learning techniques that are commonly used in self-care programs.

Case studies are used to apply analytical skills or communication techniques that have been presented in a class. In the Consumer Health Skills Program,[22] participants learned how to question a physician about the risks and benefits of a medical treatment plan. Participants then analyzed a case study featuring a harried businessman with heart disease who has difficulty communicating with his doctor. The subsequent discussion allowed participants to see the link between principles of communication learned in the class session and a realistic medical situation.

Simulations are reconstructions of lifelike situations for learning purposes. In the Griffin Hospital "Lay Health Advisor Program," participants learned how to diagnose a minor illness at home and select nonprescription drugs as part of their treatment plan. In the ensuing simulation they were asked to make a selection of the best and most cost-effective cough syrup from a tabletop display of nonprescription drugs. After the choice was made, the facilitator reviewed the process of reading labels and comparing ingredients and prices, using drug reference materials.

Medical self-care classes have helped clients acquire mechanical skills in using medical equipment and techniques. In Griffin Hospital's "Home Treatment of Minor Illness" course, the instructor demonstrated the use of the sphygmomanometer, the otoscope, and bandaging techniques while participants observed and later practiced themselves.

Role plays are also used effectively to practice behavioral skills in self-care learning. In a session on a doctor-patient communication, participants learned the basic techniques of assertiveness. They also viewed a videotape showing patients using a pleasantly assertive manner to obtain information. In a subsequent role play they acted out a scene where a patient requests a second opinion from a reluctant physician using the previously learned assertiveness techniques. An analysis of the dialogue and body language used in the role play followed.

CLIENT INVOLVEMENT IN PROGRAM MAINTENANCE

Self-care programs seek to incorporate the best elements of professional and lay health care into a functional partnership. As the Yale Self Care Program matured, it promoted advisory committee members to positions as teachers, group leaders, and lay health advisers. Working advisory groups, client-written materials, peer teaching, and leadership training were all methods used in self-care to maximize the client contribution.

The Kellogg Self Care Program began its process of leadership training by inviting participants in classes to become members of working advisory groups. Some members of these groups chose to attend writing seminars and to submit stories to the program newsletter on an ongoing basis. Others assisted in the design of promotional materials and new class curricula. Those with an interest in leadership training attended workshops on group facilitation. Some of these participants were later hired by the project as group leaders and program assistants.

Whenever possible, peer teaching was used in the self-care program as another form of leadership training. One group of clients taught each other simple anatomy and physiology through poetry, home-built models of muscles and joints, and colored transparencies of the cardiovascular system. The same group researched alternative health practices by interviewing naturopaths, chiropractors, and other types of healers and presented their findings and opinions about the usefulness of these disciplines to the class.

EVALUATION OF SELF-CARE LEARNING

The most important type of evaluation in self-care is the one that measures achievement of clients' goals and objectives. In the Yale/Kellogg Project, questionnaires were used to measure clients' opinions of instructional methods and content. Oral evaluations at the end of programs, using open-ended questions, provided even more intense and meaningful data. Other evaluation approaches included asking clients to describe the applicability of techniques learned in class to their personal health situations. Dissemination of self-care information was measured by asking if the information gained in the program was considered valuable enough to share with family and friends.

As previously noted, organizational integration equals long-term survival for self-care programs. Levels of funding, allocation of staff, materials, and space, and the status level of the project director are indicators of this integration. Numbers of referrals from sponsoring facility staff also provided a measure of the credibility of the program within the organization.

Facilitator satisfaction was measured through questionnaires and interviews. Program facilitators were asked how valuable the experience had been for their personal and professional development. Stability of instructor participation was considered an indirect measure of satisfaction.

Although not used in the Kellogg Self-Care Project, in certain self-care programs, an estimate of cost effectiveness and impact on utilization patterns might be an integral part of the evaluation process. For example, an industrial consumer health education program should be able to document an increase in the use of outpatient medical services, second opinions, and home treatment of minor illness, as well as increased employee satisfaction with medical care. A chronic disease self-care program in an HMO might need to demonstrate a decrease in referrals to specialists and a reduction in the length of hospital stay.

THE PEOPLE PUZZLE IN SELF-CARE

Self-care is a movement that emphasizes personal empowerment, critical analysis of medical alternatives, and more caring interactions between health professionals and patients. Such a philosophy has strong adherents and opponents among both lay people and professionals.

Research has yet to uncover the factors that determine a preference for personal empowerment in medical care interactions. Age, severity of illness, previous experience with the health care system, family health beliefs, and economic circumstances are all factors that may influence the adoption of a self-care philosophy.

The Yale/Kellogg Self Care Project was able to make some general observations about the characteristics and motivations of program participants. The largest pool of clients were well-educated, middle-class, and aged 30–55. Home treatment of minor illness in children, decision making about services for elderly parents, and an interest in better communication with health professionals were the motivating factors for program participation.

Contrary to prior predictions, all of the program sites recruited sizable populations of lower-income and minority clients. Stress management, exercise, weight reduction, and other health promotion programs, not readily available in poorer communities, were the drawing cards for these clients. Child care, limited numbers of sessions, and class sites that were accessible by public transportation were all factors that facilitated participation.

"Health hobbyists," or persons with an avocational interest in nutrition, exercise, or medicine, were a small but enthusiastic segment of the client population. In all of the sites, their names appeared again and again on class lists. Advisory committee members and program assistants were most frequently recruited from the ranks of this group.

The medical care "avoiders" were at the other end of the self-care continuum. Frequent unhappy experiences with the health care system involving poor interpersonal interactions with physicians, withholding of medical information, or development of iatrogenic illness were precipitating factors in keeping them away from formal medical care. People in this category participated in self-care enthusiastically but often expressed a desire to abandon self-care for "a family doctor who would really care about me." For these clients, self-care would always be a less desirable choice than a strong relationship with a concerned health provider.

Many people with serious medical problems participated in the Self Care Program. Almost all of them expressed some degree of ambivalence about self-care because of the confusion, denial, and regression that normally accompanies a diagnosis of cancer or some other life-threatening illness. In the early stages of the disease process, a more dependent role and extra confidence in health professionals are a necessary part of the therapeutic process.

Family members often participated in self-care programs as a way of providing support to the ill person and gaining some sense of control over a stressful situation. For example, a cancer self-care program attracted as many family members as patients, since many patients felt too ill or depressed to summon up the interest in self-care.

Another group of cancer patients with a strong need for control and participation in their own healing were observed. Active self-help groups that featured training in self-hypnosis, relaxation, and positive mental visualization better met their self-care needs.

Health professionals were, understandably, ambivalent about self-care. Nurses, especially, expressed concern about legality and lawsuits. Other professionals expressed a need to behave as authoritative experts and described feeling uncomfortable with a program that encouraged assertiveness and questioning by patients.

The expected resistance of physicians to self-care never materialized during the course of the project. A minority of facility physicians participated as guest speakers or authors of articles. A majority ignored it as irrelevant to their medical practice.

Personal concerns, job burnout, and a search for new areas of expertise seemed to be the major motivating forces for health professionals who became instructors or advisers to the self-care program. Instructors, such as the operating room nurse who led exercise groups or the coronary care supervisor who taught first aid classes, were seeking relief from the life or death tension and highly technical functions of their respective positions.

PROBLEMS AND OBSTACLES IN SELF-CARE

Self-care is a movement that inspires considerable controversy. Power, responsibility, and access issues are at the heart of this controversy. Any health education effort that proposes unrestricted access to medical information, critical examination of medical "fashions," and an equal relationship between patient and provider is bound to be somewhat unpopular in a medical care system based on hierarchical authority patterns.

Institutions that sponsor self-care programs often find themselves in an economic and philosophical dilemma. Hospitals, for example, survive economically by admitting more patients and performing more diagnostic procedures. Since self-care postulates a critical analysis of medical treatment options and emphasizes adoption of preventive health practices, a successful program could conceivably have an adverse economic effect on its institutional sponsor, although this was not demonstrated in the course of the Kellogg Self Care Project.

Health maintenance organizations, on the other hand, are well served economically by self-care. Since HMOs receive no extra money for office visits, diagnostic services, and hospitalization, the patient who practices self-care and utilizes health services selectively can be very helpful to the bottom line. Paradoxically, the prepayment concept, with its easy access to formal medical care without economic incentives for reduced use, tends to make even normally self-reliant people more likely to seek medical advice for minor illnesses.

Some critics of self-care describe it as a philosophy that "blames the victim." These critics consider illness a multifaceted phenomenon, much of which is not under the patient's control, so attempts to help patients take a more active role give an illusory sense of empowerment. If the illness worsens, the patient then blames his or her own defective self-care abilities.[23]

Because of the complex interplay between emotions and health, there may be some validity to this charge. However, those patients who choose an active self-care approach to serious illness report that their increased sense of self-esteem and control helps them cope with life-threatening disease more positively.[24]

Self-care efforts in low-income communities have come under attack as poor substitutes for access to adequate professional health care.[25] There is currently no evidence to support the theory that self-care programs have any effect on the allocation of medical care services. In fact, self-care programs, with an empowerment focus, provide participants with the knowledge and skills to more assertively demand adequate care. Self-care programs can even serve as a focus for community organization efforts around access to care issues.

SELF-CARE AND THE FUTURE

It is generally agreed that the American health care system is experiencing a period of revolutionary change. Government, corporations, and insurance companies have served notice to providers that the unlimited use of expensive, highly technological, hospital-based care must be curbed. It seems likely that the new delivery system that is slowly arising out of the current turmoil will support the development of self-care education programs.

Health care cost-containment efforts by corporations will create effective financial barriers to the use of professional health services. Self-care education is a logical step for corporations that want to avoid the hazards of employees forgoing needed medical services. The Travelers Insurance Group, for example, provides clients with a home treatment manual, a self-care newsletter, and telephone advice by nurses on alternatives to surgery.[26]

Shorter hospitalizations and widespread use of ambulatory surgery will force families to care for newly discharged but still ill relatives. Self-care classes, telephone advice lines, audiotapes, and booklets will probably be developed by health facilities to fill in the gap between professional and home care.

Advances in home medical and communications technology will provide resources and the impetus for home self-care in the future. Programs to teach home blood pressure measurement[27] and blood glucose monitoring[28] are already being offered to patients with hypertension and diabetes. It is likely that self-care classes and educational materials will develop as more home diagnostic tools come on the market.

The widespread popularity of audio and videotapes for home entertainment is beginning to spread into the area of self-care education. Large book stores offer videotapes on postpartum exercises, low back care, and stress management. Customized self-care audiotapes featuring provider instructions for presurgical relaxation care of low back pain at home are being developed to meet consumer demands and improve recovery rates.[29]

The use of the computer for medical self-care is still in its infancy. It is possible to predict that software will be developed to give consumers advice about home medical treatment, drug side effects, and personal assessments of health risks.

Increased competition among health facilities and physicians will force consumers to educate themselves about delivery alternatives. Self-care materials and classes about evaluating the quality of health services may emerge as competition becomes more ferocious and advertising more misleading.

Self-care will provide both a theoretical base and practical tools for people struggling to take control of their own health in the face of monumental change. Many will express nostalgia for the "old days" when the physician managed all their health care needs. Many more will be grateful for the opportunity to find care and cure on their own terms.

NOTES

1. G.B. Risse, R. Numbers, J.W. Leavitt, *Medicine Without Doctors: Home Health Care in American History* (New York: Science History Publications, 1977), 11–30.

2. *Peoples' Medical Society,* 14 East Minor Street, Emmaus, PA. 18049.

3. John Williamson and Kate Dahaher, *Self Care in Health* (London: Croom Helm, 1978).

4. U.S. Department of Health and Human Services, Public Health Service, Office of Disease Prevention and Health Promotion, *Prevention 84/85* (Washington, D.C.: Government Printing Office, 1985).

5. Molly Laughlin, "The Burgeoning Self Care Industry," *Medical Self Care,* Fall 1983, 32–34.

6. Steven Schroeder, "Curbing the High Costs of Medical Advances," *Business and Health,* July/August 1984, 7–11.

7. P. Nazemetz, "Health Benefit Redesigns to Stay Atop the Competition," *Business and Health,* July/August 1985, 40–42.

8. Boston Womens' Health Collective, *Our Bodies, Ourselves* (New York: Simon & Schuster, 1969).

9. Jane Zapka and Barry Averill, "Self Care for Colds: A Cost Effective Alternative to Upper Respiratory Infection Management," *American Journal of Public Health* 69, no. 8 (August 1979): 814–816; and American Hospital Association, "Patient Education Plays Integral Role in Innovative Acute Care Unit," *Promoting Health* 2, no. 6 (1981): 46.

10. Center for Medical Consumers, 237 Thompson Street, New York, NY 10012, Planetree Health Resource Center, 2040 Webster Street, San Francisco, CA 94115.

11. D. Kemper, K. McIntosh, and T. Roberts, *Healthwise Handbook* (Boise, Idaho: Healthwise Inc., 1976).

12. B. Caporael-Katz and L.H. Kaplan, *Consumer Health Skills: A Handbook for Participants* (New Haven, Ct.: Reach Out for Health Program, Southern New England Telephone Company, 1985).

13. American Red Cross, *The Lowdown on High Blood Pressure Instructors Manual* (Washington, D.C.: American Red Cross National Headquarters, 1984).

14. Interface, 552 Main St., Watertown, MA 02172.

15. Lowell Levin and Ellen Idler, *The Hidden Health Care System—Mediating Structures and Medicine* (Cambridge: Ballinger, 1981).

16. Towers, Perrin, Forster and Crosby, Inc., "I'm in Charge," 600 Third Avenue, New York, NY 10016.

17. Charles Inlander and Ed Weiner, *Take This Book to the Hospital with You* (Emmaus, Pa.: Rodale Press, 1985).

18. T.G. Gutheil et al., "Malpractice Prevention through the Sharing of Uncertainty," *New England Journal of Medicine* 311 (1984): 49–51.

19. *Promoting Health/Preventing Disease,* Department of Health and Human Services, Public Health Service (Washington, D.C.: Government Printing Office, 1983).

20. E. Bartlett and B. Manzella, "Innovative Solutions to PPS: Focus on Patient Education," *Patient Education Newsletter,* Birmingham, AL, University of Alabama School of Public Health, 1985.

21. Lowell Levin et al., *Yale University/ W.K. Kellogg Foundation Self Care Education Project Final Report* (New Haven, Ct.: Yale University School of Medicine, Department of Epidemiology and Public Health, 1982).

22. B. Caporael-Katz and L.H. Kaplan, *Consumer Health Skills.*

23. R. Crawford, "You Are Dangerous to Your Health: The Ideology and Politics of Victim Blaming," *International Journal of Health Services* 7, no. 4 (1977): 663–679.

24. American Hospital Association, *Strategies to Promote Self Management of Chronic Disease* (Chicago: Center for Health Promotion, American Hospital Association, 1982).

25. A. Deria, "Self Care Puts the Onus on People Themselves," *World Health Forum* 2, no. 2 (1981): 194–195.

26. Patient Advocacy Program, The Travelers Insurance Companies, 1 Tower Square, Hartford, Ct.

27. "Vital Signs Module" (Washington, D.C.: American Red Cross National Headquarters, 1984).

28. Charles Kilo and J. Dudley, *Self Blood Glucose Monitoring* (St. Louis: Kilo Diabetes and Vascular Research Foundation, 1984).

29. "Presurgical Instruction Tape" (New Haven, Ct.: Community Health Care Plan).

SUGGESTED READINGS

American Hospital Association. "Patient Education Plays Integral Role in Innovative Acute Care Unit." *Promoting Health* 2, no. 6 (1981): 4–6.

American Hospital Association. *Strategies to Promote Self Management of Chronic Disease.* Chicago: AHA, 1982.

Belsky, Marvin, and Leonard Gross. *How to Choose and Use Your Doctor.* Greenwich, Ct.: Fawcett, 1975.

Berman, Henry, and Diane Burhenne. *The Complete Health Care Advisor.* New York: St. Martins/Marek, 1983.

Boston Women's Health Collective. *The New Our Bodies, Ourselves.* New York: Simon & Schuster, 1984.

Bursztajn, Harold, Richard Feinbloom, Robert Hamm, and Archie Brodsky. *Medical Choices Medical Chances.* New York: Delta/Seymour Lawrence, 1981.

Caporael-Katz, Barbara. "Health, Self Care and Power—Shifting the Balance." *Topics in Clinical Nursing,* October 1983, 31–41.

Cornacchia, Harold, and Stephen Barnett. *Shopping for Health Care.* St. Louis: C. V. Mosby, 1983.

Levin, Lowell, and Ellen Idler. *The Hidden Health Care System: Mediating Structures and Medicine.* Cambridge: Ballinger, 1981.

Mager, Robert. *Analyzing Performance Problems.* Belmont, Calif.: Pittman Learning, 1984.

Medical Self Care Magazine. Inverness, Calif., published monthly.

Napoli, Maryann. *Health Facts.* New York: Center for Medical Consumers, published monthly.

Rados, William, ed. *FDA Consumer.* HHS Publication No. (FDA)86-1001. Rockville, Md.: Department of Health and Human Services, published monthly.

Vickery, Donald. *Lifeplan for Your Health.* Reading, Mass.: Addison-Wesley, 1978.

Chapter 11

Evaluation of Medical Information: The Role of Health Educators

Arthur Aaron Levin, MPH

To use a word is not to define it. Health and education are Humpty Dumpty words: whoever we are, we all think that we know what they mean, more or less, until we talk about them carefully; when that happens, we discover that agreement on their meaning, except in the most general and imprecise terms, is difficult.[1]

—*Ian Sutherland*

Combining all the varied activities that occur in hospitals, clinics, practitioners' offices, etc., under the heading of "health care" is misleading. A more accurate description would be "illness care." The focus of these settings, and of the great majority of those who labor in them, is the provision of "medical care"—more precisely, intervening to help the sick, wounded, and disabled. To help us understand what "health care" might be, one analyst suggests that it be seen as the continuum of concerns illustrated below:[2]

1. health promotion
2. disease prevention
3. cure
4. disease control
5. rehabilitation of the sick
6. palliation

While few medical practitioners actively engage in health promotion, the other points on the continuum more or less describe medical practice. The majority of medical energy and resource is focused on points 3 and 4: the cure and control of disease. Health educators, on the other hand, traditionally view themselves as removed from the practice of medicine and concerned mainly with points 1 and 2.

209

OBJECTIVES

This chapter argues for greater expansion of health educators' activities to include all points on the continuum and has several objectives:

- to demonstrate why the responsible health educator must become involved in evaluating medical practices
- to encourage health educators to become advocates for all citizens' rights to informed consent
- to suggest some skills that can help educators become better evaluators and advocates

Many methods in health education are derived from education theory and behavioral science.[3] Most of its curricula, however, are built on information derived from medicine and public health (epidemiology). In addition, the daily work of health educators is frequently interwoven with that of medical practitioners and providers who regulate what is to be taught.

Learning to evaluate medical information has two potentially direct benefits for health educators: (1) it can validate the curricula used in health education and (2) it can strengthen the educator's role as advocate for both sick and well citizens. Health educators, however, may find it difficult to become critical evaluators of medical practice for several reasons. As professionals, health educators have been socialized by their own education and training into believing in their own expert abilities. This may make it difficult for them to critique the "expertise" of another profession, particularly medicine, which occupies such a powerful place in our social structure.

Since health education relies primarily on medical and public health science to demonstrate a relationship between health interventions and better health; educators have little firsthand exposure to the research literature that is supposed to provide justification for clinical practice. It is likely that the frequent disagreement about etiology, diagnosis, safety, and efficacy of treatment would be startling. That there is *no* scientific evidence to justify certain medical practices is probably even more unsettling. Worse still would be the revelation that some practices continue long after their efficacy and/or safety has been disproven.

For those health educators who doubt that such problems exist, the following remarks made a decade ago in the *Journal of The American Medical Association* are instructive:

> Therapeutics is essentially practical. It seeks to alter the patient's way of life or the structure or chemical composition of his body so

he will live longer more productively or more happily. In so ancient a profession as medicine, it is natural that a code of practice has been built up and is constantly changing. This code is based partly on knowledge and partly on belief. Medicine, like theology, cannot tolerate ignorance. If it does not know the answer, it must invent it.[4]

INFORMED CONSENT

We have discussed how understanding medical and health care practices benefits the health educator. An important benefit to *society* is achieved if the understanding encourages health educators to become advocates for informed consent. Analysis of the numerous moral, ethical, and legal imperatives supporting the doctrine of informed consent is compelling and need not be discussed here. In addition, there is evidence of public support. A 1982 poll conducted by Lou Harris revealed that the majority of the public is in favor of complete disclosure.[5]

Even though there may be little argument about the importance of informed consent, the question might still be asked, what has it to do with health education? The 1973 President's Commission on Health Education concluded that:

Health education is a process which bridges the gap between health information and health practices. Health education motivates the person to take the information and do something with it—to keep himself healthier by avoiding actions that are harmful and by forming habits that are beneficial.[6]

If health educators accept the role of change agent, it is their responsibility to find out the benefits and risks of the changes *they* recommend. Educators can then work to make sure their "clients" understand the consequences of any action. Advocacy for informed consent should be viewed as a primary ethical and professional obligation.

EMPOWERMENT

George Bernard Shaw said that *all* professions are a conspiracy against the laity.[7] One of the ways that professions may "conspire" is through controlling access to information. Political tyrants seize control of a "free" press in order to maintain control of a population. Limiting citizen access to information fixes the locus of decision making with those who have the information. Assuring access helps decentralize control thereby empowering citizens and permitting democratic action.

In the case of the professions and sciences, access is hampered by an additional impediment—special languages, which further serve to concentrate power. Health educators must help translate the language of science as part of the process of facilitating informed consent.

Is empowerment of the laity in medical encounters a legitimate concern? Eliot Friedson, the sociologist, wrote:

> The medical system, like many another professional system, is predicated on the view that the layman is unable to evaluate his own problem and the proper way it may be managed; this justifies the imposition by the profession of its own conception of the problem and management. . . . This I believe is improper.[8]

Some observers believe that historically the physician-lay relationship has been predicated on this unequal, potentially oppressive footing since Hippocrates. As Friedson implies, many other kinds of practitioners also promote inequitable relationships with clients. In the last decade, however, it has become evident that many people want to reassert their basic right of informed free choice.

INFORMATION OVERLOAD

Where science is concerned, people find it increasingly difficult to achieve a degree of technical literacy basic to making informed choices. There are ways to bridge the gap between the "consumer-generalist" and the "scientist-specialist." Environmentalists, as an example, encourage debate about the complex alternatives involved in decisions affecting the quality of how and where we live. Part of this educational process includes opening up public discussion of scientific controversies. In other areas of science, there is less timidity about airing disagreement among professionals than that displayed by doctors. The environmental press, and to a lesser extent the news media, produces critical analysis of issues written for a general audience. This approach is rarely used in discussion of medical and health issues. Instead, most health information is expressed in the form of advice about disease prevention and health promotion.

As medicine and health care become more reliant on technology and specialization, the amount of information that is required for informed decision making grows. Not only is the amount increasing, but also the ability to keep information current is being constantly challenged. Some experts have estimated that the "shelf life" of a medical fact is about five years. But many practitioners base their practice on the validity of that fact for years *past* its "shelf life."

Consumers, faced with an overwhelming amount of information whose timeliness and validity may be questionable, need help. With specialists in medical practice generally unwilling to explore controversies in public view, the public persona of medicine is that of the wise advice giver and *possessor* of truth, not the *searcher* for truth.

The print media, radio, and television have recognized the public's appetite for information. Almost every magazine has at least one regular column or feature on health; science magazines such as *Science 86* or *Discover* devote a major share of space to these subjects. Publications devoted entirely to medicine and health, for example, *American Health* and *Prevention,* have prospered in recent years. Radio talk shows regularly discuss medical and health topics. Many TV news departments have a practitioner-expert or health reporter or editor on staff; some stations have weekly broadcasts devoted to these subjects.

Unfortunately, the quality of much of this information is questionable. In many cases what the public hears and reads is little more than a public relations campaign for a particular technique, drug, or theory. Medical and health reporting often lacks comprehensiveness and the critical analysis needed to make coverage valuable. Information is presented in a facile manner, contradictions go undiscussed, and there are sometimes serious factual errors. This serves to hinder rather than enhance informed consent. The media need drama—even if public hysteria is sometimes the result. The effects of these shortcomings are seen vividly in regard to the problem of AIDS and have resulted in depriving some citizens of their civil liberties.

The level of misinformation is such that a 1986 CBS poll showed that over 30 percent of Americans thought they could get AIDS by donating blood.[9] Blood banks are experiencing acute shortages, although there is absolutely no evidence—laboratory, clinical, or epidemiological—to support this belief. Use of disposable needles and other equipment makes *donors* safe from any blood-borne infectious disease.

LACK OF AGREEMENT

The principal justification for the interventions of doctors, nurses, herbalists, nutritionists, health educators, etc., should be the improvement of personal or community health. Unfortunately, health outcomes are neither easily defined nor measured. The discussion of how to measure and confirm such a causal relationship is ongoing and contentious.

A review of the literature of quality assessment reveals many different approaches but little or no *replication* of either method or result. There is currently no agreed upon method of quality assessment. Practitioners often disagree among themselves as to what is best for a particular person or community. Even the simplest medical problem may have a wide range of possible interventions, each of different benefit and risk for a particular individual at a particular time. For the inquiring health educator to learn about the degree and depth of such disagreement may be more important than finding where agreement exists.

The October 24, 1985, issue of the *New England Journal of Medicine*, the country's most influential medical publication, contained two articles reaching exactly opposite conclusions. The researchers were attempting to determine whether postmenopausal women who used estrogens had any untoward cardiovascular effects. One study found that hormone use increased death and disability from cardiovascular causes, while the other found it protected women from such outcomes. The only unusual thing about this disagreement was that it appeared in the pages of one journal issue.[10]

There are numerous examples of practices that are perceived as efficacious by some healers and quackery by others. Chelation therapy for heart disease, laetrile for cancer, macrobiotic diets for both are but a few examples. Even perceptions by the same speciality or organization will dramatically change over time. For example, The American Cancer Society maintains an advisory committee on quackery and publishes a list of "unproven" therapies for cancer. Hyperthermia, or use of high levels of heat to treat cancer, was on this list for years. It is now an intervention receiving attention from established cancer researchers and has been removed from the "unproven" list.[11] The treatment and condition did not change, but perceptions of so-called medical "experts" did—though it is not clear why. This allowed the procedure to be tested in clinical trials to see if it was of value.

SUBJECTIVE DECISIONS

The problem is further complicated by the subjectiveness of practitioner decisions about appropriate health and medical interventions. This in part results from a lack of practitioner concordance as to what are appropriate and achievable health goals. It is also because the objectives of individuals or communities frequently are different from one another as well as from those of professionals.

There is possible tension between the views of practitioners and consumers. For example, a doctor urges a person with elevated blood pressure to continue to take medication. The person refuses because the side effect of impotence resulting from medication is of greater concern than risk of heart problems.

There can be disagreement between a sick person and well family members or friends. Consider a person with a recent heart attack who doesn't want to undergo coronary bypass surgery but is urged or even begged to do so by family members. It can also occur between the individual and his or her community, for example, a person who believes that childhood immunization (DPT) is of greater risk to his or her child than benefit and therefore doesn't think it should be required for school attendance (as it is in most communities). Objectives may differ among communities as well.

This unique subjectivity makes the attempt at assessment painfully difficult. But informed consent, by definition, involves the exercise of personal preference even if that requires all parties to work harder to resolve disagreements.

> Self-determination (sometimes called "autonomy") is an individual's exercise of the capacity to form, revise and pursue personal plans for life. Although it clearly has a much broader application, the relevance of self-determination in health care decisions seems undeniable. A basic reason to honor an individual's choices about health care . . . (is that) under most circumstances the outcome that will best promote the person's well-being rests upon a subjective judgment about the individual.[12]

In our context the word "community" is interchangeable with "individual" in the above statement.

INFORMED CONSENT AS THERAPY

Much about illness and cure is still poorly understood, particularly with regard to the process of healing. Why do some people survive a particular illness and others succumb, when all of the other known factors appear to be the same?

One concern that emerges from discussion of informed consent is that some practitioners believe it may not enhance the process of cure and recovery. There is no research to support this view. In fact, there is evidence to support the opposite, i.e., that informed consent and active participation in medical encounters helps people get well.[13]

The benefit of information exchange can be seen in specific areas. For example, one study demonstrated that an unrushed and informative visit between anesthesiologist and patient prevented or reduced preoperative anxiety more than drugs administered for that purpose.[14] Another showed that postoperative pain was reduced when patients were fully informed in advance about its anticipated severity and duration.[15] Other research demonstrates reductions in hospital admissions for persons with chronic diseases when they are educated about and encouraged to participate in management of their condition.[16] There is some evidence as well that good communication reduces malpractice suits.[17]

THE RISKS OF PROGRESS

Perhaps the most compelling argument for consumer equity in medical decision making has to do with the risk of iatrogenic disease—disease caused by the treatment itself. The risks of medicine are not unique; almost all of the so-called "progress" of a technologic and scientific nature is double-edged. Nuclear power is one example—promising freedom from the limited supply, high cost, and politically vulnerable fossil fuel. Three Mile Island and Chernobyl vividly portray the risk side: death for some and lifetimes of illness and despair for others.

Unfortunately, there is a sense of the imperative attached to "progress"; a technology *discovered* is one that is going to be *used*. The individual rarely has the opportunity to choose whether or not to pursue progress. Such decisions are made at governmental and corporate levels, although citizens may find that the consequences of such decisions on their lives are inescapable.

Where personal health is concerned there does exist opportunity for choice. Health educators should encourage consumer understanding that it is the individual's to make. This is not to say that forces described above are not at work to shape, influence, and limit it.

MEDICATIONS—HELPFUL *AND* HARMFUL

Medicine has two basic clinical interventions: pharmacology and surgery. The risks of drugs include those inherent in the chemical(s) themselves. It has been said that there is no such thing as a drug that is not potentially toxic.[18] Therefore, the evaluation of benefit and risk is always an appropriate activity. Risks can range from annoying side effects to fatal consequences and can be immediate, short, or long term. An example of immediate risk is the allergic reaction to penicillin known as anaphylactic shock, which can kill an allergic person within minutes. An example of short-term risk but with long-term consequences are drugs that adversely affect fetal development when taken by a pregnant mother. Accutane, used to treat severe cases of acne, is a recent case in point.[19]

Drugs with risks that become evident only after the passage of time include examples like DES, which has been found to cause genitourinary cancers and anomalies in the offspring of women who took the drug during their pregnancy. These often do not become symptomatic until well past the child's first or second decade of life. (The DES story is particularly sad since the drug was not only not safe, but ineffective as well.) An example of long-term risk is the frequent occurrence of the motor disorder called tardive dyskinesia in those taking antipsychotic medications such as thorazine and phenalzine for many years.

All the possible short- and long-term risks of drugs are difficult to discover until large numbers of people are exposed for several decades after the drug is marketed. This is because the premarketing clinical trials required by the FDA involve limited numbers of participants (1,000 to 3,000) and take place over a relatively short period of time—often a year or less. The small number of participants means that only risks of very high frequency will be seen; the short time span of the trials means that longer-term risks are not seen. There is, therefore, considerable reliance on laboratory and animal data in predicting the risk of human injury. Such reliance has not always been proven justified and people have been injured.

Drugs can also have paradoxical effects. For example, penicillin can cause gastrointestinal problems since "good" stomach bacteria necessary for digestion are killed; antianxiety drugs can produce symptoms of rage and agitation; drugs to treat heart disease can precipitate heart attacks.

Despite these cautions, drugs have produced many, if not most, of the substantial medical gains of the last 50 years. The discovery of penicillin and the development of succeeding families of antibiotics may have made the single greatest contribution toward improving medical outcomes. Drugs to lower blood pressure have played an important part (along with nutritional and behavioral changes to modify risks) in producing the dramatic decreases in death from stroke and the somewhat more modest decline in death from heart attack among middle-aged males.

The presence of risk should not discourage the rational use of "appropriate" pharmacologic interventions of proven effectiveness. However, the decision about appropriateness should be made by the individual and practitioner jointly, with both having access to all available relevant information.

SURGERY—THE DOUBLE EDGED SCALPEL

The well-known chances of dying during or immediately after surgery, the risk of serious complications, and the possibility of less than optimal recovery underscore the importance of citizen involvement in decision making about these medical interventions. Participation at all levels—the decision to operate (as opposed to receiving other treatment), the specific kind of procedure, the surgeon and the setting—is critical. Many people are probably aware that there are risks to surgery because the "drama" of surgical procedures has been incorporated into our entertainment—television series, soap operas, documentaries and movies about doctors and hospitals. But in these depictions, risks exist because of the urgency and life threat of the disease or accident; they are neither portrayed as inevitable nor as the result of physician incompetence and impairment.

The risks inherent in surgery are many. One 1982 study showed that more than 30 percent of more than 800 consecutive admissions to a major New England teaching hospital contracted a treatment- or doctor-caused problem; 9 percent of admissions suffered life-threatening iatrogenesis, and 2 percent actually died.[20] Hospital environments are notorious for nuturing so-called nosocomial infections and this is a major concern.[21] For certain kinds of "dirty" surgery, such as that involving the bowel, there is a higher risk of wound infection.

It has been estimated that as many as one in ten physicians are seriously impaired as a result of substance abuse, mental state, or inability to keep up with the skill and information required of their speciality. Most continue to practice.[22] Some of them are surgeons.

Studies have shown geographical differences in surgical rates that cannot be explained by patterns of disease.[23] Other research finds different national surgical rates among countries that appear more the result of the number of surgeons than medical necessity.[24] More surgery is done in the United States than in England but the health status of the two populations is similar. What is different is that there are more surgeons per capita in the United States.

The implementation of peer review and educational efforts to optimize surgical performance has been shown to reduce the incidence of some procedures.[25] This reduction is enhanced by second opinion programs. These experiences have led some experts to conclude that up to 30 percent of all surgery may be "unnecessary."[26] Unnecessary surgery which cannot be medically justified makes any risk unacceptable. Examples of procedures that are thought to be abused are tonsillectomy, hysterectomy, hernia repair, and cataract surgery.

Surgeons, like all professionals, like to practice their craft. They may resist change even when there is substantial evidence suggesting they should do so. For example, the standard treatment for breast cancer remained the Halstead radical mastectomy long after there was evidence that supported other, less invasive techniques.[27] Coronary bypass surgery (CABG) has become a growth industry with over 200,000 procedures, costing approximately $60 million for 1986.[28] A less invasive and less costly procedure, appropriate for up to 15 percent of those recommended for bypass, is transluminal percutaneous angioplasty (PCTA), also known as balloon catheterization. Although it is estimated that as many as 30,000 of those recommended for a bypass could benefit from this option, analysts suggest that far fewer will be done. This is due to several factors, not the least of which is professional lack of information about the newer procedure and unwillingness to change established and more remunerative patterns of practice.[29]

All these are examples of potentially *avoidable* risk. Unfortunately, even with the most competent surgeon doing the most appropriate procedure, there will always be some incidence of *unavoidable* death or serious injury.

The information necessary for an informed surgical decision is usually not available to the public. Operative morbidity and mortality rates for specific procedures, as well as for specific surgeons and hospitals, have not usually been made public. The Department of Health and Human Services ruled in 1985 that aggregate data for each hospital be made public under the Medicare program. It is not clear how helpful this ruling will be. Without access to information, surgical decision making is problematic. Second opinions can be helpful. However, if the second opinion doctor is another surgeon, the bias of the specialty and professional reluctance to criticize peers may limit their value.

RISKS OF HEALTH PROMOTION AND DISEASE PREVENTION

Even health promotion and disease prevention efforts present risks as well as benefits. It cannot be assumed that all such activities are of sufficient benefit and so little risk that they need not entail informed consent.[30]

Health educators are often involved in health "fairs," some of which try to encourage screening asymptomatic people in order to make an "early" diagnosis of illness. Some of the screening procedures can result in actual harm. For example, a small number of people taking stress tests have heart attacks and die. The long-term cumulative effect of low-level radiation, such as is used in mammography screening, is still not well understood and may actually promote tumor growth.

Screening tests also represent problems with regard to false-positive and false-negative results. A false positive means that the test shows the presence of disease when there isn't any. False negative means that the test shows no disease when it really is present. There are two risks associated with false-positive results: first, people are likely to be subjected to further, even more invasive diagnostic or curative procedures; second, they will be labeled as "sick," which can negatively affect function. False-negative results may mean that a truly sick person does not get treatment.

Here again the health educator can benefit from researching the literature. Some of what is generally understood to be "good" preventive activities have not been shown to improve outcomes in clinical practice. Because of this, previous recommendations of a regular annual physical exam or multiphasic screen of healthy adults have generally been dropped in favor of age-, sex- and symptom-specific workups.

The current enthusiasm for health promotion and wellness activities has no doubt produced health benefits, but it is difficult to determine exactly what, how many, and for whom. There is still much to learn about the strength of any hypothesized relationship between the alteration of certain behavior and specific health outcomes.

It is understandably difficult to ask health educators to be less than enthusiastic in encouraging the public's acceptance of health-promoting self-care. But these activities have risk; of the millions of runners in this country, for example, a high percent are injured each year, some seriously. Weight loss that is too rapid or of too great a degree can produce health problems. Concentration on self-improvement when carried to excess may desocialize people and make them less involved in those citizen activities that make for "healthy" communities.

SKILLS FOR ASSESSING MEDICAL INFORMATION

Besides an open mind, a critical eye, and common sense, a health educator can benefit from employing skills for judging the research foundations of medical and health education practices. Familiarity with the basics of study design and epidemiology is helpful. Knowing exactly what a study proves and does not prove and the strength of any proof are important.[31] Professional practices should be critiqued before they are widely adopted. Retrospective evaluations may be of intellectual interest but are little value in changing already diffused practices.

RANDOMIZED CONTROLLED TRIALS

There is a so-called "gold standard" of research design to evaluate the efficacy or benefit of interventions. Called the Randomized Controlled Trial (RCT), it has two key elements: (1) the randomization of participants to minimize selection bias and (2) the use of a control group to eliminate the "placebo" effect. A placebo effect occurs when the goal of the intervention is achieved without the person ever having been exposed to the intervention. In drug trials this means people take a sugar pill (placebo), thinking that they are getting active medication. It has been estimated that as many as 30 percent of any group will react positively to placebo. In order to minimize the risk of observer bias, there is often "double blinding." Research staff evaluating subject responses do not know who is getting active medication and who is getting placebo. The blind is "broken" at the conclusion of research.

In an RCT, participants are randomly assigned either to an experimental group, which is exposed to the intervention being studied, or to a control group. The latter can be exposed to no treatment (placebo pill, for example), an older standard treatment (in the case of testing a new drug), or a variation of the experimental treatment. The members of both groups are randomly drawn from a pool of persons having been selected on the basis of their similarities.

The RCT asks the basic question, Does what is observed in the experimental group differ from what is observed in the control group? Statistical tests ensure that the difference is not just due to chance. If the results pass this test, then the effect(s) observed in the experimental group can be said to be caused by the experimental intervention. New drugs and medical devices must go through clinical RCTs before FDA approval. RCTs are used less often to assess medical procedures in part because of ethical, logistic, and cost considerations.

VALIDITY

The terms *valid* and *invalid* refer to the best available approximation as to the truth or falsity of a proposition about cause. Discussions of validity in medical and social science are usually divided into four categories:

- Internal
- External
- Statistical conclusion
- Construct

Internal Validity

Internal validity refers to the approximate validity with which we infer that a relationship between two variables is causal or that the absence of a relationship implies the absence of cause.

Experiments examine the effect of an *independent* variable on a *dependent* variable. The independent variable is the intervention, and the dependent variable is the outcome. In health care, the independent variable might be a diagnostic test, a drug or surgical procedure, or a health education program. The dependent variable would be some measurable outcome, such as function, blood pressure level, or understanding of good nutritional practices.

Unfortunately, proving the presence or absence of a relationship between independent and dependent variables is difficult because so-called "threats" to validity exist. Good study design attempts to minimize these threats by keeping them within accepted parameters. Threats to internal validity include:

- History—There is often a time spread between pretest and post-test. Therefore the observed effect may really be due to something other than the independent variable under study.
- Maturation—The observed effect might be the result of a subject getting older during the study.
- Testing—The testing process itself is known to change outcomes. Put another way, being a participant in a research project may produce an effect.
- Instrumentation—A change in the instrument(s) used to measure effect could bias results.
- Selection—Randomized trials go a long way toward achieving equivalent groups for study and controls. However, there are still problems that may emerge, and in quasi-experimental research, selection bias remains troubling.
- Mortality—Despite the best efforts to achieve equivalent groups at the start of a trial, people die or drop out. The result can be that groups are less equivalent as the trial progresses.
- Statistical Regression—What is being studied may be at the extreme value of a given measure. This is sometimes called the regression to the mean (of the population). Studies often look at subjects that are included because they are at the extremes of whatever is being measured. When followed over time they tend to regress to the mean of the general population. This can be mistaken as proof of causal relationship.

External Validity

External validity is concerned with the degree to which study results can be generalized. According to Cook and Campbell:

External validity refers to the approximate validity with which we can infer that the presumed causal relationship can be generalized to and across alternate measures of the cause and effect and across different types of settings and times.[32]

The Office of Technology Assessment of the U.S. Congress defines the problem in a slightly different way.

Efficacy refers to the probability of (usually health) benefit to individuals in a defined population from a medical technology applied for a given medical condition under ideal conditions of use. *Effectiveness* is similarly defined, except that it refers to the probability of benefit under average conditions of use . . . Because information concerning the efficacy of medical technologies often cannot be generalized to wide populations, receiving medical care in diverse settings, information on the effectiveness of such technologies is also needed.[33]

Unfortunately, the setting, sample population, and atmosphere of many research projects may not be replicable in everyday practice. Thus the possibility exists that a causal relationship observed in a study environment would not exist in a practical setting. Ways to minimize this threat include doing numbers of smaller studies in varied clinical settings, adapting the research setting to more closely resemble clinical practice, or at the very least, aggregating data from all existing studies before reaching a conclusion.

Statistical Conclusion Validity

Statistical conclusion validity has to do with the proper analysis of data. It focuses on whether the statistical tests used in the study are appropriate for ensuring that the observed result was or was not due solely to chance. In research, the goal is to show that the dependent and independent variables "covary," a term used to describe the relationship between the dependent and independent variable. A study is usually thought to prove covariation if there is less than a 5 percent chance the observed result was due solely to chance. In some studies this standard of proof is as low as 2 percent.

Construct Validity

Construct validity deals with conceptual issues and depends on two factors: the adequacy of the hypothesis about *why* the intervention has a certain effect and the *adequacy of the measures* used to observe these effects. The use of the Halstead radical mastectomy to treat breast cancer was based on the theory that breast cancer was localized disease, not systemic. It therefore seemed logical that if all of the host tissue and nodes were removed, there could be no further disease. However, the fact many women died from breast cancer even after having Halstead procedures gave rise to a new hypothesis: that at least some breast cancer was systemic disease. This led the way to experimenting with localized minimal tumor excisions coupled with adjuvant systemic treatment.

Studies comparing the Halstead with less invasive techniques showed that the newer minimal procedures were as efficacious as the older ones, and today women with breast cancer have many more treatment options to choose from.[34]

The definition of outcome measures in health has also been problematic. As previously discussed, this has led to continuing controversy over appropriate evaluation and assessment techniques. For example, one study looked at evaluating the value of bypass surgery by using the measure of postsurgical work status.[35] Researchers found that a considerable percentage of those having had bypass surgery did not return to work, even though they reported themselves to be physically much improved as compared with their presurgery condition. Does this prove or disprove the value of bypass surgery? Because there is disagreement over the value of postoperative work status as an outcome measure, the study is interesting but cannot be said to prove anything.

CONCLUSION

Hopefully, this chapter will both encourage and improve the development of health education practices. The work of health educators should be guided by respect for the rights and desires of each individual. The elitism of professions can be destructive of such respect. The role of educator and adviser necessarily involves responsibility and is well served by use of available scientific principles to validate advice.

Health educators should serve as models for consumers through their own efforts to critically evaluate health information. To be effective they must learn what resources are available and how to access them.

Unfortunately, there are few health information resources designed specifically for consumers (see Appendix 11-A). The Center for Medical Consumers in New York City operates a free health library and publishes a newsletter, *HealthFacts*. Planetree, based in San Francisco, California, also has free library services and will do a computer search and provide other information for a fee. The Boston Women's Health Collective answers inquiries by mail at low cost. The U.S. Office of Disease Prevention and Health Promotion supports the National Health Information Clearinghouse, which offers access to its computerized health information database by telephone.

There are information hotlines available for many conditions and diseases. The National Health Information Clearinghouse can provide access to these and other resources. Hospitals have begun to set up consumer-oriented libraries for patients and visitors or have opened up medical libraries to the public. Despite progress, information resources for consumers are still few in number and limited in accessibility.

Technological "progress" in medicine continues to accelerate. New and far-reaching discoveries in genetic research may soon have profound effects on the human condition. Meanwhile, more sophisticated mechanical technology such as the artificial heart poses as many questions as it answers. The possibility of "bionic" body parts that can be used when originals malfunction is no longer considered pure fantasy.

Where these changes will lead health educators is not yet clear. But we can guess that the issues surrounding protection of informed consent will become even more critical. The role of health education in facilitating assessment of health care options by consumers is an exciting and promising one. It is founded on the belief that empowerment is a major objective of educators. In matters of health, access to information is the prerequisite to making informed choices. The complexity and uncertainty of medical practice make informed choice by consumers an issue not only of rights, but also of good health. If doctors are first "to do no harm," health educators should "advise no harm." Developing the skills to assess available medical information is a prerequisite of that mission.

NOTES

1. I. Sutherland, *Health Education. Perspectives and Choices* (Boston and Sydney: George Allen and Unwin, 1979), 1.

2. G. Rosen and E. Balmuth, "A Conceptual Framework and a Code for the Analysis of Preventive Services in Medical Care" (Undated paper from the Columbia University School of Public Health and Administrative Medicine Archives).

3. L.W. Green et al., *Health Education Planning. A Diagnostic Approach* (Palo Alto: Mayfield, 1980), 7.

4. Sir G. Pickering, "Therapeutics: Art or Science?" *Journal of the American Medical Association* 242, no. 7 (1979): 649–653.

5. *Making Health Care Decisions,* vol. II, President's Commission for the Study of Ethical Problems in Medicine and Biomedical and Behavioral Research, Appendices, Empirical Studies of Informed Consent (Washington, D.C.: Government Printing Office, 1982).

6. L.W. Green et al., *Health Education Planning,* 7.

7. G.B. Shaw, *The Doctor's Dilemma* (Baltimore: Penguin, 1954).

8. E. Friedson, *Professions of Medicine: A Study of the Sociology of Applied Knowledge* (New York: Dodd, Mead, 1970), 353.

9. CBS Evening News (National), 9 January 1986.

10. P.W.F. Wilson, R.J. Garrison, and W.P. Castelli, "Postmenopausal Estrogen Use, Cigarette Smoking, and Cardiovascular Morbidity in Women over 50: The Framingham Study," *New England Journal of Medicine* 313, no. 17 (1985): 1038–1043; M.J. Stampfer et al., "A Prospective Study of Postmenopausal Estrogen Therapy and Coronary Heart Disease," *New England Journal of Medicine* 313, no. 17 (1985): 1044–1049.

11. V. Cowart and J. Henahan, "Medical News: Cautiously Optimistic Researchers Study Hyperthermia's Potential Uses." *Journal of the American Medical Association* 252, no. 24 (1984):3341–3348.

12. President's Commission, *Making Health Care Decisions.*

13. B. Starfield et al., "The Influence of Patient-Practitioner Agreement on Outcome of Care," *American Journal of Public Health* 71, no. 2 (1981): 127–131.

14. L.D. Egbert et al., "The Value of the Preoperative Visit by an Anesthetist," *Journal of the American Medical Association* 185 (1963): 553.

15. L.D. Egbert et al., "Reduction of Postoperative Pain by Encouragement and Instruction of Patients," *New England Journal of Medicine* 270 (1964): 875–827.

16. P. Levine and A.F. Britten, "Supervised Patient Management of Hemophilia," *Annals of Internal Medicine* 78 (1973): 195–201; and L. Miller and J. Goldstein, "More Efficient Care of Diabetic Patients in a Country Hospital Setting," *New England Journal of Medicine* 286 (1972) 1388–1391.

17. J.P. Geyman, "Malpractice Liability Risk and the Physician-Patient Relationship" (editorial), *The Journal of Family Practice* 20, no. 3 (1985): 231–232.

18. M. Silverman and P.R. Lee, *Pills, Profits and Politics* (Berkeley: University of California Press, 1974).

19. P.E. Pochi, "Isotretinoin for Acne: The Experience Broadens," *New England Journal of Medicine* 313, no. 16 (1985): 1013–1014.

20. K. Steek et al., "Iatrogenic Illness on a General Medical Service of a University Hospital," *New England Journal of Medicine* 304, no. 11 (1981): 638–642.

21. W.E. Stamm, "Nosocomial Infections: Etiologic Changes and Therapeutic Challenges," *Hospital Practice,* 1981, 75–88.

22. R. Sullivan, "Physician's Misconduct Said to Be Rife," *New York Times,* 24 February, 1983.

23. B.A. Barnes et al., "Report on Variation in Rates of Utilization of Surgical Services in the Commonwealth of Massachusetts," *Journal of the American Medical Association* 254, no. 3 (1985) 371–381.

24. J.P. Bunker, "What Makes Americans so Operation Happy?" *Medical Economics* (January 8, 1973): 67.

25. F.J. Dyck et al., "Effect of Surveillance on the Number of Hysterectomies in the Province of Saskatchewan," *New England Journal of Medicine* 295, no. 23 (1977): 1326–1328; and E. McCarthy and G.W. Widmer, "Effects of Screening by Consultants on Recommending Elective Surgical Procedures," *New England Journal of Medicine* 291, no. 25 (1974): 1331–1335.

26. House Subcommittee on Oversight and Investigations, *Cost and Quality of Unnecessary Surgery* (Washington, D.C.: Government Printing Office, 1976).

27. M. Napoli, "Breast Cancer," *HealthFacts* 8, no. 44 (1983): 1–6.

28. Personal Communication. National Hospital Discharge Survey of the National Center for Health Care Statistics.

29. P. Doubilet and H.L. Abrams, "Percutaneous Transluminal Angioplasty for Peripheral Vascular Disease," *New England Journal of Medicine* 310, no. 2 (1984): 95–102.

30. A.B. Bergman, "The Menace of Mass Screening" (editorial), *American Journal of Public Health* 67, no. 7 (1977): 601–602.

31. S.S. Ellenberg, "Studies to Compare Treatment Regimens: The RCT and Alternative Strategies" (editorial), *Journal of the American Medical Association* 246, no. 21 (1981): 2481–2482.

32. T.D. Cook and D.T. Cambell, *Quasi-Experimentation: Design and Analysis Issues for Field Settings* (Boston: Houghton Mifflin, 1979).

33. Office of Technology Assessment, *Strategies for Medical Technology Assessment* (Washington, D.C.: Government Printing Office, 1982).

34. Napoli, "Breast Cancer," 1–6.

35. G.K. Barnes et al., "Changes in Working Status of Patients Following Coronary Bypass Surgery," *Journal of the American Medical Association* 238, no. 12 (1977): 1259–1262.

Appendix 11-A

Resources

Center for Medical Consumers
237 Thompson Street
New York, NY 10012
(212) 674-7105

Planetree
2040 Webster Street
San Francisco, CA 94115
(415) 346-4636

National Health Information Clearinghouse
(800) 336-4797
(703) 522-2490 in Virginia

The Boston Women's Health Book Collective
465 Mt. Auburn Street
Watertown, MA 02172

Part IV

Strategies for Specific Populations

Chapter 12

A Healthy Old Age: Health Education with Older People

Stephanie FallCreek, DSW

This chapter will identify several of the reasons that health education/ promotion with older persons is emerging as a concern for health care professionals. Some of the common barriers and challenges to effective program development and delivery will be suggested and discussed. Descriptive examples of health education/promotion programs with older adults will be provided and a variety of resources to assist with program planning and development will be identified. Finally, some trends in health, health care, and family caregiving patterns that have implications for future health education/promotion activities with older adults will be presented. In this chapter health education promotion is defined as any combination of learning opportunities designed to facilitate voluntary adaptations of behavior that enhance health.

For many years almost all health education activities involving older persons occurred somewhat accidentally. If older persons "happened" to enroll in a health education program, or if they happened to be watching, reading, or listening when health information was presented, they might have benefited from the experience. The practice of deliberately undertaking health education activities with older adults as a target population has become more common only within the past ten years.

For many years, the clear majority of health education efforts and public funds available for health education in this country focused on childbearing, childrearing, children, and infants. In the past twenty years, developing interest in and concern for the health and well-being of young and middle-aged adults has resulted in a proliferation of both public and private sector health education programs. This emphasis on youth in health education programming reflected the prevailing societal myth that later life was primarily a period of loss and decline, rather than an opportunity for continuing activity, health maintenance, and even health improvement and personal growth.

Historically, reducing risk factors for premature death has been a primary objective of health education programs. Many elders who were prime candidates for health promotion/education had already lived beyond the risk of premature death in terms of average life expectancy. They simply did not "fit" well into the existing traditional educational programs. The term "Youth Society" was coined in response to prevailing values. Those values and priorities seem to be changing, at least in the area of health education and health promotion activities with older adults.

ADDRESSING ELDER NEEDS IN HEALTH EDUCATION/HEALTH PROMOTION

Perhaps the most readily identifiable cause of this shift to address elder needs in health education/promotion is seen in simple numbers. In the past, the number of people living beyond age 65 was very small, and hence did not seem to merit much attention, compared with the numbers and needs of children and younger adults. Most people died before the multiple chronic health conditions, which today limit function in old age for many people, were fully evident. The population of older adults, however, is now mushrooming. In 1900, older adults accounted for about 4.1 percent of the population while today persons over 65 account for about 12 percent of the population, and by 2020, approximately one in five Americans may be over the age of 65.[1] Even more important, approximately 12 percent of the population accounts for more than 30 percent of all health care.[2]

The mortality rate decline among the very old is particularly dramatic. Between 1968 and 1978, for those 75–84 years of age, the decline was 13 percent and for the 85 and older group, there was a 25 percent decline, compared with a 3 percent decline during 1958–1968.[3] These figures suggest that older persons can expect to live for many years beyond the traditional age of retirement. The quality of those years often depends directly upon the individual's health. As the popular commercial says, "If you've got your health, you've got just about everything." Health education and promotion activities thus have a clear and logical place in the lives of older adults.

The disproportionate expenditure of health care dollars can be expected to continue or even increase unless other forces intervene, because the fastest-growing group of the older population are those over 85. These are also the people most likely to need high-cost, high-technology health care. Life expectancy at age 65 increased only 2.4 years between 1900 and 1960, while just since 1960, 2.5 more years have been added. Most of the increases in life expectancy between 1970 and 1983 were due to decrease in mortality among middle-aged and elderly populations (65–84). Life expectancy at age 65 in 1983 was approximately 14.5 years for males and 18.8 years for females.[4]

The incidence of poverty among elders is significant. Although many older adults are economically self-sufficient, others are not. Out-of-pocket expenditures for health care consume a substantial share of the income of older persons, averaging $93.00 per person per year.[5] These expenditures represent an economic strain for many individuals.

Similarly, the economic burden of health care expenditures for this portion of the population borne by the taxpayers is also great. In 1981 the total expenditures of the Medicare program amounted to $44.8 billion. Although few would argue with the provision of some health care services through taxpayer-supported programs such as Medicare and Medicaid, the potential long-term consequences of continuing and even increasing outlays is staggering. Given current population projections, by 2040, the amount spent for personal health care of those 65 years of age and older will rise to $416.75 billion, approximately 44 percent of which would be borne by Medicare, under existing rules and regulations.[6] Health education programs can have a significant impact on health care expenditures.

Consider medication management. Older adults are prescribed more drugs than any other age group in the population. For example, among those enrolled in Supplemental Medical Insurance under Medicare, an average of 17.9 prescriptions are obtained annually. This extraordinarily high figure may be somewhat deceiving, since it includes both new prescriptions and refills. Nevertheless, it reflects the pattern of prescription drug usage among older persons. Unfortunately, consistent findings about the number of different medications that elderly persons take are not available. A conservative estimate suggests that, on an average, older persons take from two to four prescription medications at any one time. Nursing home residents, in contrast, appear to take between four and seven.[7] Freese[8] estimates that on the average, the elderly person spends over $100.00 per year on prescriptions and may use as many as 13 prescriptions. Pfeiffer[9] suggests that approximately 80 percent of all drugs prescribed and paid for are not actually consumed for that purpose at that time. Those prescriptions that are not paid for by the individual are paid by either insurance or government subsidy, an enormous burden no matter who pays.

The high cost of care associated with accidents among elders is also directly related to issues of medication management. Falls are the primary cause of accidental death among persons over 65, and about 90 percent of nighttime falls are attributed to the use of sleep-inducing drugs.[10] Some health education strategies that may directly reduce the economic burden of medication-related health care costs are:

- increased compliance with necessary drug regimens
- elimination of unnecessary or duplicated drugs
- decreased reliance on drugs where behavior changes such as improved diet and exercise can effectively assist in the management of some health problems (e.g., mild hypertension, diabetes)
- substitution of generic therapeutic equivalents, where clinically appropriate, for name brand drugs

In addition to demographic and economic arguments supporting increased health education programs with older adults, there are social and cultural values that would encourage such efforts. This age group requires access to the information, support, and skills needed to promote health, independence, and well-being. With retirement often lasting a quarter of a century, there can be many years for individuals to continue to enjoy a high quality of life and also continue to contribute to the family and community in which they live.

OBSTACLES AND OPPORTUNITIES FOR HEALTH EDUCATION

In addition to their relatively small numbers in the overall population and other factors discussed above, several obstacles influenced and continue to influence the scarcity of health education activities with older adults. A whole package of "myths" about aging and the aged needed debunking before health education/promotion with older adults could be perceived as viable. Some of the most destructive of these myths that create and reinforce stereotypes include:

- Older persons are not interested in health education activities.
- Older persons cannot/will not undertake attitudinal and behavioral change.
- Lifestyle changes in late life often are dangerous.
- Health-enhancing behavioral change in older persons usually does not result in improved health status.
- In terms of health, aging is inevitably associated with frailty and decline.

The widespread acceptance of these stereotypes meant that few health education/promotion programs with older adults were planned, and those that were planned were likely to be based on false assumptions. Another problem has been a failure to recognize or acknowledge these myths and dispel them when working with both consumers and providers, even when program developers have been aware of their potential influence.

Fortunately, this set of commonly held beliefs among both service providers and consumers is finally beginning to fade with both experiential and quantifiable evidence from older persons, health educators, and other service providers delivering programs to older adults. Numerous pilot and model projects (see model project descriptions, Appendix 12-A) have demonstrated that:

- Older adults are interested in health education.
- They will and can change health-related behaviors and attitudes.
- They can actively participate in most health education activities with little or no danger to their health status.
- They report improved health (although hard research evidence of significantly improved health status is still minimal) and enhanced sense of well-being.

A recent market study clearly indicates that older adults are very interested in health information.[11] They may in fact be more interested in the evaluation of one health education effort, the Healthstyle Campaign.[12]

Research suggests that not only are they interested in health information, they are also able to undertake and successfully accomplish desired changes in knowledge, attitude, and behavior as a result of well-designed program interventions. Results from the Wallingford Wellness Project[13] and the Dartmouth Self-Care project demonstrate this clearly.[14]

About 80 percent of older persons have one or more chronic conditions. The most common of these are arthritis, hypertension, hearing impairment, heart conditions, sinusitis, visual impairments, orthopedic impairments, arteriosclerosis, and diabetes. Approximately 46 percent of those over 65 experience some limitations in activity due to one or more of these conditions. For most people, these conditions are at least partially the result of lifestyle choices and thus are appropriate subjects for health education interventions. Hypertension and diabetes, for example, may both be partially prevented and/or controlled through interventions that include improved physical fitness and nutrition behaviors. Others, such as vision and hearing impairment, may have little or no relation to lifestyle, being associated with normal physiological changes of aging, but their impact on limiting individual independence frequently may be lessened through proper management and the development of compensating skills. Contrary to the myth, appropriate health education/promotion activities are not dangerous for those older adults with health problems but may be in fact critical to maintaining health status.

For those elders not yet afflicted with these or other limiting health conditions, risk-reduction programs may offer an opportunity to contribute directly to a prolonged period of independence and good health. Finally, health education/promotion programs that move beyond health maintenance and disease management to strive for high-level wellness in late life are appropriate. For many people, it is reasonable to expect actual improvement in capacity or ability, even in late life.

PROGRAMS FOR OLDER ADULTS

Health education/health promotion programs for older adults have been increasing in number for the past decade. Fortunately, a greater number of education resources such as books, curriculum guides, audiovisual materials, and pamphlets available to support such programs are also finally being distributed. While many existing programs focus only on one particular content or intervention area, such as physical fitness or accident prevention, others are more comprehensive and designed to influence the total lifestyle of participants.

Several topic areas that are important to improved health and well-being for older adults have emerged as particularly popular among program developers and participants. These include:

- physical fitness
- nutrition
- stress management
- accident prevention
- safe use of drugs/medication management
- communication skills, especially with health care providers

The content that is addressed in these areas is similar to what would be covered for other age categories; the differences are primarily in content emphasis or presentation style. For example, in a cardiovascular risk reduction program, a lower target heart rate or more caution related to the frequent brittleness of older bones is a consideration in an exercise program. Individual and group physiological, educational, cultural, and experiential characteristics are more important when shaping the program. In the future, as the scientific knowledge base of older adults grows, guidance in areas such as nutrition, medication strength, dosage, and frequency, and fitness routines may increase and be more specific.

Although the structure, content, and methodology of health education/ promotion programs with elders differ widely, several qualities seem to characterize successful models. These include:

- An approach to content based on common sense and application-oriented knowledge rather than complex or technical information because it is useful to a wider audience
- The use of a participatory learning model involving participants in the classroom educational experience, program planning, development, simulation, and dissemination
- The development of peer advocate/trainer roles
- Initial delivery of the program in community-based organizations where older people already congregate, such as senior centers, churches, housing projects, etc.
- Focus on empowering the total person by integrating information and skills that are broadly applicable to enhancing daily life as well as to addressing a specific topic or concern.

The differences among programs are vast, of course. Diversity of sponsors, sources of funding, and delivery sites characterize the field. Some of the more interesting distinctions include the kinds of trainer/educator/facilitators used to deliver the program, an intergenerational approach, and innovative or unusual approaches to a particular content area (e.g., Tai Chi for fitness, massage for stress management, environmental assertiveness for communication skill development and community health enhancement). Health education/promotion programs for older adults are offered in a variety of settings, including:

- senior centers
- churches
- public and private hospitals
- outpatient clinics
- health maintenance organizations
- adult day care centers
- park and recreation and community centers
- colleges and universities
- restaurants
- department stores
- public health departments and clinics
- health care provider offices

Leadership in Aging Programs

Program sponsorship is usually, though not always, closely related to delivery sites. Public health departments are beginning to be more active in health education with older adults, particularly in providing traditional public health services, e.g., screening, diet, and fitness programs associated with hypertension screening clinics.

The kinds of professionals who are currently involved in health education and promotion efforts are also diverse: health educators, nurses, nurse practitioners, social workers, nutritionists, dieticians, physical therapists, occupational therapists, adult educators, exercise physiologists, community health workers, physicians, and psychologists. In the hospital setting, public relations staff often have primary responsibility for the health promotion program with older adults. Another kind of professional, the private sector entrepreneur, who may run a franchised weight loss "clinic" or a holistic fitness center without formal educational training in any health related field, is increasingly seen.

The roles of professionals in health education and promotion programs vary widely. In some programs, all leadership, teaching, training, and program development activities are exclusively the domain of professionals. Some programs provide training to peer leaders, volunteer facilitators, or health advocates, who then assume primary responsibility for program delivery. In others, professionals act as initiators but turn over the entirety of program delivery to peer facilitators, lay volunteers, or staff persons who have no formal training related to health education but who are "located" in the program organizational structure in a way that facilitates their assuming program delivery responsibility. In a few programs, older people themselves have organized programs and called upon professionals strictly as consultants to assist with specific areas of program development, delivery, or evaluation. The range of possibilities is obviously great.

Common Challenges

A host of challenges and problems are common to many health education/ promotion programs with older adults. These are not unique to working with older adults, but many of them simply are encountered more frequently with this age group. Some of the most common situations requiring special consideration are described briefly.

Today's older adults typically were socialized strictly in the medical model when it comes to use of the formal health care system. The myth of the "doctor god" lingers longer and stronger among this age group because it is the myth they grew up with and usually encountered in their contacts with the health care system. For many, this experience, related experiences, and perceptions pose barriers to appropriate use of health education resources and the health care system. Special efforts may be needed to help participants accept appropriate self-responsibility for their health rather than solely relying on their physician. Most older adults require assertiveness or communication skills training to increase their effectiveness in patient/ provider communication.

Also, some culturally distinct groups of elders place considerable reliance on health care and treatment practices that lie outside today's conventional health care system. Herbal medicine among mountain folk, curanderismo among Hispanics, acupuncture among Asian elders, and shamanism among some American Indian tribes are just a few examples of belief systems that strongly influence the health practices and behaviors of many elders. It is important to recognize them in health education/promotion programming, because many elders will continue to use or rely on such approaches as an important source of health information and care. It is also a good idea to keep in mind that practices that today are considered unconventional may represent mainstream healing practices tomorrow. Acupuncture, for example, though still considered unconventional or unproven by some, is reimbursable today by many health care plans.

A higher degree of illiteracy presents special challenges to health education/promotion with some groups of older adults, particularly those more likely to be in poor health, such as the very old, minority group elders, rural elders, and those in the lowest income groups. Educational materials, therefore, must be developed to respond to the educational levels of participants, with perhaps greater reliance on audiovisual supports. A lack of familiarity with the health and social services system may require emphasis on understanding options and alternatives in disease management and prevention.

Poverty afflicts many older adults. Although most older persons live independently and are relatively self-sufficient economically, many are not. Those with the fewest financial resources are likely to be in the poorest health, frequently as a result of a lifetime of deprivation. A program with high fees or one requiring expensive equipment or accessories (e.g., costly running shoes) will not be accessible to this population.

Strategies for Developing Health Education Programs

Two recent studies identify another important strategy for developing effective health education/promotion programs, the market study discussed earlier and the most recent data from the Health Promotion and Disease Prevention Supplement to the National Health Interview Survey. The studies both suggest that older adults need more accurate information about appropriate health behaviors stated in a positive manner, rather than what behaviors to avoid. For example, 45 percent of adults over 65 in the HIS sample said they did not know how many minutes a person should exercise on each occasion to strengthen heart and lungs, while only 10 percent believed that less than 15 minutes is sufficient. Similarly, in the market study, more people could cite examples of what was nutritionally less desirable behavior than could identify components of a balanced diet.[15]

In the 1970s, health fairs proliferated and, indeed, in many communities they still constitute the only organized educational (and screening) effort undertaken with older adults at the poverty target group. Unfortunately, many of the early health fairs did not have mechanisms for referral or followthrough with participants, only problem identification. Although today's health fairs are usually better organized to deal with this, there are often still gaps in the system. The large numbers of participants typically result in a minimum of time being spent with individuals, referral is spotty, and the scrap of paper handed out with the blood pressure reading or the cholesterol level seldom finds its way to the participant's health care provider.

The health fair approach typifies programs that rely upon screening or risk assessment and transfer of information, assuming that these activities are sufficient to generate behavioral changes that will be maintained. Unfortunately for most people, there is little evidence to support this assumption. In addition, many health education/promotion programs neglect to plan for followthrough and ongoing support for participant attitudinal and behavior changes. A series of classes to inform and educate participants may be useful, but without some type of continuing support, many of the gains made during the sessions are likely to be lost.

This support can take many forms, depending upon the group, the sponsor, and the resources available. Some examples of effective approaches to this challenge include:

- peer support or self-help groups
- periodic consultation with providers (in person, by phone, or letter)
- enlisting the informal support system in the maintenance of change effort (as participants, or as "encouragers")
- ongoing support "events" (formal or informal)
- incorporating a self-recording and reinforcement component into the educational program
- enlisting participants as facilitators or advocates (paid or volunteer) with successive health education programs

Networking among providers of health education/promotion programs with elders appears to be minimal, though growing. The development of shared communications, coalitions for action, and joint programming activity offers many benefits to providers. Shared resources, greater visibility, backup personnel, moral support, and encouragement are among the key advantages.

Research and evaluation efforts in health education/promotion with older adults have been sparse. Typically, resources for program delivery are scarce and, consequently, it is difficult for many providers to justify diversion of resources into evaluation. However, it is very important to have an evaluation component for both individuals and programs. Some of the benefits include:

- Providing documentation needed for securing ongoing program support
- Providing individuals with a baseline from which to measure their progress
- Providing program planners/developers with information needed to revise, adapt, and improve programs
- Contributing to the knowledge base of health education/promotion with older adults

There are numerous possible evaluation strategies. Previous evaluation activities in early programs suggest some of the available approaches that can be tailored to the resources of the program.[16]

The solution to these challenges and related dilemmas typically is very creative programming and an in-depth understanding of the target participant and provider populations, which usually requires a substantial investment in planning and development activities.

FUTURE IMPLICATIONS

Several changes in the health care industry support the need for increased health education efforts with older adults. Most of these, of course, affect people of all ages, but they are identified here because the incidence and prevalence of both chronic and acute conditions among older adults give them particular relevance. The use of Diagnostic Related Groups (DRGs) with reimbursement caps for Medicare patients, for example, should increase demand for good patient education. With the need to release patients as quickly as prudent from the institutional setting, patient (and family) education is essential for an effective and smooth recovery and transition to other care arrangements. Patient teaching by nurses in home health care has been a reimbursable service, within the skilled nursing visit limits. With the advent of DRGs and earlier discharge, patient and family education could become an integral and economically viable discharge activity, with support and reinforcement through health services after discharge.

"Medicine on the Mall," storefront health care providers, diagnostic clinics, ambulatory care clinics, etc., may offer lower-cost, more accessible medical care to older adults. At the same time, appropriate use of this diversity of service options requires better consumer skills, which could be acquired most readily through health education/promotion programs.

The proliferation of self-care and self-diagnostic tools similarly suggests an urgent need for health education. Used appropriately, these tools can play an important role in the person's overall care plan. Used inappropriately, they can be costly and/or dangerous. The market study discussed earlier suggests that one of the prevalent fears of many older adults is loss of independence through illness and disability. When self-care and self-diagnostic tools are used inappropriately, they may result in unnecessary fears and inappropriate, excessive use of health care providers, causing both psychological and economic hardship. Similarly, a failure to understand the sensitivity or lack of sensitivity of a particular test may influence an older adult to avoid or delay screening or treatment that is appropriate and necessary. However, with proper education individuals can use these tools wisely, benefiting themselves and the health care system.

The Role of Family

The role of the family and its changing nature are also relevant to health education/promotion program development. Several aspects deserve mention:

- increase in families containing three, four, or even five generations
- changing role of women in elder care
- importance of older persons as models, information givers, etc.

The decrease in mortality among the oldest age groups means that many families are now responsible, at least in part, for support, be it economic, social, emotional, or personal care, of more and older family members. Families have traditionally provided the majority, perhaps as much as 80 percent, of personal health care to older persons, and indeed this pattern seems not to have changed. However, increased numbers of partially dependent older adults and frail elderly cause caregiving to be more difficult, placing major demands upon younger family members.

These "younger" family members may themselves be persons past retirement and in need of some support. On the other hand, it is not unusual to find members of the oldest living generation caring for less healthy adults and children. The most common situation would appear to be that of middle-aged adults facing simultaneous demands from their children, their marriage, and their employment as well as the visible need for help from elderly parents or other kin.

The health education/promotion needs of individuals and family units in these situations are not well-defined, but at a minimum clearly include information and skills needed to provide mutual aid and assistance in coping with any chronic health problems being experienced by one or more members. The decision to seek health care and the compliance or noncompliance with recommendations for disease or problem management may be directly related to family encouragement. The expectations of family and friends often have an important influence on the older individual's decision to undertake preventive health practices.

Shared responsibility and authority in the family unit also plays a strong role in determining whether or not an individual feels powerful or in control enough to try preventive health behaviors. This suggests the importance of debunking stereotypes about the inevitability and irreversibility of many health changes that often are associated with aging. It also indicates the critical nature of an individual's perception of control over his or her environment, which is strongly influenced by the way the family unit perceives older adults and their capacities.

As more women have entered the full-time labor force, this expectation, in many cases, has become more difficult to fulfill. In addition to the obvious needs for information and skills related to managing particular health conditions, stress management and communication skills for both caregivers and receivers seem critical for families in long-term caregiving situations. For example, time management skills may be most valuable for the working woman who has caregiving demands at home. Communication skills are essential for all family members if relationships are to be maintained and responsibilities are to be equitably shared in a high stress situation.

A good realistic assessment and understanding of the functional abilities, capabilities, and possibilities of all family members will be important for planning that supports the maximum personal independence and contribution for those in dependent roles. While the methodology for this type of assessment is not yet developed, it will certainly become a priority in the future.

Peer Models

The importance of older persons as models/teachers/supporters of healthy lifestyles should be emphasized. Despite some good health education programs in some school settings, patterns of health care utilization and life-style behaviors are learned and reinforced primarily in the family. Older persons can provide either good or bad examples of health responses to aging for other members of the family. If the oldest family members develop or maintain healthy lifestyles throughout life, it is more likely that age peers and younger family members will make healthier choices and better age/stage life transitions.

In many cultures, older adults provide a significant portion of child care. It appears that this trend may be increasing, even among those groups who have not traditionally relied on this type of care. Older adults who are well-educated in terms of health and lifestyle issues can certainly provide a better foundation for both children and adults in their caregiving units.

DEMOGRAPHIC TRENDS

Health promotion/education programs of the future will be affected by a variety of changes, including an increased population of older adults, particularly those over 75, migratory trends of elders, changes in financing and service delivery mechanisms of the health care system, and increases in high-tech, high-cost medical care.

Geographic trends and projections suggest that different areas of the United States will experience the "graying of America" differently. Heavy migration of elders to specific states (e.g., Florida, Arkansas, Arizona, New Mexico, etc.) will place unique demands upon the health care systems located there. Many elders are moving because they are already experiencing chronic health problems that are better managed in a different climate and others are moving because they are in good health and wish to maintain it. In either case, a particularly strong market for health education/promotion programs seems likely to develop in those regions.

Also, in the "sunbelt" there is the increasing phenomenon of seasonal migration, elders coming to live during the cold months and returning north for the rest of the year. Both opportunities and challenges for health education accompany this trend. For example, followthrough and the development of ongoing support for behavioral changes are made more difficult by the seasonal departure of the client, who may live in an area only three to five months of the year. Creative strategies for addressing this challenge must be devised.

In addition, although the precise nature of some of these changes is unpredictable, it is reasonable to anticipate important changes in the incidence and prevalence of existing illnesses and disease as well as the emergence of new health problems. For example, it is relevant when considering the future of health education/promotion with older adults to look at the increased incidence of Alzheimer's and related diseases among the very old. As the very old population increases, and without a major medical breakthrough, the increase in the numbers of persons with Alzheimer's can be expected to increase as well. Although there currently is no treatment for this disabling and eventually deadly disease, there is certainly benefit to be obtained from educational strategies directed toward disease management, both by the patient and the caregivers.

Another disease that appears to be on the rise, which has implications for health education/promotion, is diabetes. At least one prominent gerontological health promoter is predicting a startling increase in the number of adult onset diabetics, partially due to lifelong excess consumption of sugar.[17] Health educators can respond to these trends by designing innovative education and environmental interventions as well as by planning for coping with the problems of disease management.

Estes has suggested that the medical care system will become increasingly stratified and characterized by increased inequalities in access to health care.[18] She identifies several factors that contribute to this trend:

- increasing emphasis on price competition to solve the problems of cost, access, and quality health care
- shifting of the burden of financial responsibility from the federal government to state governments and from the state to local governments and to individuals
- increasing fragmentation of third party reimbursement policies, aimed at controlling costs rather than assuring equity, access, or quality
- the fact that the government is increasingly acting as simply another interest group in defending industry interests in health[19]

If one accepts Estes' arguments, it becomes even more critical that elders be empowered in the area of health. A high priority must be given disseminating those educational tools and political skills that can be used to prevent disease, manage chronic and acute health problems, and enhance well-being.

Health Care Delivery System

Other changes in the health care delivery system, such as a combination of agency competition, empty beds (and associated falling revenues), and, in some cases, corporate good will, are compelling hospitals actively to develop and encourage health education/promotion activities with older adults. Dozens of hospitals throughout the country have programs, ranging from the simple public lecture series to the elaborate senior health care centers with primary care provision in conjunction with lifestyle assessment and educational interventions. The American Hospital Association's commitment of funds and staff to materials development, teleconferences, and training conferences on the subject clearly reflects this interest.

Proactive planning for these future needs in health education/promotion should be occurring now to avoid ineffective, costly, fragmented programming. Environmentally based interventions also support the goals of health education/promotion strategies since access to health-enhancing choices often determines whether or not an individual will make healthy or unhealthy choices. For example, if the local pharmacist does not make generic drugs easily available, then the older individual is less likely to choose or obtain them. Or, in cities where air pollution is dangerously high, it would be foolish to suggest that older adults with respiratory problems develop "fresh air" walking as their form of cardiovascular exercise.

The Media

The role of the media is increasing rapidly. Both the public and private sectors in health care are recognizing the importance and influence of the media in reaching older adults. The Healthy Older People Campaign of the Office of Disease Prevention and Health Promotion represents the kind of coordinated public/private effort that may come to characterize health education/promotion strategies with older adults. This campaign developed public service announcements for television, scripts for radio, and press releases and magazine and journal articles for the print media related to diet, exercise, and safe use of drugs with older adults.

The campaign was part of the joint initiative of the U.S. Public Health Service and the U.S. Administration on Aging on health promotion with older adults. The American Association of Retired Persons, as well as volunteer consultants from a variety of disciplines assisted with the development of the public service announcements, and coalitions or task forces were developed in most of the states to assist in the distribution of the media materials. The primary purpose of this campaign is to create awareness of health promotion possibilities with elders and to increase knowledge about potential areas of risk reduction.

It is impossible, pending evaluating results, to discuss the effectiveness of this massive media campaign. It may represent an approach to media utilization in health education/promotion programming that offers promise for the future, since a large number of people can be reached relatively inexpensively. However, without followup and support, such a media "blitz" has many of the disadvantages of the health fair approach to health education/promotion. Clearly, a variety of intervention strategies are necessary and available for health education/promotion efforts. The challenge is choosing the best intervention or combination of interventions for any particular target population.

Reimbursement

Changes in the financial reimbursement mechanisms for health care also suggest a demand for more and different health education/promotion programs. Although there is little direct financial reimbursement for preventive services today, this picture may be changing. Already some insurance companies are lowering premiums for those who practice preventive health behaviors. With increasing Medicare-Medicaid expenditures, it is likely that third-party reimbursement will at least be tried and evaluated in experimental programs. The experience, to date, with the reimbursement strategy of Diagnostic Related Groups (DRGs) suggests that some patients are being released sooner and sicker than previously.

Insurance companies are beginning to recognize the benefits of a well-educated client population and several have instituted educational programs targeted directly to older subscribers and prospective subscribers. Blue Cross/Blue Shield of New Mexico has created a senior citizens department and developed the "Health Partners" program—a project that trains and supports older volunteers to do peer education on health-related subjects as well as encourage new subscriptions. Businesses already pay more for the health benefits of retired employees than for working employees. As the retired workforce increases, which it surely will, given current trends, the incentives for business to institute health education and promotion programs for older employees and retirees will also increase.

It is impossible to predict reliably what the reimbursement mechanisms of the coming decades will be. It is clear, however, that there will be changes and that these changes will have significant implications for health education. The proliferation of Health Maintenance Organizations (HMOs) and the more comprehensive Social HMOs (HMOs targeting the elderly) now being developed and evaluated should provide increased roles for health educators, since the economic well-being of these types of health care delivery systems depends directly upon maximum appropriate client self-care.

WHERE ARE WE NOW?

Recent and projected demographic changes have propelled older adults into the spotlight for both medical care and health promotion education planners and providers. Not only is the over-65 population multiplying at more than twice the rate of the rest of the population, but the over-86 group is increasing the fastest. The acute infectious diseases that limited lifespan throughout history until this century largely have been replaced by chronic degenerative diseases that linger and gradually disable rather than kill quickly. Older adults, therefore, as they live longer, are also living with multiple chronic conditions, perhaps for decades. The development and later optimal management of these conditions are associated with a complex of lifestyle-related health behaviors, as well as social, cultural, and economic factors.

It is increasingly important to include this age group in health promotion/ education activities. Further, market research and the experience of program providers suggest that older adults are receptive and responsive when offered the opportunity to participate, and when appropriate information, skill development, and support are incorporated into a health promotion/ education program.

We must remember that knowledge and lifestyles develop and are maintained in an economic, social, and cultural context. Health is conditioned and influenced, for example, by income, genetics, availability, and accessibility of services. The older person's motivation toward health-enhancing behavior changes may be affected by the images of aging held by health and human service providers, or grocery store clerks, or adult children and grandchildren. Their support or lack of support can easily make the difference between undertaking and maintaining change or simply resigning oneself to the status quo.

The impact of governmental and corporate health policy similarly influences the development and implementation of health promotion/education programs with older adults. A rhetoric of support for disease prevention/ health promotion without legislative and financial support for people and programs inappropriately places all the responsibility for health on the elder consumer. In many cases the result is no access to the benefits of health promotion/education for subgroups of older adults, e.g., the poor, rural elders, ethnic minorities, or the disabled.

Developing health promotion/education programs and services that effectively address the needs, interests, resources, and abilities of adults through transfer of knowledge and skill development is an important role for health professionals. Education and advocacy to improve social and health policies that address underlying issues such as the still unrelenting emphasis on developing and reimbursing high-cost, high-technology, and end-of-life medical care services, agism, and poverty are an equally critical component of responsible health promotion/education programs with older adults.

NOTES

1. American Association of Retired Persons, "A Profile of Older Americans: 1984" (Washington, D.C.: American Association of Retired Persons, 1984).

2. B. Bladeck and J. Firman, "The Aging of the Population and Health Services," *Annals* 468 (1983): 132–148.

3. Alan Pardini et al., "Health Promotion for the Elderly: Program and Policy Issues" (San Francisco: Aging Health Policy Center, University of California, Policy Paper No. 11, 1984).

4. National Center for Health Statistics, "Health, United States, 1984," Public Health Service, DHHS Pub. No. (PHS) 85-1232 (Washington, D.C.: Government Printing Office, December 1984).

5. American Association of Retired Persons, "A Profile of Older Americans: 1984."

6. Pardini et al., "Health Promotion for the Elderly."

7. William Simonson, *Medications and the Elderly: A Guide for Promoting Proper Use* (Rockville, M.D.: Aspen Publishers, 1984).

8. A.S. Freese, *The End of Senility* (New York: Arbor House, 1978).

9. Eric Pfeiffer, "Pharmacology of Aging," in *Health Care of the Elderly,* ed. Gari Lesnoff-Caravaglia (New York: Human Sciences Press, 1980).

10. International Center of Social Gerontology, "Medical and Social Aspects of Accidents Among the Elderly" (Paris, 1983).

11. Susan K. Maloney, Barbara Fallon, and Clarissa Wittenberg, "Executive Summary— Aging and Health Promotion: Market Research for Public Education" (Washington, D.C.: Office of Disease Prevention and Health Promotion, U.S. DHHS, Public Health Service, 1984).

12. J. J. Hersey, J. Probst, and B. Portnoy, "Evaluation of a Natural Health Promotion Media Campaign," *Final Report to the Office of Disease Prevention and Health Promotion* (Washington, D.C.: U.S. Public Health Service, Office of Disease Prevention and Health Promotion, 1982).

13. Stephanie FallCreek and Sue Stam, eds., "The Wallingford Wellness Project: An Innovative Health Promotion Program with Older Adults," Center for Social Welfare Research, University of Washington, Seattle, 1982 ($7.00, available from TIGRE, 3TG, Las Cruces, NM 88003).

14. National Council on the Aging, "Health Promotion for Older Persons: Group Program Models," *Proceedings of the Seminar: Wellness—A Community-Based Approach* (Washington, D.C.: National Council on the Aging, June 1982).

15. National Center for Health Statistics, "Provisional Data from the Health Promotion and Disease Prevention Supplement to the National Health Information Survey," *January–March, 1985—Advance Data from Vital and Health Statistics, No. 113* (Washington, D.C.: U.S. DHHS, Public Health Service, November 15, 1985).

16. National Council on the Aging, "Health Promotion for Older Persons."

17. Ken Dychtwald, ed., *Wellness and Health Promotion for the Elderly* (Rockville, M.D.: Aspen Publishers, 1985).

18. Carroll J. Estes et al., *Political Economy: Health and Aging* (Boston: Little, Brown, 1984).

19. Ibid., 114.

SUGGESTED READINGS

There are many pamphlets, brochures, books, and films for health promotion/education with older adults and more are produced daily. Below is a small sample of some of the types of materials available in addition in those mentioned as references.

AAHPERD. *Health, Physical Education, Recreation and Dance for the Older Adult: A Modular Approach* (1900 Association Drive, Reston, VA 22091).

Addison, Carolyn, and Eleanor Humphrey. "Fifty Positive View Exercises for Senior Citizens." *AAPERD Practical Pointers* 3, no. 6 (1979).

Aging Health Policy Center. "Lifetime Fitness and Exercise for Older People." San Francisco: Aging Health Policy Center, University of California in San Francisco, 1984.

"Aging in Action" (video). (Education Department, Baycrest Centre for Geriatric Care, 3560 Bathurst Street, North York, Ontario, Canada).

American Association of Retired Persons. *A Profile of Older Americans: 1984.* Washington, D.C.: American Association of Retired Persons.

American Hospital Association. "Health Promotion for Older Adults: Planning for Action," *Live Interactive Satellite Video Teleconference* (December 12, 1985).

American Hospital Association. "Promoting Health." 55, no. 5 (September-October, 1984). Four articles: "The Aging of America and the Implications for Health Promotion"; "Filling the Gap: Programs Offer Ideas for Meeting Special Needs of Older Persons"; "Hospitals Tailor Health Promotion Efforts to Fit Special Needs of the Elderly"; "Study of Senior Identifies Attitudes, Barriers to Promoting Their Health."

American Hospital Research and Education Trust. *Health Promotion and Wellness Programs for Older Adults: Opportunities for Hospitals to Serve Their Communities.* Chicago: American Hospital Association, 1983. ($8.00)

American Red Cross. *Health Series for Senior Citizens: 10 Curriculum Modules on Health Issues* (Pittsburgh-Allegheny County Chapter, 225 Boulevard of the Allies, P.O. Box 1764, Pittsburgh, PA 15230).

Ayerst Laboratories. *Osteoporosis: The Impact of Exercise.* New York: Ayerst Laboratories, April, 1985.

Becker, Gay, et al. *The Management of Hearing Impairment of Older Adults.* San Francisco: Aging Health Policy Center, University of California in San Francisco, 1984.

———*Vision Impairment in Older Persons.* San Francisco: Aging Health Policy Center, University of California in San Francisco, 1984.

Bladeck, B., and J. Firman. "The Aging of the Population and Health Services." *Annals* 468 (1983): 132–148.

Bogaert-Tullis, Marjorie. *A Resource Guide for Nutrition Management Programs for Older Persons.* San Francisco: Aging Health Policy Center, University of California in San Francisco, 1985.

———*A Resource Guide for Drug Management Programs for Older Persons.* San Francisco: Aging Health Policy Center, University of California in San Francisco, 1985.

Burkhart, Audrey, and Lois Aronson. *Nutrition for Seniors Mini-Lesson Kit.* New Brunswick, N.J.: Rutgers University, 1983.

Butler, Robert, and Myrna Lewis. *Sex After Sixty: A Guide for Men and Women in their Later Years.* New York: Harper & Row, 1976.

Caplow-Linder, Erna, et al. *Therapeutic Dance/Movement: Expressive Activities for Older Adults.* New York: Human Sciences Press, 1979.

Consumer Reports. *Eating Right for Less: For Older People.* Mt. Vernon, NY: 1977.

Coppard, Larry, et al. *Self/Health/Care and Older People.* Schergifsvej O., Denmark: World Health Organization, Regional Office for Europe, 1984.

Dible, Leah, Alan Pardini, and Marjorie Bogaert-Tullis. *A Resource Guide for Injury Control Programs for Older Persons.* San Francisco: Aging Health Policy Center, University of California in San Francisco, 1985.

Estes, Carroll L., et al. *Political Economy, Health and Aging.* Boston: Little, Brown, 1984.

FallCreek, Stephanie, with Beverly Allen and Dolores Halls. *Health Promotion and Aging: A National Directory of Selected Program.* San Francisco: Aging Health Policy Center, University of California in San Francisco, 1985.

FallCreek, Stephanie, and Patricia Franks. *Health Promotion and Aging: Strategies for Action.* San Francisco: Aging Health Policy Center, University of California in San Francisco, 1984.

FallCreek, Stephanie, and Molly Mettler. *A Healthy Old Age: A Sourcebook for Health Promotion with Older Adults.* New York: Haworth Press, 1984.

FallCreek, Stephanie, and Sue Stam, eds. *The Wallingford Wellness Project: An Innovative Health Promotion Program with Older Adults.* Seattle: Center for Social Welfare Research, University of Washington, 1982. ($7.00, available from TIGRE, 3TG, Las Cruces, NM 88003).

Freese, A. S. *The End of Senility.* New York: Arbor House, 1978.

Gaarder, Lorin, and Saul Cohen. *Patient Activated Care for Rural Elderly.* (P.O. Box 6756, Boise, Idaho 83707, Mountain State Health Corporation). ($7.50)

Garnet, Eva. *Chair Exercise Manual: An Audio Assisted Program of Body Dynamics.* Princeton, N.J.: Princeton Book Company, 1982.

Harris, Ray, and L. Frankel. *Guide to Fitness After Fifty.* New York: Plenum Press, 1977.

Health Promotion/Disease Prevention School of Allied Health Professions. *HPDP Health Promoter.* Stony Brook, NY: State University of New York at Stony Brook.

Health Promotion for the Elderly, A Resource Manual. (Catholic Health Corporation, 920 South 107 Avenue, Omaha, NE).

Hospital Research and Educational Trust. *Caring for Older Adults: A Resource Guide.* Chicago: American Hospital Association, 1984.

International Center of Social Gerontology. *Medical and Social Aspects of Accidents Among the Elderly.* Paris, 1983.

Lee, Phillip R., and Helene Lipton. *Drugs and the Elderly: A Background Paper.* San Francisco: Aging Health Policy Center, University of California in San Francisco, 1983.

Lehman, Frank. *Positive Living for Older Americans.* Center for Health Promotion, 2727 McCelleland Blvd., Joplin, MO 64801.

Longe, Mary, and Janet Tedesco. *Health Promotion and Wellness: Services for Older Adults.* Chicago: Hospital Research and Educational Trust, American Hospital Association, 1984.

Lorig, Kate, et al. *The Arthritis Helpbook: What You Can Do for Your Arthritis.* Reading, Mass.: Addison-Wesley, 1980.

Maloney, Susan K., Barbara Fallon, and Clarissa Wittenberg. *Executive Summary: Aging and Health Promotion: Market Research for Public Education.* Washington, D.C.: Office of Disease Prevention and Health Promotion, U.S. DHHS, Public Health Service, 1984.

Mason, Nancy, Ellen Roberts, and Eugene Nelson. *The Self-Care Planner.* Hanover, N.H.: Dartmouth Medical School, Dartmouth Institute for Better Health, 1980.

Medicine Education Program. *Program Development Guide.* (3519 Crenshaw Blvd., Gardenia, CA 90249).

National Association for Human Development. *Basic Exercises for People Over 60; Moderate Exercises for People Over 60; Exercise Activity for People Over 60;* and *Exercise, Diet, and Nutrition for People Over 60* (NAHD, 1620 Eye Street, NW, Washington, DC 20006).

National Center for Health Statistics. *Provisional Data from the Health Promotion and Disease Prevention Supplement to the National Health Information Survey: United States* (January-March, 1985), Advance Data from Vital and Health Statistics. Public Health Service. Washington, D.C.: Government Printing Office, November 15, 1985.

National Center for Health Statistics. *Health, United States, 1984.* DHHS Pub. No. (PHS) 85-1232 (Public Health Service). Washington, D.C.: Government Printing Office, December, 1984.

National Council on the Aging. *Health Promotions for Older Persons: Group Program Models.* NCOA Publication No. 298. Washington, D.C.: National Council on the Aging, 1982. ($4.00)

———"Health Promotion for Older Persons: Group Program Models," *Proceedings of the Seminar: Wellness—A Community-Based Approach.* Washington, D.C.: National Council on the Aging, June 1982.

National Health Information Clearinghouse. *Healthfinder.* (P.O. Box 1133, Washington, DC 20013-1133).

National Safety Council. *Safety of the Elderly Program Kit.* Washington, D.C., ND.

Nestle, Marion, et al. *Nutrition and the Elderly.* San Francisco: Aging Health Policy Center, University of California in San Francisco, 1983.

Pardini, Alan. *A Resource Guide for Fitness Programs for Older Persons.* San Francisco: Aging Health Policy Center, University of California in San Francisco, 1985.

Pardini, Alan, and Deborah Lerner. *Health Promotion for Older Persons: A Selected Annotated Bibliography.* San Francisco: Aging Health Policy Center, University of California in San Francisco, 1984.

Pardini, Alan, et al. *The Health of Older People: A Framework for Public Policy.* San Francisco: Aging Health Policy Center, University of California in San Francisco, 1983.

Pardini, Alan, et al. *Health Promotion for the Elderly: Program and Policy Issues.* Policy Paper No. 11. San Francisco: Aging Health Policy Center, University of California in San Francisco, 1984.

Pfeiffer, Eric. *Pharmacology of Aging.* In *Health Care of the Elderly,* edited by Geri Lesnoff-Caravaglia. New York: Human Sciences Press, 1980.

Pizer, Hank, ed. *Over Fifty Five, Healthy and Alive: Health Resources for the Coming of Age.* New York: Van Nostrand Reinhold, 1983.

Procino, Jane. *Growing Older, Getting Better.* Reading, Mass.: Addison-Wesley, 1983.

Raynor, Margot. *AHOY: Add Health to Our Years.* Raleigh, N.C.: North Carolina Division on Aging, 1980.

———*North Carolina Senior Games Planning Guide.* (708 Hillsborough Street, Suite 200, Raleigh, NC 27603). ($10.00)

Rosenberry, Magda. *Sixty-Plus and Fit Again: Exercises for Older Men and Women.* New York: Evans, 1977.

Ross, Lorraine N. *Compendium of Health Promotion-Related Initiatives for Older Americans.* National Voluntary Organization for Independent Living for the Aging. (NVOILA).

Senior Medication Education Project. *Preventing Geriatric Medication Misuse.* (SRX, 101 Grove Street, Room 204, San Francisco, CA 94102).

Simmons, Richard. *Reach for Fitness.* New York: Warner Books, 1986.

Simonson, William. *Medications and the Elderly: A Guide for Promoting Proper Use.* Rockville, Md.: Aspen Publishers, 1984.

Skeist, Robert. *Growing Older: Staying Healthy: A Senior's Health Program Manual.* (2035 North Lincoln Avenue, Chicago, IL 60614, Augustana Hospital, Senior's Health Program, 1985). ($25.00)

————"Healthy Times." *Newsletter of the White Crane Senior Health Center.* Chicago.

————*To Your Good Health.* Chicago: Chicago Review Press, 1980.

Sobel, David S., and Tom Ferguson. *People's Book of Medical Tests.* New York: Summit Press, 1985.

Spectrum Films. *Staying Active: Wellness After Sixty.* Carlsbad, CA, 1985.

Switkes, Betty. *Senior-cize: Exercise and Dancing in a Chair.* Washington, D.C., 1982.

Tedesco, Janet, and Mary Longe. *Health Promotion and Wellness: Services for Older Adults.* Chicago: The Hospital Research and Educational Trust, 1984.

USDHHS. *Locating Funds for Health Promotion.* Washington, D.C.: National Health Information Clearinghouse, 1984.

————*Public Health Service, Towards a Healthy Community.* Organizing Events for Health Promotion. DHHS (PHS) 80-50113, 1980.

U.S. Government Printing Office. *Staying Healthy: A Bibliography of Health Promotion Materials.* (Stock No. 0–47–913:QL 3, 1983).

Warner-Reitz, Anne. *Healthy Life-Styles for Seniors: An Interdisciplinary Approach to Healthy Aging.* New York: Meals for Millions/Freedom from Hunger Foundation, 1981.

Wells, Thelma, ed. *Aging and Health Promotion.* Rockville, Md.: Aspen Publishers, 1982. ($24.95)

Western Gerontological Society. "Wellness and Health Promotions for Elders." *Generations* (Spring 1983).

Yelin, Edward, et al. *Arthritis Policy and the Elderly.* San Francisco: Aging Health Policy Center, University of California in San Francisco, 1983.

Appendix 12–A

Health Education/Health Promotion Models

Sketches of a few of the many health education/promotion programs and projects are provided below. These suggest the breadth and depth of current activities in the field and may provide those who wish to initiate or expand health education/promotion activities with ideas and sources of additional information.

- Health Promotion Programs—NCOA
Susan Abbott, Health Promotion Programs
National Council on Aging
600 Maryland Avenue, SW
Washington, DC 20024
202-479-2002

The National Council on the Aging has established a Center for Health Promotion and Aging in conjunction with its other programs and materials on health education/promotion. The Center will collect and make available information about programs and resources in health education/promotion with older adults and will offer consultation and training as appropriate.

- Health Promotion—Private Consultant
Ken Dychtwald,
Age Wave
1900 Powell, Suite 700
Emoryville, CA 94608
415-652-8881

Dr. Dychtwald and his associates offer consultation in health and productivity in the workplace and in the field of aging and have a special emphasis on health promotion with older adults. Dr. Dychtwald has been active in gerontology and health promotion for the past decade and was one of the directors of the pioneering SAGE project.

- The Live Better Longer Project
Stephanie FallCreek, Director
The Institute for Gerontological Research and Education, 3 TG
New Mexico State University
Las Cruces, NM 88003
505-646-3426

The New Mexico State Agency on Aging and The Institute for Gerontological Research and Education (TIGRE) at New Mexico State University in cooperation with statewide senior program sites sponsor health education/promotion activities for older adults. Health Advocates, older persons who are employed under Title V of the Older American's Act, work in settings such as senior centers, nursing homes, and nutrition sites. They coordinate programs that other community-based providers implement or may themselves offer information and experiential training in physical fitness, nutrition, stress management, communication skills, medication management, and other topics identified locally. Advocates vary widely in their educational level, their background in health, and their program development skills and, consequently, programs differ from site to site.

In addition to the Health Advocate Project, the statewide Live Better Longer Task Force works to incorporate a health education/promotion perspective in all statewide training activities sponsored by the aging network. Representatives from several state agencies, voluntary organizations, and the private sector serve on the Task Force, which is staffed by TIGRE. Activities have included dissemination of the Healthy Older People media materials, a statewide "Brown Bag" medication awareness campaign involving about two-thirds of the pharmacies in the state and 50,000 brown bags! Consultation and training materials are available at cost from TIGRE.

- Growing Younger/Growing Wiser
Don Kemper, Director, Healthwise Wellness Center
Molly Mettler, Project Director, Growing Wiser
Healthwise, Inc.
P.O. Box 1989
Boise, ID 93701
208-345-1161

Growing Younger and Growing Wiser are neighborhood-based health education/promotion programs operated by Healthwise, Inc. Growing Younger, which began in 1981, provides educational training to older adults in nutrition, physical fitness, stress management, and medical self-care, in a basic series of four two-hour workshops. The program has been replicated in sites nationwide and a complete training package including materials is available. Growing Wiser is an educational program similar in many ways to Growing Younger in organization and methodology, which focuses on mental health/wellness. It grew from the needs and interests expressed by participants in earlier Growing Younger training workshops.

• The Healthy Older People Campaign
Susan Maloney, Project Officer
Office of Disease Prevention and Health Promotion
U.S. Public Health Service
Room 2132 Switzer Building
330 C Street, SW
Washington, DC 20201
202-472-5660
800-626-5433 (Healthy Older People Hotline)

The Healthy Older People Public Education Campaign is being implemented by the Office of Disease Prevention and Health Promotion in cooperation with a variety of public and private national organizations, including, for example, the American Association of Retired Persons, the American Hospital Association, the National Council on the Aging. Media materials such as public service announcements, press releases, magazine articles, etc., are being developed and disseminated through health promotion coalitions in most of the states. Information and training materials for service providers are also being developed and should be available for distribution through the designated state contact in each state. Also, the U.S. Administration on Aging and the Public Health Service are cooperating in a multiyear continuing joint initiative in health promotion for older persons, and information is available through state and area agencies on agency and state and local health departments in many settings.

Another program of the Healthy Older People National Public Education Campaign currently includes a hotline. The hotline offers assistance to health and social service professionals developing state or local health promotion programs for older adults. Hotline staff can provide callers with tips on quick and often inexpensive program ideas, identify resources, as well as provide technical assistance on how to market a program and work with the media.

• Wisdom Project
Paul O'Brien, Acting Director
American Red Cross
150 Amsterdam Avenue
New York, NY 10023

The Wisdom Project is a preventive medicine and health education project undertaken by the Red Cross in cooperation with Queens Hospital and the Bronx Lebanon Hospital Center. The program provides primary health care as well as education. The education component aims to enhance individual self-reliance in health and improve lifestyle factors related to health. Participants are provided with health education modules on wellness-illness issues. Curriculum materials are available at cost.

• AHOY/LIFE
Margot Raynor, North Carolina Division on Aging
N.C. Department of Human Resources
Division on Aging #20
700 Hillsborough Street
Raleigh, NC 27603-1691
919-733-3983

The North Carolina Division on Aging sponsors a variety of health education/promotion programs for older adults. Add Health to Our Years (AHOY) emphasizes fitness for older persons. Training is provided for health professionals, senior volunteers, and community leaders to enable them to deliver a program in their own settings. Depending on the ability or capacity of the target participant population, training for fitness activities focuses on stretching and flexibility, strength, cardiovascular endurance, or a combination of these. More than 4,000 persons have received training in settings as diverse as nursing homes, YMCA/YWCAs, senior centers, churches, retirement communities, etc.

Living Independently for Elders (LIFE) is a statewide health education/promotion program that emphasizes the development of community-based coalitions to deliver educational programs in nutrition, stress management, physical fitness, and community involvement. Health professionals and other community leaders receive training and support in the areas of networking and program development to supplement materials and training in specific health-related content areas. Both of these programs are coordinated by the Health and Recreation Specialist in the Division on Aging, in collaboration with staff of the Division of Health Services and local Area Agencies on Aging.

The *AHOY Manual* and the LIFE training materials are available from the North Carolina Division on Aging.

- Staying Healthy After 50 Project
Jeanette Simmons, Department of Family and Community Medicine
Dartmouth Institute of Better Health
Dartmouth Medical School
2 Maynard Street
Hanover, NH 03755
603-646-7846
Zora Salisbury, American Red Cross
202-639-3088
Edna Kane-Williams, Health Advocacy Services
202-728-4450

This cooperative project is funded by the W.K. Kellogg Foundation to disseminate a health education/promotion program in 57 communities nationwide. Based upon materials developed in the Dartmouth Self-Care Project, this program will provide training to older persons as participants and potential instructor/facilitators. Approximately 114 trainer teams will be developed for ongoing delivery of the 11-session educational program. Educational focus is divided into three areas: medical self-care, lifestyle, and independent living. Since AARP and Red Cross currently have active chapters across the country, this model can be expected to have a significant impact on health education/promotion with older adults. Consultation and training materials will be available from project staff after the pilot programs are completed.

- Quality Aging Program
David Turner, Director
Salt Lake County Aging Services
135 East 2100 South, Building 3
Salt Lake City, UT 84115
801-488-5764

Quality Aging, begun in 1983, is a prevention and education program serving Salt Lake City older persons. The curriculum focuses on medications, stress management, personal and community self-help, physical fitness, and nutrition. Educational programs are offered in senior centers, libraries, hospitals, churches, community centers, and residential buildings. Funds from the State Division of Alcoholism and Drugs are used to support materials and staff. Staff consists of a program manager, partial secretarial support, student interns, and volunteer group leaders. A program brochure and description are available at cost.

• The White Crane Senior Health Center
Rob Skeist, Director
Illinois Masonic Medical Center
836 West Wallington
Chicago, IL 60657
312-883-7151

The Illinois Masonic Medical Center, in cooperation with the Senior Caucus of the Jane Addams Center, has developed a model for the delivery and financing of comprehensive medical services for older adults. Health education and promotion services are an integral part of this program. This project began in July 1985, and is supported with funds from Illinois Masonic, individual donations, and other sources as available. In a summer health series, consisting of six sessions that are 90 minutes each, topics include Staying Healthy; Body Awareness, Movement, and Massage; Food Is the Best Medicine; Don't Just Do Something—Sit There; A Pill for Every Ill?; and Now What? Also included in the Center's wellness educational activities are men's and women's discussion groups, and Tai Chi fitness activities.

Chapter 13

Community Health Advocacy

Sally Kohn, MPH

Health programs that promote social change are vehicles for advocacy. To write a chapter on community health advocacy in the mid-80's is a challenge. A conservative political outlook in the nation and limited funding are not conducive to developing new programs or activities to address community health problems. For an organization, maintaining adequate funding and meeting the requirements of the funders, certifiers, and licensers can use all available personal and programmatic resources. The concepts and even the language in this chapter may seem outdated, but the increasing magnitude of community health problems is very current.

Community health advocacy has no specific definition but it does have several characteristics. It is a *process*, which involves the members of a community in identifying symptoms, diagnosing causes, and developing strategies to prevent unnecessary illness at the community level. Community health advocacy can take the form of community organizing, coalition building, or educating and lobbying public officials on behalf of the public's health. Making an advocacy approach work requires skill, persistence, and ingenuity. Examples from two case studies illustrate the complexities and process of advocacy approaches. This chapter will:

- Present two projects to illustrate the types of programs that have aimed to promote social change while simultaneously offering health services.
- Identify factors that can facilitate and/or prevent an advocacy approach. These factors include the type of agency, funding, political climate, and support of other organizations.
- Examine the roles programs and individual staff members play in making an advocacy approach work.

In previous decades, efforts to improve the health and well-being of the poor, chronically ill, minority, and other nonmainstream groups have taken

261

many forms. In the last 25 years, we have witnessed rapid and broad changes in ideas and programs that attempt to determine what combination of community involvement, public funding, private funding, professional staff, community workers, administrative structure, and sponsorship will be most effective in promoting improvements in health for a community.[1]

The following statistics illustrate the severity of public health problems today. Fourteen million children, 20 percent of the children in the United States, live in poverty, a number that is greater than before the War on Poverty.[2] The infant mortality rate for blacks in nine cities is at least twice the national rate for whites, 10.1 per thousand live births.[3] Over 100,000 hazardous waste sites exist in America.[4] Lead poisoning, a totally preventable disease, continues to plague children in urban areas. Migrant workers still do not have access to running water and toilets in their living accommodations. The number of homeless people in the United States has increased dramatically in the last five years. The list of health problems whose solutions require more than a curative, medical approach is still growing. Many of these health problems can be addressed adequately only if health professionals join with community groups in advocacy efforts to draw attention to their causes and to create solutions.

People seek care at health centers and hospitals for the health problems that result from community and environmental health conditions. These include toxic dumps, transportation and storage of hazardous materials, nuclear tests and potential disasters including war, occupational hazards, lack of access to family planning and abortion services, untreated or undiagnosed sexually transmitted diseases including AIDS, and inadequate or inaccessible primary health care. Health professionals who come into contact with these individuals can be instrumental in focusing public attention on the nature of such problems.

This chapter is based on two basic beliefs. First, health programs have an obligation to go beyond traditional service delivery in order to adequately meet the needs of clients. Solving some health problems on a case-by-case basis may work for individuals, but it does little to address causes or to improve the health of others in a community. Second, a long-standing American belief, education is a vehicle for social change. Health programs or services often overlook the opportunity to educate the clients, the community, the sponsoring agency, and public officials because of the necessity of keeping up with the day-to-day demands of patients and the requirements of funding agencies.

HEALTH ADVOCACY PROGRAMS: TWO CASE STUDIES

Two urban-based health programs that have incorporated the concept of community advocacy into their activities are presented below. The first, the

Montefiore Medical Center's Community Health Participation Program in the Bronx, New York, relies on trained lay volunteers to act as advocates on behalf of their neighbors. The second, The Hub, A Center for Change for South Bronx Teens, is co-sponsored by Bronx Lebanon Hospital Center and Planned Parenthood of New York City. The Hub has a dual mission of providing health services and advocating for additional services for adolescents.

The Montefiore Medical Center Community Health Participation Program

The Community Health Participation Program (CHPP) was developed in 1975 by the Department of Social Medicine, a Montefiore Medical Center department devoted to teaching and research in community health and social medicine. Based on models of utilizing trained indigenous health workers to deliver primary care in Third World countries, the CHPP adapted the role of the community worker to a diverse, working-class, urban neighborhood in an industrialized country. The essential aspect of the model adapted was development of a special role for community residents in caring for their own and their neighbors' health.

This idea went beyond a concept of "self-care," that is, "a process whereby a layperson can function effectively on his or her own behalf in health promotion and decision-making, in disease prevention, detection, and treatment at the level of the primary health resource in the health care system."[5] The CHPP is a program that, though initiated by Montefiore Hospital, responds to the health concerns of community residents. Along with other professionals working in similar endeavors, the original staff recognized the inherent danger in assigning all responsibility for health to the individual.

> If self-care is going to measurably contribute to the health of the people, especially central city populations, . . . it cannot be conceived as an individualistic or even family enterprise isolated from the community infrastructure and its need for resources. Self-care must be seen as a community concept to be effective.[6]

From the outset, the Community Health Participation Program aimed to:

1. Teach people about health so that they could learn how to maintain and improve their own health and prevent specific illnesses.
2. Encourage people to be more responsible for their own and their neighbors' health by developing a support network for advice and referral and for practical nonmedical help in various stages of illness.

3. Teach people how to utilize local health and social services more appropriately and effectively.
4. Develop and evaluate a model, replicable in other urban neighborhoods, for involving people in decisions affecting their health and their medical care.

The specific nature of the role of Health Coordinators has evolved over time, but they were never expected to be paraprofessionals or the first medical care contact in the community. Instead, they have become health educators, counselors, organizers, and advocates for their neighbors. Once program funding and a community advisory board for the project were in place, two staff members—a community organizer and a coordinator—started implementing the Health Coordinator program. Recruiting volunteers for the program from tenants' groups, parent associations, and senior citizen centers, and training the first group of volunteer community Health Coordinators started in 1976.

For each training group Health Coordinators have participated in a 12-session program in which the following topics are covered: interviewing skills, survey techniques, the health care system, community resources, mental health, nutrition, CPR and first aid, measuring blood pressure, child health, and the changing community.

The primary health-related problems of the community, as identified by staff and Health Coordinators are:

1. An increasing sense of fear, isolation, and alienation, particularly among the elderly and non-English-speaking groups
2. Neighborhood problems such as poorly maintained housing and sanitation, an increase in crime, and a lack of programs for youth
3. Health problems such as obesity, smoking, high blood pressure, fatigue, depression, and minor accidents that do not always receive the attention they need from the medical profession
4. Confusion about and misuse of existing health and social services[7]

The numerous activities reflect this concern. Some of the problems, projects, and outcomes of the Health Coordinators' work are outlined in Table 13-1.

In another part of the country, Dr. Eva Salber in the Department of Community and Family Medicine at Duke University Medical Center developed a similar program. In rural North Carolina, "health facilitators" were trained in many of the same areas as Bronx health coordinators, and their work with their neighbors was quite similar. Dr. Salber, thinking along the same lines as the Montefiore group, wrote,

Table 13-1 Activities Sponsored by the Montefiore Medical Center Community Health
Participation Program

Health-Related Problem	*Health Coordinators' Activity*	*Outcome*
Poor sanitation	Organization of block associations	Street clean-ups, block fairs, flower planting
Littered parks	Park clean-ups	Neighbors cleared litter
Unmet needs of adolescents	Organization of teenage group	Training program and rap group for teens
Mental health	Organization of mothers' groups	Regular meetings of mothers
Housing	Organization of tenants' groups	Locked doors on buildings, improved housing conditions

The Health Facilitator concept was conceived in an attempt to improve the health of people through better use of their own and other resources and in response to some major problems in the delivery of health services to communities.[8]

The factors that contributed to the development of the CHPP will be discussed later.

The Hub, A Center for Change for South Bronx Teens

The Hub, developed in 1982 by two long-standing institutions in the South Bronx, was created in order to counteract high rates of teenage pregnancy and early childbearing. The leadership of the two institutions, Bronx Lebanon Hospital Center (BLHC) and Planned Parenthood of New York City (PPNYC), were intent on building a new program which, by providing high-quality comprehensive services, would improve the health and well-being of South Bronx adolescents and, ultimately, prevent adolescent pregnancy. A four-year seed grant was awarded to the Hub in 1982.

The Hub is based on the assumption that primary prevention of pregnancy includes helping adolescents to improve their life options; that is, helping them to remain in school, have a positive self-image, be able to make good life decisions, and have access to contraception. The direct services at the Hub include comprehensive health services—family planning, abortion, general health care, counseling, prenatal care, well-baby care—as well as educational programs—tutoring, counseling, and advocacy; recreation; and community education for parents and teens on human sexuality. A staff of health professionals, educators, and youth workers provide these services to over 3,000 adolescents each year.

From the outset, the sponsors and senior staff of The Hub put equal emphasis on providing health services for adolescents and on advocacy regarding barriers adolescents face in obtaining services. PPNYC has a long tradition of public education and advocacy on behalf of women's rights to reproductive health care, and protecting the rights of minors has always been a high priority.

The uniqueness of the Hub stems not only from the comprehensiveness of services, but also from the commitment to use the program to educate public officials and legislators about the need for improved services for adolescents.

Figure 13-1 illustrates the many constituencies with whom the Hub interacts in improving services for all high-risk adolescents.

The Hub has been effective in these efforts. Congressional hearings on The Prevention of Adolescent Pregnancy, Parenting and Poverty were held at the Hub, and were the basis for legislation introduced into Congress in February 1985.[9] Governor Mario Cuomo initiated a statewide comprehensive pregnancy prevention program in New York, which was partially based on the service model of The Hub. Minors' access to reproductive health care in public hospitals, regardless of ability to pay and parental consent, continues to be a concern with which The Hub is involved.

The CHPP and The Hub were developed in response to different community needs—to involve residents in a working-class neighborhood in improving the health and medical care of their neighbors and to advocate for the rights and future well-being of "high-risk" adolescents. The type of organization, funding, political climate, and support of other organizations, while different in these two cases, has had an impact on their respective development and their accomplishments. The following section identifies the common factors that encourage community advocacy in health programs, based on these and other experiences.

FACTORS THAT PROMOTE ADVOCACY

There are many ways to advocate for change. Several factors facilitate or encourage the use of a variety of community resources for social advocacy.

Type of Institution

When analyzing an organization's capacity and/or willingness to take on community advocacy, its mission and sponsorship must be examined. Pro-

Figure 13–1 Health Advocacy Services

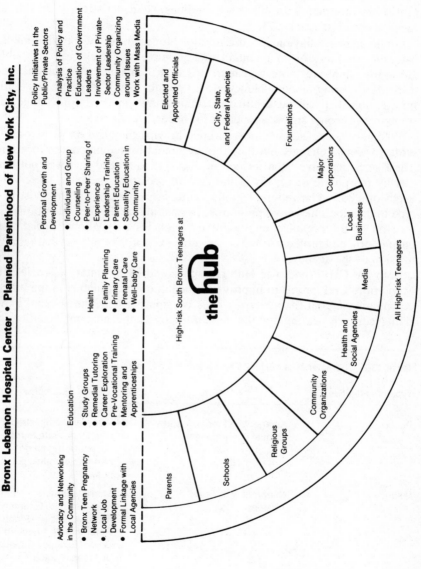

Bronx Lebanon Hospital Center • Planned Parenthood of New York City, Inc.

the**hub**

Advocacy and Networking in the Community
- Bronx Teen Pregnancy Network
- Local Job Development
- Formal Linkage with Local Agencies

Education
- Study Groups
- Remedial Tutoring
- Career Exploration
- Pre-Vocational Training
- Mentoring and Apprenticeships

Health
- Family Planning
- Primary Care
- Prenatal Care
- Well-baby Care

Personal Growth and Development
- Individual and Group Counseling
- Peer-to-Peer Sharing of Experience
- Leadership Training
- Parent Education
- Sexuality Education in Community

Policy Initiatives in the Public/Private Sectors
- Analysis of Policy and Practice
- Education of Government Leaders
- Involvement of Private-Sector Leadership
- Community Organizing around Issues
- Work with Mass Media

High-risk South Bronx Teenagers at

the**hub**

Parents
Schools
Religious Groups
Community Organizations
Health and Social Agencies
Media
Local Businesses
Major Corporations
Foundations
City, State, and Federal Agencies
Elected and Appointed Officials

All High-risk Teenagers

Source: Used with permission of Planned Parenthood of New York City, Inc.

viders of health services, whether hospitals, health departments, ambulatory clinics, or health education programs, are either public, voluntary (nonprofit) or proprietary. Table 13-2 outlines characteristics of health and medical care institutions.

Public agencies have a specific mission, for example, to provide medical care for veterans, or to maintain and promote the health of the public. Generally, they are large bureaucracies in which innovation or change is difficult to bring about. Nonetheless, public health departments gather information that can be useful in documenting the need for change, and sometimes become strong advocates for needed services.

Voluntary agencies have more latitude in what they can do to advocate or work for social change, but they too are bound by bureaucratic procedures. These agencies have been formed in response to a need that was not being met by the public sector or, in the case of sectarian agencies, to serve the needs of a particular religious group. Voluntary agencies are the most likely type to develop innovative programs. Depending on the size, flexibility, and mission of the organization, voluntary agencies may allow special social change-oriented projects to move forward, even if they are not central to the mission of the agency.

Both the CHPP and The Hub are sponsored by voluntary agencies. The Montefiore CHPP aims to improve the health of the residents in the hospital community, a goal that certainly does not conflict with the hospital's overriding concern—caring for the sick. Moreover, the hospital benefits from

Table 13-2 Characteristics of Health and Medical Care Institutions

Type of Institution	Structure	Examples
Public	An agency of federal, state, or local governments	Veterans Administration Hospitals, state mental hospitals, health departments, municipal hospitals
Voluntary	Nonprofit with Board of Trustees	Medical centers, community hospitals, voluntary health agencies (Planned Parenthood, American Red Cross, Epilepsy Foundation of America, etc.)
Proprietary	For Profit	Community hospitals, medical groups, health maintenance organizations

the positive public relations and from better-educated health care users. The CHPP, a small project in a large institution, has the support of the senior staff of the hospital. The goals of The Hub exemplify the mission of Planned Parenthood of New York City, a voluntary agency with a long history of advocacy for women's and minors' rights to reproductive health care.

Proprietary agencies such as for-profit community hospitals are the least likely type of institution to launch or support working for social change.

Funding

New funding is often the crucial factor that gets a community advocacy project off the ground. In Table 13-3 the positive and negative features of various sources of funds (excluding fee-for-service income, from third party payers or clients) are described.

In the two cases described above, grants from private foundations were received. Once initial funding is secured, a substantial amount of time and

Table 13-3 Funding for Community Advocacy Projects

Source	How To Obtain	Comments
Public Grants and Contracts	Respond to a Request for Proposals (RFP)	The availability of new funds is announced in the *Federal Register* and funding bulletins. The following are useful: knowledge of the agency, personal contact with agency officials and with politicians.
Private Foundation Grants	Submit proposal	Research foundation interests, and guidelines; personal contact is helpful; procedures vary greatly; best source of funding for special projects, but general support is difficult to obtain.
Corporations	Submit letter or proposal	Relatively small grants are available; research as for foundations.
Donors	Direct appeal via mail or special events	Time and cost are considerable; funds are unrestricted.

energy is devoted to looking for more funding. Fund raising is very time consuming. Moreover, foundations will fund projects for a time-limited period, which requires that new program initiatives be developed on an ongoing basis. By funding a project, a foundation may influence it directly or indirectly. Awareness of the ways in which this happens and how that can affect the mission of the project or organization is important.

Political Climate

While not always accounted for, the political climate has a strong influence over the development of change-oriented health projects. The development of over 150 Neighborhood Health Centers between 1965 and 1971 provides the best recent example in health care history of change-oriented health programs stemming from a widespread political movement, the War on Poverty.[10] According to Hollister, Kramer, and Bellin, "The [health] centers are not merely projects that implement a series of improvements in primary health care. They also express and carry a social movement defined by several impulses toward change that converged in the 1960's. . . . It is important to analyze the health centers at least in part in terms of the extent to which they represent a playing out of larger political themes."[11]

The early '70s, when the CHPP was initiated, was a time of serious questioning about the effectiveness of the U.S. health care system. The upsurge in medical costs focused governmental attention on the ever-expanding health care industry. The growing demand for some kind of national health insurance or health service led to legislative proposals for these types of programs. A demystification of medical practice and a dedeification of physicians were taking place, allied to demands for a lessening of the control resting in the hands of the health care industry. The time was ripe for programs that sought to put the responsibility for the maintenance of people's health back into their own hands. Mutual support groups for those with chronic health problems, health screening programs, exercise groups, and nutrition study groups are examples of programs that emphasized self-reliance in disease care and the importance of individual effort in health maintenance.

The beginning of the '80s was a time of funding cutbacks for community health programs and of particular threats to family planning agencies. The development of The Hub occurred at a time when teenage sexuality was a very timely topic. New projects to teach adolescents to abstain from sex were funded through "the chastity bill," which established the Office of Adolescent Pregnancy Prevention. There was an all-out effort to institute the "squeal rule," which would have required federally funded family planning programs to inform parents when their children received contraceptive services.

For both the CHPP and The Hub the political environment has influenced the programs' development. The CHPP was an approach to addressing health care problems that appeared to be increasing in urban areas. Something had to be done to curb costs and make health care more accessible for inner-city residents. Developing an active role for community residents in their own and their neighbors' health was a logical next step at a time when expansion and innovation of health services was supported politically.

The Hub has responded to a recognized need—for additional services for adolescents—but the political climate is less hospitable now than in the 1970s. The Hub's role in educating a variety of constituents, including legislators, about the needs of adolescents is ongoing and important.

Support of Other Organizations, Clients, and Community Leaders

A community advocacy project can gain needed legitimacy if other organizations support the effort. Support can take many forms. As in the case of the CHPP, an advisory board might be established, with members from the community and other agencies who are interested in the project. Interagency networks or coalitions can be either formed or joined, to give strength to the issues for which the project is advocating. In the case of the Hub, the Bronx Teen Pregnancy Network was formed to advocate for pregnant, parenting, and at-risk teens in the Bronx. Letters of support or understanding can document that other agencies support the effort.

THE ROLE OF HEALTH PROFESSIONALS IN ADVOCATING FOR A COMMUNITY GROUP

Health professionals can choose from several approaches to health advocacy. Specifically, they are documentation, education and training, research, and working with elected officials and legal strategies. (For a list of organizations involved with various health related activities, see Appendix 13-A.)

Documentation

Incidents in which services are denied or grossly inadequate or prevalent health problems that appear to be preventable should be documented and eventually reported either within the agency or externally. Anecdotal material can be powerful if it is carefully and accurately recorded. Patterns may emerge that can lead to specific recommendations for correction. Local publicity of a well-documented problem often attracts the attention of influential people. A problem-solving attitude is more likely to yield positive results than a blaming one.[12]

Education and Training

Clients, staff, the community and elected officials are among the groups who can be educated about the need for addressing problems more effectively. Often the "victims"—those who, for example, are suffering from exposure to toxic materials, lack of access to health services, lead poisoning—are most effective in educating others about the need for change. Education about the nature and cause of the problem that has been identified, approaches other groups have taken to address it, legislation or funding that exists to remedy it, and, most important, the impact of the problem on the community can be very instrumental in beginning to build support for change.

Both the CHPP and the Hub utilize a training program to actively involve community residents. In the CHPP, community problems are identified and solved by trained health coordinators, with the support of the staff. At the Hub, trained adolescents work as community surveyors, tutors, and youth workers. Their involvement as more than recipients of service has been an important factor in the Hub's relevance to South Bronx teenagers.

Research

While not easy to undertake, research into a problem may shed new light on a long-standing situation and thereby lead the way to a new solution. Unfortunately, most community-based health agencies do not possess the expertise or resources necessary to do credible research. However, action-oriented research that helps develop an understanding of the nature or cause of a problem is within reach of a nonacademic "technically unsophisticated" agency by means of the following techniques:

- *Analyzing occurrences of health problems by mapping them geographically*—Two examples: (1) The CHPP mapped negative birth outcomes in three Bronx areas to pinpoint where more education and outreach were needed and to preliminarily investigate if environmental conditions in Bronx neighborhoods had an effect on birth outcomes. (2) Automobile accidents in Chicago were mapped for a community group. "From the map the people could see, for example, that within three months six people had been injured, and one person killed. . . . They were then ready to act. . . ."[13]

- *Conducting a survey of individuals affected by a health problem—* While the data may not be sound epidemiologically, they might suggest a cause-and-effect relationship and pave the way for further investigation by more sophisticated research methods.
- *Undertaking a community survey—*The survey conducted by The Hub participants served the program well. Their efforts and the survey results both convinced the Hub staff that the overall program was headed in the right direction and focused more community attention on adolescent sexuality and drug abuse.

Networking

Forming a coalition can be one of the most effective means of attracting attention and marshaling resources to attack a health problem. Other agencies that are likely to be addressing similar health problems are likely to join a coalition. Grass-roots organizations, social service agencies, and public agencies can give a group the legitimacy that is derived from broad-based support. One danger is that the focus of the coalition becomes diluted and the ability to advocate is hampered by internal squabbles or divergent opinions for which no consensus can be reached.

Working with Elected Officials and Legal Strategies

Getting to know the elected officials in the area served by an agency or project is crucial. It is best to establish a relationship with elected officials prior to seeking support on an issue or help in solving a problem. An office visit to introduce the program and its key staff is the best way to start.

The legislative process is a long and cumbersome one (see Figure 13-2).

The process at the state and local level is more accessible than at the federal level, but it is still complex and politically driven. Elected officials are motivated by votes and publicity. If it can be demonstrated that the constituents support the project or its goals, endorsement is more likely to be gained.

The Hub has been active in the legislative arena. For example, Planned Parenthood of New York City was instrumental in the development of the Adolescent Pregnancy Prevention and Services Act of 1984 in New York State. Meetings with highly placed elected officials and their staff and lobbying with local representatives helped to create a bill that was acceptable to PPNYC and to ease its passage. Largely as a result of Congressional hearings held at the Hub in October 1984 Congressman Robert Garcia introduced HR 947, The Comprehensive Adolescent Pregnancy Program

Figure 13–2 Lobbying at the Federal and State Level

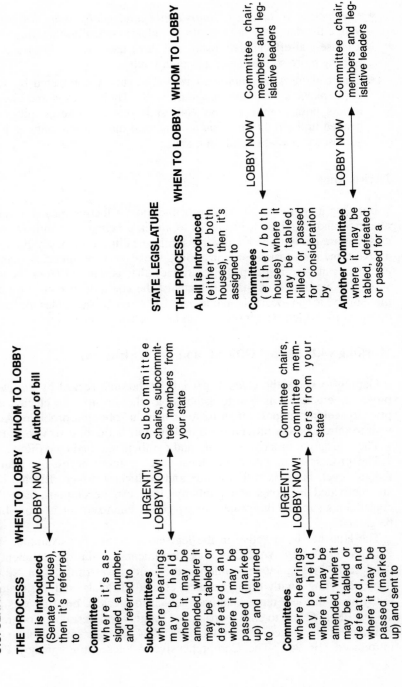

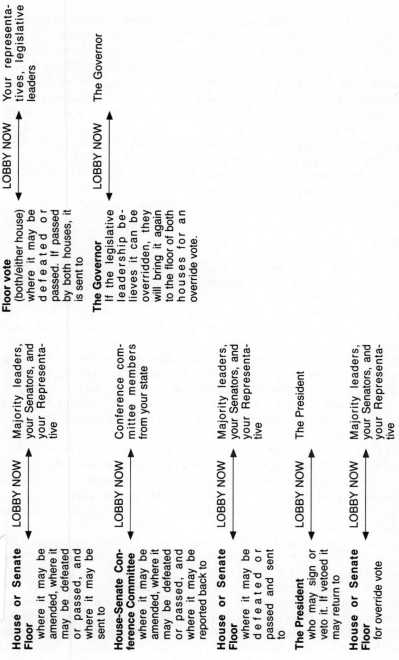

Source: Adapted from *Planned Parenthood's Guide To Your Elected Officials* with permission of Planned Parenthood of New York City, Inc., © 1985.

Amendments of 1985, which proposed amendments to pending or existing federal legislation affecting comprehensive services to adolescents.

Lobbying is a legitimate activity of a nonprofit organization. Exactly what constitutes lobbying, as opposed to public education, on the one hand, and participating in a political campaign, on the other, is open to some interpretation. Lobbying includes writing letters, making telephone calls, and visiting legislators to express opinions on legislation and issues of concern to an organization.

Although very costly and lengthy, lawsuits are effective in bringing about change. However, legal fees add up quickly. Finding a case that will not be struck down because of technicalities and that will test a particular issue can be difficult. Years can pass before an issue is resolved in the courts. Nonetheless, in some instances there may be no other recourse.

SUMMARY

As the solutions to health and medical care problems become more elusive and complex and as funding becomes more scarce, the necessity to advocate for a greater emphasis on eliminating the causes of health problems and for changes in the delivery of services will increase. The CHPP and The Hub have both incorporated the concept of working for change into their mission. The results have been beneficial.

The CHPP staff and volunteer health coordinators have been responding to the needs of a changing community for over ten years. Through training programs for Health Coordinators, educational forums for the community at large, and the neighbor-to-neighbor provision of health information and services, the community surrounding the Montefiore Medical Center has been strengthened.

Health Coordinators can be found in every community organization. They are known to the Montefiore Hospital administration. They actively participate in health campaigns in the community such as screening programs for hypertension or lead poisoning. Health Coordinators who were trained ten years ago and those trained six months ago sit together on the CHPP Coordinating Council to plan activities. The CHPP is one of the few voluntary organizations in the North Bronx in which people of diverse ages and cultural backgrounds work closely together to promote the health of their community.

The Hub, a much younger program, has also developed a role for adolescent community residents in the delivery of services. Peer teachers and youth service workers become advocates for all of the adolescents at the Hub. In addition, the Hub has been instrumental in creating new legislation designed to improve services for adolescents at the state and federal level.

Several roles an individual can assume in promoting advocacy within a health care organization have been described. The potential benefits include better service delivery, new legislation, additional funding for existing services, or new funding for new services and strengthened community organizations.

Developing nontraditional programs or roles for individuals can be challenging, however. Programs that work for change by responding to the needs of the community or a particular population are evolutionary, by definition. Goals and objectives change in response to changing community pressures. Creative funding strategies are required. For individuals, identifying a support network is essential. To develop programs that advocate change without jeopardizing the well-being of an organization can be a delicate balancing act.

Advocacy on behalf of a constituent group—clients, the local community, or a target population—can be appropriately incorporated into the mission of health care agencies. Resources, both financial and human, can be harnessed to document problems, educate the public, and join with community residents to prevent unnecessary health problems and to improve access to services.

NOTES

1. Victor Sidel and Ruth Sidel, eds., *Reforming Medicines: Lessons of The Last Quarter Century* (New York: Pantheon Books, 1984), 1–8.

2. Congressional Research Service, Congressional Budget Office, "Strategies for Reducing Childhood Poverty," Report prepared for the United States Congress, Committee on Ways and Means, U.S. House of Representatives, Washington, D.C., 1985.

3. Children's Defense Fund, *The Data Book: The Nation, States and Cities* (Washington, D.C.: Children's Defense Fund, 1985), 10, 191.

4. Nicholas Freudenberg, *Not in Our Backyards!* (New York: Monthly Review Press, 1984), 9.

5. Lowell S. Levin, "Forces and Issues in the Revival of Interest in Self-Care: Impetus for Redirection in Health," *Health Education Monographs* 5, no. 2 (Summer 1977): 115.

6. Nancy Milio, "Self-Care in Urban Settings," *Health Education Monographs* 5, no. 2 (Summer 1977): 138.

7. Department of Social Medicine, Montefiore Hospital and Medical Center, "Evaluation of the Montefiore Hospital Community Health Participation Program," A Report to the New York Community Trust Fund, New York, 1980.

8. Eva J. Salber, "Introduction to the Health Facilitator Concept," in *Community Health Education: The Lay Advisor Approach,* ed. Connie Service and Eva. J. Salber (Durham, N.C.: Community Health Education Program, Department of Community and Family Medicine, Duke University Medical Center 1977), 5.

9. H.R. 947, "Comprehensive Adolescent Pregnancy Program Amendments of 1985," February 6, 1985, introduced by Congressman Robert Garcia.

10. H. Jack Geiger, "Community Health Centers: Health Care as an Instrument of Social Change," in *Reforming Medicine,* ed. Victor Sidel and Ruth Sidel (New York: Pantheon Books, 1984), 19.

11. Robert M. Hollister, Bernard M. Kramer, and Seymour S. Bellin, "Neighborhood Health Centers as a Social Movement," in *Neighborhood Health Centers,* ed. R. M. Hollister, B. M. Kramer, and S. S. Bellin (Lexington, Mass.: Lexington Books, D.C. Health, 1974), 13.

12. John L. McKnight, "Politicizing Health Care," *Social Policy,* November/December, 1978, 38.

13. Hollister, Kramer, and Bellin, "Neighborhood Health Centers," 13.

SUGGESTED READINGS

Boufford, Jo Ivey, and Pat Shonubi. *Community-Oriented Primary Care: Training for Urban Practice.* New York: Praeger, 1986.

Ewles, Linda, and Ina Simnett. *Promoting Health: A Practical Guide To Health Education.* New York: John Wiley, 1985.

Freudenberg, Nicholas, ed. *Not In Our Backyards! Community Action For Health and The Environment.* New York, Monthly Review Press, 1984.

Joffe, Justin M., and George W. Albee, eds. *Prevention Through Political Action and Social Change.* Hanover and London, University Press of New England, 1981.

Kark, Sidney. *The Practice of Community-Oriented Primary Health Care.* New York: Appleton-Century-Crofts, 1981.

Levin, Lowell S., and Ellen Idler. *The Hidden Health Care System: Mediating Structures and Medicine.* Cambridge, Mass.: Ballinger, 1981.

Levitan, Sar A. *Programs in Aid of the Poor.* Baltimore: The Johns Hopkins University Press, 1985.

Ryan, William. *Blaming the Victim.* New York: Vintage, 1971.

Shellow, Jill R. *The Grantseekers Guide.* Chicago: National Network of Grantmakers, 1981.

Sidel, Ruth. *Women and Children Last.* New York: Viking, 1986.

Sidel, Victor, and Ruth Sidel, eds. *Reforming Medicine.* New York: Pantheon Books, 1984.

Appendix 13-A

Organizations

Center for Science in the Public Interest
1501 Sixteenth Street, NW
Washington, DC 20008
(202) 332-9110

Citizens Clearinghouse for Hazardous Waste
P.O. Box 926
Arlington, VA 22216

The Foundation Center
79 Fifth Avenue
New York, NY 10003
(212) 620-1400
(Also offices in Washington, Cleveland, and San Francisco)

Health Policy Advisory Center
17 Murray Street
New York, NY 10007
(212) 267-8890

Health Research Group
2000 P Street, NW, Suite 708
Washington, DC 20036

League of Women Voters of the United States
1730 M St., NW
Washington, DC 20036
(202) 429-1965

National Women's Health Network
224 7th St., SE
Washington, DC 20003
(202) 543-9222

Physicians for Social Responsibility
639 Massachusetts Avenue
Cambridge, MA 02139
(617) 491-2754

Chapter 14

Workplace Health Promotion

Michael P. Eriksen, ScD

The involvement of corporations in employee health and well-being is an issue of increasing interest. Many leading-edge companies are beginning to manage their health care costs more aggressively because of their visible impact on the corporate bottom line. Corporate executives are expanding their involvement beyond cost containment and are addressing other employee health issues such as performance, attendance, and risk-based medical management. Workplace health promotion programs are becoming increasingly seen as an integral part of a comprehensive employee health management program.

This chapter will review the current interest in corporate health care cost containment and the emerging role of workplace health promotion. Emphasis will be placed on reviewing the rationale for establishing workplace health promotion programs, their current status in U.S. business, and the critical issues and future trends facing this growing movement.

The goal of many corporate health care cost-containment strategies is to ensure that employees, retirees, and dependents continue to have access to quality health care, delivered in a cost-effective manner, achieving the greatest possible value for the health care dollar. Wellness programs are an integral part of a comprehensive health care cost-containment strategy for the following reasons:

- Many of the traditional cost-containment efforts such as utilization review and selected hospital contracting affect health care costs in the short term by improving the management of either the cost, length, or appropriateness of the service. Effective wellness programs are a long-term strategy, which can either totally prevent the need for the service or result in the service being provided earlier at a substantially lowered cost. Thus, wellness programs offer the promise of long-term cost savings through early detection and disease prevention. The combination of both short- and long-term tactics ensures a sustained impact on health care costs.

- Wellness and health promotion programs are popular with employees and often make the other components of a cost-containment program more acceptable. A 1985 survey conducted by Louis Harris for the Equitable Life Assurance Society[1] found that the introduction of wellness programs was the most accepted of all health plan changes introduced by employers.
- Wellness programs emphasize the personal responsibility of the employee to ensure his or her own health. The attitudes and skills associated with personal responsibility are valuable for other employee health care behaviors, such as requesting a second opinion, using the utilization review system, choosing appropriate self-care techniques, and managing one's own health care.
- Medical expenditure databases are providing the information needed to develop wellness programs targeting preventable disorders and allowing for the documentation of the effectiveness of such programs.

Many leaders in the health cost management field believe that it would be irresponsible to attempt to contain health care costs without becoming aggressively involved in disease prevention and health promotion programs.

WHY WELLNESS IN THE WORKPLACE

Why are wellness programs appropriately included in a comprehensive health care cost-containment strategy? Research evidence is accumulating which shows that lifestyle plays an increasingly important role in the development of chronic diseases such as heart disease, cancer, and stroke.[2] In fact, the Centers for Disease Control recently estimated that of the ten leading causes of death, 51 percent are attributable to lifestyle, with human biology accounting for 20 percent, environment 19 percent, and health care delivery 10 percent. Additional analysis indicates that 16 percent of all mortality is caused by smoking, 10 percent is due to hypertension, 8 percent to obesity, and 7 percent to drinking.

Research has not only firmly established the link between lifestyle behaviors and chronic disease, but has also shown that when these behaviors are changed, the risk of chronic disease decreases accordingly. In fact, the recent decline in cardiovascular disease mortality over the last decade is believed to be due more to lifestyle changes than to advances in medical care delivery.[3] Medical research convincingly shows that smoking, cholesterol, and blood pressure levels can be reduced and when this is done, the risk for chronic disease, especially heart disease and cancer, is correspondingly lowered.

Besides helping to contain health care costs, wellness programs also benefit a company in other ways. For example, major corporations have established wellness programs for one or more of the following reasons:

- reduce medical expenditures
- reduce absenteeism
- prevent accidents
- reduce stress claims
- prevent disability cases
- improve job performance
- improve job satisfaction
- improve employee morale
- enhance external relations

Until recently, it was not clearly understood why corporations established worksite health promotion programs. Recognizing the need to better understand these factors, the Office of Disease Prevention and Health Promotion of the Department of Health and Human Services sponsored a National Survey on Worksite Health Promotion Activities.[4] The results of this survey provide the first national assessment of what worksites are doing and why they start workplace health promotion programs. This survey clarifies and expands the earlier work done in California[5] and Colorado,[6] as well as the surveys conducted by benefit consulting firms.

The national survey revealed that "to improve employee health" was the leading reason (28 percent) corporations offered worksite health promotion programs. The next most common response was "because management wanted it" (17.6 percent). Other responses are as follows:

- To improve employee health
- Because management wanted it
- To increase output/production quality
- To reduce health insurance costs
- To improve employee morale
- Because employees wanted it

THE STATUS OF U.S. WELLNESS PROGRAMS

Many of the leading Fortune 500 companies, such as General Motors, AT&T, Ford, Tenneco, IBM, XEROX, Johnson & Johnson, Campbell

Soup, Honeywell, General Electric, and DuPont, are actively engaged in workplace wellness programs. These companies believe that their investment in prevention is good business and that a "wellness commitment" to employees will become an indicator of "excellence" in business.

A number of national surveys also have documented the growth in workplace wellness programs. A 1984 survey by Hewitt and Associates[7] indicated that approximately one-third of major companies were conducting health promotion and preventive health care programs. These findings were confirmed by a similar survey conducted by the Business Roundtable.[8] A recent survey conducted by the National Association of Employers on Health Care Alternatives[9] found that the implementation of wellness programs has increased 100 percent since a similar survey done in 1979.

While these benefit consulting firm surveys provided an indication of the prevalence of workplace health promotion programs, no national data were available on the topic. However, the recently completed National Survey of Worksite Health Promotion Activities[10] provides the first national view of what is being done and why in workplace health promotion.

The national survey found that 44 percent of private employers with more than 50 employees had health promotion programs. A health promotion program was defined as meeting the following criteria: (1) active within the past 12 months, (2) covering one or more of nine identified health program areas, (3) at least one component offered on an ongoing basis or more than once per 12-month period, (4) active employee participation, and (5) paid in whole or part by the employer.

Health promotion programs were most likely to be offered in larger worksites and among larger companies. Smoking cessation and health risk assessment programs were the most common program activity and nutrition and off-the-job accident education programs were least prevalent. The national survey concluded that worksites that have implemented a health promotion program can be characterized as:

- being significantly larger
- having a lower percentage of male employees
- being more likely to have on-site health professionals
- being more likely to have implemented a health care cost management program within the last three years

Not only are major corporations increasingly adopting wellness programs, but the evidence that these programs are effective is also increasing. A 1983 survey by TPF&C[11] found that 60 percent of both employers and unions felt that wellness programs improve overall employee health and that specific risk-factor reduction programs have a long-term cost-containment impact. The 1985 Equitable Life Assurance Society survey[12] found that two-thirds of benefit officers rated wellness programs to be very or somewhat effective in controlling health care costs.

In attempting to evaluate the effectiveness of workplace health promotion programs, the Business Roundtable survey[13] found that employers feel that their wellness efforts are somewhat or very successful or that the impact is unknown. Less than 5 percent of the respondents felt that their programs had no impact or were unsuccessful. A 1985 survey by Mercer-Meidinger[14] revealed that more than 90 percent of chief executive officers believe that health promotion programs can help control costs and that these programs are underused by corporations.

In addition to the support given wellness programs through corporate surveys, there is increasing evidence from corporations themselves on the cost effectiveness of wellness programs. Companies such as AT&T,[15] Johnson & Johnson,[16] and Control Data Corporation [17] have all recently published reports documenting the effectiveness of their programs.

The next section will describe the common elements of workplace health promotion programs, discuss reasons why they are initiated, and provide examples of model programs with documented results.

CURRENT LEVEL OF PRACTICE: OVERVIEW

As the National Worksite Health Promotion Survey[18] results indicate, health promotion programs are becoming popular throughout American businesses. Nearly one out of every two worksites is engaged in some type of organized health promotion effort for its employees. Not only do the specific activities vary, but so do the reasons why companies become involved in workplace health promotion.

To better understand the different ways workplace health promotion activities are organized, it is necessary to develop a classification scheme or conceptual model. A number of researchers have conceptualized health promotion programs along different dimensions. Parkinson and Fielding[19] differentiate three models on the basis of program scope: (1) comprehensive, (2) physical fitness, and (3) single-component. It is their view that the comprehensive model, which offers a wide variety of health promotion activities and attempts to influence the corporate culture and organizational environment, is the most sophisticated and most likely to have the greatest impact on employee health status and costs. The physical fitness model focuses primarily on exercise and often has a workplace fitness facility as the core of its program. The single-component model often focuses on information dissemination, although it may include an occasional behavior change program.

Nay[20] has identified four major strategies for implementing workplace health promotion programs: (1) problem-focused, (2) employee-focused, (3) comprehensive/risk-focused, and (4) comprehensive/preventive-focused. These four approaches vary according to the number of employees that are affected by the program—ranging from the most limited to the most expansive.

The problem-focused model attempts to reach only those employees who are at high risk of chronic disease. It provides an intensive intervention for a subset of the workforce. This traditional "medical model" approach is likely to benefit those at risk but does little for the majority of employees or has any impact on the corporate culture. The employee-focused approach is similar to the problem-focused one except that rather than focus on health problems, it focuses on employee characteristics—most typically age and/or sex. The strengths and weaknesses for these two approaches are similar.

The comprehensive/risk-focused model suggests health screening for all employees and then selected chronic disease risk-reduction interventions for all employees, whether they are at high risk or not. This model begins to reach out to the entire workforce and can have an impact on the corporate culture. The comprehensive/preventive model is similar to the previous one but is not limited in the type of wellness and health promotion programs that are offered. Nay[21] concludes that the right approach for a company should be based on the corporate objectives and available resources.

A third approach, proposed by Kiefhaber and Goldbeck,[22] differentiates on the basis of type of intervention: (1) control of disease and biological risk, (2) control of high-risk behavior, and (3) influence on corporate culture. The first model places emphasis on screening and the early detection of disease and usually requires some element of medical intervention. The second model focuses on lifestyle and behavioral risk factors and suggests interventions that help individuals modify their personal risk behavior. The third model focuses on strategies that attempt to influence the corporate culture and the physical environment such as corporate policies, leadership, and management style.

Thus, various researchers have proposed distinctly different ways of conceptualizing workplace health promotion programs. Parkinson and Fielding differentiate on the basis of program scope; Nay focuses on the number and type of employees involved; and, Kiefhaber and Goldbeck distinguish among the types of intervention conducted. Each of these models has value and can be used effectively in designing a workplace health promotion program.

Because of the different models available and lack of consensus on the preferred approach, the remainder of this chapter will review seven of the most common workplace health promotion program elements which can then be assembled into any of the models. The elements that will be reviewed are smoking control, nutrition education, fitness programs, weight control, high blood pressure control, stress management, and cancer screening programs. There are many other workplace health promotion activities that are not reviewed but that are integral to many programs: health risk appraisal, employee assistance programs, accident prevention programs, among others. The review of the following health promotion activities is organized according to the significance of the health problem, current prevalence and trends, workplace implications, and model programs.

SMOKING CONTROL

Health Issues

The Surgeon General has stated, "Cigarette smoking is the chief, single, avoidable cause of death in our society and the most important public health issue of our time." Cigarette smoking is responsible for 83 percent of lung cancer—the leading cause of cancer death for both American men and women. Overall, it is estimated that cigarette smoking is responsible for 30 percent of all cancer deaths—cancer of the larynx, head, neck, esophagus, bladder, kidney, pancreas, and stomach—in addition to cancer of the lung. Thus, cigarette smoking accounts for approximately 130,000 cancer deaths annually.[23]

In addition to the cancer burden, smoking is responsible for 30 percent of all coronary-heart-disease-related deaths[24] and is associated with gastric ulcers, chronic bronchitis, emphysema, and a host of other chronic and debilitating disorders. All told, it is estimated that over 300,000 people die each year from cigarette smoking—the equivalent to three jumbo jet crashes a day.[25]

The adverse health effects of cigarette smoking are directly related to the amount smoked, the duration of the smoking habit, the tar yield of the cigarette, the absence of filters, and the depth of inhalation. Surprisingly, while most Americans are aware of the health risk of smoking, 40 percent of the public is not aware that smoking causes lung cancer and 20 percent do not know that it can cause cancer at all.[26]

Fortunately, quitting smoking decreases the risk of smoking-related disease. When an individual stops smoking, the mortality ratio declines as the years of nonsmoking increase.[27] It is estimated that after 15 years of nonsmoking, mortality ratios for ex-smokers resemble those of individuals who never smoked.[28] The risk of lung cancer for smokers who quit is reduced by at least half within 10 years after cessation[29] and after 15 years or more the risk of lung cancer is only slightly higher than that of nonsmokers.[30]

A related but distinct issue with particular relevance to the workplace is the health effects of secondhand smoke. While the data are not conclusive, preliminary evidence seems to indicate the potential of a health risk for those nonsmokers chronically exposed to secondhand smoke, particularly for those with preexisting health conditions. Recent studies in Japan, France, Greece, and the United States all indicate an increased risk of lung cancer for the nonsmoking wives of smoking husbands. The health implications of secondhand smoke have been recently reviewed by Fielding[31] and Eriksen[32] and are the subject of the 1986 Surgeon General's Report. It is recommended that the conclusion of the 1982 Surgeon General's Report[33] be considered in developing strategies for the control of secondhand smoke in the workplace:

> For the purpose of preventive medicine, prudence dictates that nonsmokers avoid exposure to secondhand tobacco smoke to the extent possible.[34]

Current Prevalence and Trends

It is difficult to assess the exact prevalence of smoking among adults in America today; however, it is clear that the percentage of adults who are currently smokers has declined dramatically over the last 20 years. In 1965, 52 percent of men and 34 percent of women were smokers. Current estimates indicate that approximately 33 percent of men and 28 percent of women are smokers today. Overall, the percentage of adult smokers in America has dropped to at least 32 percent, according to the National Center for Health Statistics.[35] The 1983 Gallup survey[36] reported a smoking rate of 29 percent and preliminary data from the ACS Cancer Prevention Study II indicate that current cigarette smoking prevalence may be closer to 25 percent.[37]

While a smaller percentage of adults are smoking, there are more heavy smokers (more than 25 cigarettes a day) than ever before. Table 14-1 reveals the increasing percentage of heavy smokers for both men and women, white and black.[38]

Workplace Implications

The National Cancer Institute estimates that if smoking prevalence is reduced to 15 percent by the year 2000, cancer mortality will be reduced by

Table 14-1 Percentage of Smokers Smoking More Than 25 Cigarettes a Day

	1965	1976	1980
White Men	26.0	33.3	37.3
White Women	13.9	20.9	25.2
Black Men	8.6	10.8	13.8
Black Women	4.6	5.6	8.6

Source: Health Interview Survey, National Center for Health Statistics, U.S. Department of Health Services, February 1986.

at least 8 percent.[39] Given the potential of prevention and the fact that smoking is considered by many to be the greatest single threat to the public health, it makes sense for workplace smoking control to become a corporate priority.

A workplace smoking control program should include an effective corporate smoking policy, smoking cessation opportunities and technological changes, such as ventilation modification, when necessary. Orleans and Shipley feel that workplace smoking control programs can be even more effective than community efforts if the worksite exploits the unique characteristics of the business setting, i.e., a cohesive peer support network and the availability of corporate reinforcements for nonsmoking.[40]

The recent national survey on Worksite Health Promotion activities[41] revealed that nearly 35.6 percent of surveyed worksites had smoking cessation activities, making it the most prevalent type of workplace health promotion effort. Nearly 20 percent had smoking cessation programs and 27 percent had smoking policies. Furthermore, 76.5 percent that reported smoking cessation activities had a smoking policy. These results illustrate the rapid interest in workplace smoking control programs over the last few years. A previous survey[42] indicated that smoking cessation programs were one of the least common of all workplace health promotion activities in California companies in 1981.

The establishment of workplace smoking policies is also on the increase. Shipley and Orleans estimate that at least 50 percent of all U.S. companies have adopted some type of restrictive smoking policy.[43] Even research sponsored by the Tobacco Institute indicates that nearly 40 percent of America's leading corporations have formal smoking policies.[44] Workplace smoking policies are even popular with smoking employees. Over half of surveyed Pacific Bell employees who smoked were in favor of a corporate smoking policy and separate smoking and nonsmoking sections.[45] Of these smokers, 13 percent said they would try to quit and 38 percent said they would cut down if a smoking policy were implemented.

The *Decision Maker's Guide to Reducing Smoking at the Worksite*[46] provides rational and practical suggestions for implementing effective smoking control interventions. A workplace smoking control program will not only save lives, it will also save dollars. While estimates vary,[47] most researchers concur that smoking employees cost their employer several hundred dollars more a year than their nonsmoking counterparts. Rice and associates estimate that smoking accounts for 8 percent of the total economic cost of illness.[48] Add to this the cost of absenteeism, insurance, and maintenance and the cost of workplace smoking becomes substantial. Not only does smoking cost a company money, but it is also expensive for the smoker. Oster and associates analyzed the cost of smoking and the benefits of quitting to the individual smoker as opposed to the employer. These researchers estimate that the lifetime cost of smoking for the average 45-year-old, two pack-a-day male smoker is $46,334 and the benefit of quitting is $24,690.[49]

Of particular interest to business is the relationship between smoking and occupational hazards. Tobacco smoke can combine with certain hazards to create a health risk many times greater than the independent risk from each hazard. The 1985 Surgeon General's Report reviews the relationship between smoking and occupation and makes recommendations for workplace smoking control in hazardous environments.[50]

Examples of Workplace Programs

A number of major companies have distinguished themselves in providing worksite smoking cessation opportunities, corporate smoking policies, and incentives for non-smoking. Among the most well-known programs are those of Control Data Corporation, Johnson & Johnson Corporation, and Pacific Northwest Bell.

Control Data discovered that smoking employees had 25 percent higher health care costs than nonsmokers and 114 percent more hospital days. As part of "Staywell," Control Data's comprehensive health promotion program, smoking cessation programs were offered, restrictive smoking regulations were enacted, and the availability of cigarettes in vending machines was drastically limited. Control Data experienced a one-year success rate of 30 percent among employees who participated in an instructor-led class and another 43 percent were smoking an average of one-third less than when they entered the program. Thus, nearly three-quarters of all participating smokers benefited from the Control Data smoking cessation effort.[51]

As part of their "Live for Life" program, Johnson & Johnson developed a high-quality, behaviorally focused smoking cessation intervention. Combining this smoking cessation program with environmental changes and incentives for non-smoking, Johnson & Johnson has experienced a reduction of 23 percent of all smoking employees during the first two years of the "Live for Life" program.[52] This reduction was not only among smoking cessation program participants, but among all smoking employees. Such results attest to the effectiveness of a comprehensive approach to workplace smoking control.

Perhaps the most aggressive of all workplace smoking control efforts is that developed by Pacific Northwest Bell (PNB), the regional telephone operating company in the Washington-Oregon area. On October 15, 1985, PNB enacted the most stringent smoking policy in America for its 15,000 employees. As of that date, there would be no smoking on company premises. Period. No longer would smoking be permitted in private offices, cafeterias, or previously identified smoking lounges. This enlightened policy was developed in conjunction with the involved unions and has been widely accepted by both smokers and nonsmokers alike.

At the same time that PNB introduced its smoking policy it also announced a free smoking cessation program for all employees, spouses, and dependents. Approximately 28 percent (1,175) of all smoking employees availed themselves of the offer. In addition to the employees, 323 spouses and dependents participated in the program. Acupuncture was the most popular program selected by employees, followed by hypnotism, behavior modification, and aversion therapy. The average cost per participant was $142 and PNB intends to evaluate the effectiveness of the program.[53]

NUTRITION EDUCATION PROGRAMS

Health Issues

There is increasing evidence that dietary choices play a significant role in the development of major health problems, particularly heart disease and cancer—the two leading causes of death in America. The U.S. Surgeon General has identified dietary changes as a major disease prevention and health promotion priority in the prevention of chronic diseases[54] and the first Surgeon General's Report on nutrition and health is being written.

The most prevalent nutritional problems are dietary excesses and poor food choices. Poor eating patterns established during childhood and adolescence often continue into adulthood. These improper dietary habits pose a threat to good health and can exacerbate existing disease conditions.

High fat intake is the major nutritional threat facing Americans today. It is estimated that 10 percent of cardiovascular deaths are attributable to cholesterol.[55] For every 1 percent that serum cholesterol is reduced, the risk of heart attack will decline by 2 percent.[56] Not only has it been recently shown that when cholesterol is lowered, cardiovascular disease mortality declines,[57] but it has also been documented that cholesterol reduction is a cost-effective health promotion strategy, particularly when the intervention occurs early for high-risk individuals.[58] In addition to cardiovascular disease, dietary choices, particularly excessive fat, are felt to increase the risk for colon and breast cancer.[59]

Within the last few years, scientists and researchers have acknowledged that dietary habits are a major factor in cancer occurrence and that specific dietary modifications can have a major impact on cancer prevention. Some researchers feel that diet is as a significant cause of cancer as is tobacco. Doll and Peto estimate that 35 percent of all cancer is related to diet.[60] While diet and cancer estimates are based on multiple studies, the exact magnitude of the relationship and the specific biological mechanisms are uncertain.

The National Cancer Institute observes that, while it is not possible to quantify the exact magnitude of the relationship, a variety of studies indicate that excessive fat intake, inadequate dietary fiber, and inadequate consumption of certain vitamins and minerals are associated with higher rates of certain cancers.[61] Dietary factors are felt to be associated with cancers of the gastrointestinal tract (colon, rectum, pancreas, liver, esophagus, and stomach) and some sex-hormone-specific sites (breast, prostate, ovaries, and endometrium). The exact relationship is currently under study.

Current Prevalence and Trends

In America, while there are problems with undernourishment for specific populations, particularly the elderly, the major nutritional problems are due to excessive eating—too much fat, sodium, sugar, alcohol, and calories. These dietary habits have resulted in significant problems with obesity as well as a variety of degenerative health problems. However, they are of relatively recent vintage and there is evidence that American eating habits may be beginning to improve.

The dietary habits of Americans have changed dramatically over the last 75 years.[62] We are eating more meat, poultry, fish, dairy products, refined sugars and sweeteners, fats and oils, and processed fruits and vegetables. We are eating fewer grain products, potatoes, fresh fruits and vegetables, and eggs. This shift in consumption patterns has had a parallel effect on the proportion of nutrients in our diet, as shown in Table 14-2.

These data represent a 31 percent increase in the per capita use of fats and a 20 percent decline in the consumption of carbohydrates since the first decade of the century. The overall decline in carbohydrate consumption is characterized by a 36 percent increase in sugar consumption and a 50 percent drop in the consumption of grains and a 60 percent drop in potato consumption. Thus, Americans are consuming more dietary fat and fewer complex carbohydrates than were consumed at the turn of the century— exactly the opposite dietary changes that would constitute a chronic disease prevention recommendation.

While the changes in dietary habits over this time period are generally negative, there have been some encouraging changes during the last few years. In light of the findings of major clinical trials and research studies, many national health organizations (U.S. Department of Agriculture, Department of Health and Human Services, National Cancer Institute, American Heart Association, and the American Cancer Society) are promoting consistent and healthy dietary recommendations that seem to be having a positive impact on the knowledge and behavior of the American public.

Workplace Implications

Besides being an ideal site for providing nutrition education programs, the worksite can benefit directly from positive changes in the dietary behavior of its employees and dependents. We have already noted the relationship between lowered serum cholesterol levels and cardiovascular disease. In addition, the National Cancer Institute estimates that if dietary fat is reduced to 25 percent of calories and that fiber is increased to 20–30 grams per day, by the year 2000, there will be an 8 percent reduction in cancer mortality.[63]

Table 14-2 Changes in United States Dietary Nutrient Proportions As a Percent of Calories per Capita (1909 to 1980)

	1909	1980
Fat	32%	43%
Carbohydrates	56%	45%
Protein	12%	12%

Source: Journal of the American Dietetic Association, Vol. 81, pp. 120–125, American Dietetic Association, © 1982.

It is important to note that these are estimates and that it is extremely difficult to be precise in estimating the potential reduction in mortality due to dietary modifications.

The workplace is the site of at least one, if not two, meals a day and most adults spend about half their weekday waking hours at work. Research is continuing to document that the workplace can be an effective site to deliver health promotion and disease prevention programs to adults and that these messages and programs are often brought back into the home. Nutrition education programs at the worksite can help employees learn about the role of diet and disease, assist in making healthy food choices, help in maintaining one's ideal weight, and actually provide healthy food in company cafeterias and vending machines that reduces the risk of disease and promotes health.

The recently completed National Survey of Worksite Health Promotion Activities[64] revealed that nutrition education programs were one of the least frequently offered types of health promotion program. Of the surveyed worksites, 16.8 percent indicated that they offered a nutrition education activity. Despite these findings, many feel that worksite nutrition education programs have increased in popularity and will continue to do so.[65] In support of this concept, Willis Golbeck, president of the Washington Business Group on Health, has stated, "Unlike the more disease-specific worksite wellness topics, good nutrition is essential for 100% of employees, as well as their families and retirees."[66]

The *Decision Maker's Guide to Nutrition Programs at the Worksite* [67] and the special supplement of the *Journal of Nutrition Education*[68] provide specific information, examples, and resources to develop effective workplace nutrition education programs.

Examples of Workplace Programs

Because of the increasing evidence supporting the relationship between diet and health, it can be expected that the number of worksites conducting nutrition education programs will increase. A number of companies have already established effective workplace nutrition education programs. Among these companies are Control Data Corporation, Johnson & Johnson, L.L. Bean, and Metropolitan Life Insurance Co. Many other companies have established successful weight control programs, which will be reviewed in a separate section of this chapter.

As part of its overall "Staywell" program, Control Data offers four separate nutrition education programs, which include a weight control program, a general nutrition class, a diet and heart disease program, and a nutritional assessment.[69] Besides losing an average of eight pounds and keeping it off for a year, program participants reported reductions in butter, salt, and sugar consumption.

Johnson & Johnson employees at work locations offering the "Live for Life" program reported lower cholesterol, triglyceride, weight, and blood pressure levels than employees at sites that did not have the program.[70]

L.L. Bean in Freeport, Maine, offers a 15-week "Heart Club" education program that focuses on fat reduction and menu planning, among other heart disease prevention programs. Eight months after the program began, participants exhibited an 18 percent decrease in serum cholesterol levels, with a self-reported decrease in saturated fat and an increase in polyunsaturated fat consumption.[71]

As part of its Center for Health Help, Metropolitan Life Insurance Corporation offers a cholesterol reduction program to their employees with a serum cholesterol greater than 220 mg/dl. The program consists of two one-hour educational sessions with follow-up blood tests and counseling at three and six months. The nearly 700 employees who have participated reported an average decrease of over 7 percent in their serum cholesterol levels.[72]

FITNESS PROGRAMS

Health Issues

Regular aerobic and strengthening conditioning has a number of established positive benefits such as reducing the risk of coronary heart disease, lowering weight, and reducing symptoms of anxiety. Physical activity is also likely to have beneficial effects on the prevention and control of hypertension, diabetes, osteoporosis, and certain psychological conditions.[73] In addition to the established health benefits, people who exercise regularly report that they feel better, sleep better, and have more energy.[74]

Besides having a beneficial preventive effect, exercise can also have a positive rehabilitative effect. Beneficial effects from exercise have been documented in individuals who had suffered from lung disease, obesity, diabetes, hypertension, and myocardial infarctions.[75]

Current Prevalence and Trends

While it is clear that more people are exercising now than ever before, it is not clear who is exercising and in what way.[76] The National Health Interview Survey found that 41 percent of those surveyed said that they exercised or played sports regularly, although regularly was not defined.[77] Similarly, an earlier survey conducted by the Pacific Mutual Life Insurance Company found 37 percent of the public exercising regularly.[78]

In the attempt to define what constitutes appropriate physical activity, the Centers for Disease Control (CDC) identified four criteria necessary for exercise to produce cardiorespiratory fitness:[79]

- rhythmic contraction of large muscle groups
- intensity that requires 60 percent or more of maximal aerobic capacity
- frequency of three or more sessions per week
- duration of 20 minutes or more per session

While these criteria help to begin to define beneficial physical activity, virtually no survey research has been done using these criteria so that current prevalence rates are difficult to calculate. The CDC concludes that vigorous leisure-time activity has increased, but quantitative estimates are difficult to make.[80] Nonetheless, basing estimates on state behavioral risk factor data, CDC estimates that only 10 to 20 percent of adults 18 to 65 years old are currently exercising at a level that meets the CDC criteria. This compares poorly with the federal 1990 Objectives for the Nation,[81] which recommend that 60 percent of adults exercise at the criteria level.

Workplace Implications

Workplace exercise and fitness programs serve as the core for many corporate health promotion programs, although the exact prevalence of workplace fitness programs was, until recently, unknown. The 1986 National Survey of Worksite Health Promotion Activities[82] found that 21.9 percent of worksites reported exercise activities—a level of activity surpassed only by health risk assessment and smoking cessation programs. Exercise programs were more likely to be found in large worksites of relatively profitable companies that were not subject to regulatory influences.

The 1990 Objectives for the Nation recommends that more than 25 percent of employers with over 500 employees should sponsor fitness programs.[83] The results of the National Survey of Worksite Health Promotion Activities indicated that 32.4 percent of worksites with over 250 employees reported offering employer-sponsored programs. This suggests that the 1990 Objectives have been met.

Companies are interested in workplace fitness programs because of their potential. It is not uncommon for fitness programs to be billed as the corporate panacea—guaranteed to improve performance, productivity, morale, and absenteeism, lower health care costs, and otherwise positively affect the corporate bottom line.

Data are beginning to accumulate that support the benefit of corporate fitness programs. For example, a program designed to monitor the health status and improve the physical fitness of Los Angeles County firemen resulted in an increase in fitness levels, a decrease in myocardial infarction among the most fit firemen, and an inverse relationship between workers' compensation costs and fitness levels.[84] A fitness program among white-collar employees in a Texas insurance company reported, over a five-year period, a substantial reduction in medical costs and disability days before and after entry into the program.[85] Control Data Corporation found that employees who report not exercising regularly have higher annual health care costs ($437 versus $321) than those regularly involved in moderate or vigorous exercise.[86] A fitness program for employees of a Canadian insurance company found significant improvements in turnover, productivity, and absenteeism between experimental and control groups.[87]

These studies did not utilize a true experimental design; thus, the results suggest correlation, not causation. For this and other reasons, some employers still question the value and cost effectiveness of workplace fitness programs and facilities.[88]

Examples of Workplace Programs

In addition to the research examples described in the previous section, there are a number of companies with exemplary fitness programs that also have documented results. Of particular interest are the programs of Johnson & Johnson and Tenneco.

As part of its "Live for Life" program, Johnson & Johnson has an active physical fitness component in addition to other health promotion elements. The "Live for Life" program uses a "broad spectrum" effort to increase fitness levels. This includes a combination of an annual health screen, medical encouragement to initiate or maintain a fitness program, and a supportive work environment—that is, accessibility and availability of exercise programs and facilities.

Using a quasi-experimental design, Johnson & Johnson found that this approach resulted in significant increases in vigorous activity levels, which were maintained over a two-year period, when compared with activity levels of employees who had only the initial health screen.[89] The researchers conclude that this "public health" approach, which focuses on the entire workforce and changes the health environment, produces significant and sustained changes in fitness levels throughout the entire company. This model has far-reaching implications for other worksite health promotion programs.

At Tenneco's corporate headquarters in Houston, 16 percent of the 3,800 employees are working out daily at the corporate fitness facility, which includes an indoor track, weight machines, and racquetball courts. Fitness is considered part of Tenneco's corporate culture and the corporate leadership believes that fitness is positively associated with performance and negatively associated with absenteeism and health care costs. Research studies have been conducted that have supported the relationship. For instance, the number of health care claims of men and women who exercise regularly is about half of that of nonexercisers. Similarly, regular exercisers are absent about two days less a year than nonexercisers. Tenneco executives are the first to point out that these data do not show cause and effect but rather correlation. Nonetheless, they are happy with what they see.

WEIGHT CONTROL

Health Issues

The evidence is now considered to be overwhelming that obesity has an adverse effect on health and longevity. The National Institutes of Health consider obesity to be an "established health hazard."[90]

Obesity is clearly associated with hypertension, elevated cholesterol levels, certain cancers, heart disease, and other medical problems. The second National Health and Nutrition Examination Survey found that the prevalence of hypertension and diabetes is 2.9 times higher for the overweight than for the nonoverweight.[91] Elevated cholesterol (> 250 mg/dl) is 2.1 times more common in young (under 45 years) overweight people compared with the nonoverweight.[92] And weight negatively affects longevity. The greater the degree of overweight, the higher the mortality ratio.[93]

Weight reduction can be life saving and is particularly recommended for the extremely obese (twice desirable weight or 100 pounds overweight). Weight reduction is also recommended for those with lesser degrees of overweight and especially for those with non-insulin-dependent diabetes, hypertension, and elevated cholesterol levels.

Current Prevalence and Trends

The second National Health and Nutrition Examination Survey found that 26 percent of U.S. adults, or about 34 million Americans aged 20 to 75, are overweight, with overweight being defined as 20 percent or more above desirable body weight.[94] This means that one out of every five adult Americans is technically obese. Of these, 11 million are considered severely obese, that is, exceeding their desirable weight by 40 percent. Approximately the same percentages can be expected to be found among employed adults.

In the 1985 National Health Interview Survey, 37 percent of respondents indicated that they were currently trying to lose weight and that 45 percent considered themselves to be at least a little overweight.[95]

Workplace Implications

The National Survey of Worksite Health Promotion Activities found that 14.7 percent of surveyed worksites offered weight loss programs as part of their health promotion program.[96] Only nutrition education and off-the-job accident education programs were offered less frequently. However, as obesity becomes recognized as a serious health threat, corporate weight loss programs are likely to become more prevalent.

Unfortunately, successful weight control programs that result in initial and sustained weight loss are rare.[97] There is, however, the promise of effective programs from recent workplace weight control research. Research programs have shown weight loss competitions[98] and the use of financial incentives[99] to be clinically successful and cost effective. Both these approaches have shown that the use of competition or financial incentives is of more importance than the particular method of weight loss instruction.

Examples of Workplace Programs

The National Survey of Worksite Health Promotion Activities[100] indicated that the prevalence of weight loss programs was relatively low. However, many feel that weight loss programs are the most popular of all nutrition-related health promotion activities[101] and that the popularity of weight loss programs will increase because of employee interest and the interrelationship with other risk factors such as high blood pressure and elevated cholesterol.[102]

There are a number of companies with existing weight loss programs and documented results. Nutrition education and weight control activities play an integral part in Campbell Soup Company's "Turnaround Health and Fitness Program." Weight loss incentives are used as part of this program and in a recent competition, 230 participants lost over 3,000 pounds. Participants who reach their weight loss goal receive prizes and the winning "team" is the recipient of the "Fat Cup" trophy.[103]

In January 1985, John Hancock Life Insurance Company sponsored its First Annual All-John Hancock Weight Loss Competition. Twenty-two teams were established (187 employees) with an average weight loss of 6.5

pounds per person and the winning team (the one that achieved the greatest percentage of its weight loss goal) received a financial incentive.[104]

Union Carbide Corporation uses incentives, rebates, discounts, and awards as integral components of its weight control program. In "Health Plus," embedded in its overall health promotion program, weight control participants who reach their goal receive a 25 percent rebate on the cost of the course, recognition, and a discount certificate for future classes. Participants have enjoyed an average weight loss of 7.2 pounds with a one year follow-up loss of 6.8 pounds.[105]

In 1983 Lockheed Missile and Space Company offered a weight loss campaign for employees, retirees, spouses, and dependents. Its emphasis was on competition and self-responsibility, and over 14,000 pounds were lost in three months at a cost of less than a dollar per pound. Ninty-two percent of participants lost weight, with the average loss being over nine pounds.[106]

HIGH BLOOD PRESSURE CONTROL

Health Issues

High blood pressure, or hypertension, is defined as a systolic pressure greater than or equal to 140 mmHg and/or a diastolic pressure greater than or equal to 90 mmHg. Adults with uncontrolled high blood pressure experience three times as much coronary heart disease, four times as much congestive heart failure, and seven times as many strokes as do those individuals with controlled or normal blood pressure.[107]

It is estimated that approximately 29 percent of coronary heart disease mortality and 32 percent of stroke mortality are attributable to high blood pressure.[108] A reduction of systolic blood pressure to under 140 mmHg for all hypertensives and borderline hypertensives will have a significant impact on cardiovascular disease mortality, saving an estimated 292,000 deaths.[109] The Carter Center study concludes that more than 7 million cases of cardiovascular disease can be attributed to high blood pressure, which results in 10 million hospital days, 155 million disability days, and $6.3 billion in personal medical care expenditures.[110]

Fortunately, clinical trials indicate that the systematic management of high blood pressure can reduce the expected mortality, even for those with "mild hypertension." Clinical trial data have shown a 17 percent reduction in mortality among a group of hypertensives who received systematic and vigorous hypertensive treatment compared with a control group that was referred to the community for standard medical care.[111]

Current Prevalence and Trends

According to the American Heart Association, in 1983 there were nearly 55 million Americans with high blood pressure.[112] The distribution of high blood pressure varies widely by race and age, with elevated blood pressure increasing with age and being more prevalent among black men and women. The American Heart Association reports that the prevalence of hypertension among U.S. adults ranges from a low of 25 percent among white females to a high of 38 percent among black males.[113]

It is estimated that 80 percent of Americans with high blood pressure are aware of their condition and that this represents a doubling in the level of awareness over the last decade.[114] Nevertheless, many with high blood pressure do not seek treatment and as a result, only a minority of hypertensives are under control.[115]

Workplace Implications

Not only is high blood pressure control considered to be the most cost-effective workplace health promotion activity,[116] it has subsequently been shown that workplace programs can be even more effective than community blood pressure control efforts. Research funded by the National Heart, Lung and Blood Institute found that workplace programs have high blood pressure control rates ranging from 68 to 98 percent compared with the average community control rate of 31 percent.[117]

Workplace high blood pressure control programs usually combine screening with differing levels of control and follow-up. In some programs, treatment is done on-site; in others, identified hypertensives are referred to their private or community physician. However, when employees are referred to community resources, there is usually a significant reduction in compliance. One study found that only half of the referred employees actually visited a physician and, after two years, only half of these had maintained their blood pressure under control.[118] These figures do not compare favorably with the high rates of control found in workplace programs.[119]

While workplace high blood pressure control programs have been shown to be cost effective and more effective than community programs, their adoption by corporations has been somewhat limited. According to the National Survey of Worksite Health Promotion Activities, only 16.5 percent of surveyed worksites had a hypertension control program.[120]

Examples of Workplace Programs

A number of companies have sponsored and evaluated workplace high blood pressure control programs, including General Motors, Ford Motor Company, Westinghouse, Massachusetts Mutual Life Insurance Company, New York State employees, and University of Maryland employees, among others. This listing does not include the corporations with comprehensive health promotion programs where high blood pressure detection and control are one of the many program elements. Following is a brief description of two corporate programs, those of Massachusetts Mutual Life Insurance Company and the Ford Motor Company.

Massachusetts Mutual Life Insurance Company sponsored an on-site hypertension screening, referral, and follow-up program at its home office and at the end of one year saw an increase from 36 to 82 percent of employee hypertensives under control.[121] The cost of screening was estimated to be $6 per worker and a total cost for screening, referral, follow-up, and treatment amounted to $120 per hypertensive per year for the first three program years.[122]

Ford Motor Company is fortunate to have benefited from the expertise of Foote and Erfurt of the University of Michigan and the partial funding of the National Heart, Lung and Blood Institute. In 1983, Foote and Erfurt reported the relative effectiveness of four different methods of workplace high blood pressure control in Ford plants.[123] The first method provided only screening and referral; the second method provided referral to a physician and semiannual follow-up; the third method provided referral and follow-up as needed; and the fourth method provided on-site treatment or care by a family physician. The three methods (methods 2–4) that provided follow-up or treatment had a significantly higher level of control than the method without follow-up.

STRESS MANAGEMENT

Health Issues

Although some stress may be beneficial, stressful conditions can result in substantial dysfunction. Unmanaged stress is a risk factor that is highly suspected of contributing to chronic illness, although there is little research to verify this relationship.

Regardless of the weak causal evidence, stress has been associated with a large percentage of Worker's Compensation cases and is preceived by employees and the general public to be a major, if not *the* most important, personal health concern.

Excessive stress is believed to be a risk factor for heart disease[124] and contributes to mental disorders as well as alcohol and substance abuse problems. Suboptimal mental health results in substantial medical expense and is a major cause of disability absence. Stress-associated disorders relate directly to a number of the leading causes of hospitalization, use of outpatient services, sickness disability leave, and performance problems. Stainbrook and Green argue that stress is probably a contributing factor in all the major cardiovascular and cerebrovascular diseases.[125]

Current Prevalence and Trends

Stress is difficult to measure and there are few standardized indices of stress prevalence. The 1985 National Health Interview Survey showed that 52 percent of surveyed adults reported having "a lot" or "a moderate" amount of stress during the preceding two weeks and 13 percent indicated that stress had had "a lot" of effect of their health.[126] Regarding workplace stress, Herzlinger and Calkins state that in the 20- to 64-year-old age group, 7 percent of men and 23 percent of women experience a great deal of stress on the job.[127]

Workplace Implications

The National Survey on Worksite Health Promotion Activities reported that 26.6 percent of workplaces are conducting stress management activities.[128] The provision of stress management programs is also related to company size. The larger the individual worksite and the larger the company, the more likely stress management programs will be offered. In an earlier California study by Fielding and Breslow, California employers indicated that stress management was their highest priority for new programs.[129]

Although there is little evidence that documents the cost savings of stress management programs, it is widely believed that employees with high stress levels are more likely to have lower performance, increased Worker's Compensation claims, and other detrimental and hard-to-quantify work-related problems. In 1980, it was estimated that 50 percent of the Worker's Compensation cases in California were for stress-related disorders.[130]

According to Herzlinger and Calkins, most worksite stress reduction programs have reported positive physiological, psychological, and behavioral effects and have been shown to be effective in reducing blood pressure for mild hypertensives. However, the effect of stress management programs on other health problems and any effect on mortality have not been established.

While it may be difficult to quantify the benefits of stress management and positive mental health programs, there have been attempts to estimate the benefits. At the Equitable Life Assurance Company, Manuso estimated a $5.52 return on every $1.00 invested in a workplace stress management program.[131] Despite this finding, it is generally concluded that workplace stress management programs suffer from the lack of objective measures of stress, the number of factors that can influence the perception of stress, and the differences among individuals.[132]

Examples of Workplace Programs

Despite the problems associated with measuring stress and evaluating the effectiveness of stress management interventions, numerous companies have established stress management programs that attempt to influence either the individual employee, the organization, or both.

New York Telephone found that a self-taught home study course could reduce psychological and somatic symptoms six months after training.[133]

Stress management programs are integral to Honeywell's health promotion program and are available at all Honeywell locations. Honeywell's stress management program takes place two hours a week for eight weeks. The company pays half the cost of the course and over 1,000 Honeywell employees have participated.[134]

Wells Fargo has had a long history of providing stress management training for its employees. Under the direction of the Employee Counseling Program, line managers are trained to become stress management program facilitators using a modified commercially available stress management program consisting of personal workbooks and videotape presentations. To date, over 1,000 employees have participated in the program and, while there are no quantifiable results, the program has been well-received by employees and continues to be in demand.[135]

CANCER SCREENING AND EARLY DETECTION PROGRAMS

In addition to the risk-reduction areas previously described, many corporations include disease screening and early detection programs as part of their health promotion program. The purpose of early detection, or secondary prevention, is to find cancer early, before symptoms occur, and when treatment is most effective. Significant research goes into the establishment of screening recommendations for asymptomatic people; nevertheless, the effectiveness and frequency of recommended screening procedures are a major subject of debate.

The American Cancer Society recommends cancer screening procedures on an age-specific basis for the American public for three of the four major cancer sites: breast, cervical, and colorectal.

Both the National Cancer Institute and the American Cancer Society agree on the importance of cancer screening programs for breast and cervical cancer. Neither organization recommends screening programs for the early detection of lung cancer. While the American Cancer Society recommends colorectal cancer screening, the National Cancer Institute does not feel as though there is sufficient scientific evidence to prove that colorectal screening definitely reduces cancer mortality, although it recognizes the *potential* for significant reduction in mortality.[136]

Regardless of the specific recommendations, the overall level of utilization of cancer screening procedures by the American public is low,[137] with no trend toward increased utilization. The workplace can help to rectify this situation. By integrating cancer screening procedures into workplace wellness programs, educating employees about the importance of early detection, and redesigning benefit plans so as to reimburse for recommended cancer screening procedures, businesses can increase the utilization of early detection procedures among employees and their dependents. By doing so, corporations will reduce the medical costs of cancer cases, increase the probability of survival of those employees and dependents who develop cancer, and contribute significantly to the reduction of cancer mortality.

CRITICAL ISSUES AND FUTURE TRENDS

Many consider the workplace to be the ideal setting in which to conduct health education and health promotion programs. Workplace programs can be as effective as community programs and can be even more effective when the unique characteristics of the workplace are exploited.[138] First, since employees spend approximately half their working weekday hours at the workplace, workplace programs are particularly accessible and convenient for employees, and this may result in greater program participation. Second, in addition to individual intervention, the workplace has the opportunity to influence the work environment and the corporate culture, and this can subtly influence the health attitudes and practices of employees both on and off the job. In addition to these reasons, workplaces are effective sites of health promotion programs because of:

- existing communication channels
- unique peer support opportunities
- relative demographic stability
- existing personnel records to facilitate evaluation
- existing facilities and personnel to conduct and coordinate programs

The workplace health promotion movement is growing and maturing. With 44 percent of worksites already engaged in some type of health promotion program,[139] the priority need is moving away from initial program justification and toward effective program development and management. There are a number of critical issues associated with establishing and managing quality programs. These include program justification, design and management, and program evaluation.

Program Justification

Although program justification is less of a priority than it originally was, justifying and selling a program to top management, whether by internal staff or by outside consultants, is still essential and necessary for program success. All too often, top management is willing to embrace the concept of employee health promotion, but unwilling or unmotivated to commit the necessary resources to establish an effective program.

In attempting to justify a program, it is essential to determine in advance the reasons top management is interested, or is likely to be interested, in workplace health promotion. Is the primary reason employee health enhancement? Health care cost containment? Employee morale and job satisfaction? The program proposal or justification should be tailored to highlight the most likely reason, or combination of reasons, that will motivate top management.

Because top managers are first and foremost businesspeople, a program proposal that realistically documents and quantifies required resources and expected outcomes will likely meet with most success. And because top management deals daily with the economic impact of business decisions, it is recommended that the economic implications and noneconomic benefits of the proposed program be spelled out clearly so that an informed decision can be made with respect to competing proposals.

Fortunately, health and economic data are becoming increasingly available to assist in this effort. Most large companies now have access to their medical benefit utilization data, which document the cost and frequency of the leading medical problems faced by employees. These data can provide an estimate of the cost of ill health and an indication of the potential of prevention.

Some companies are attempting to determine the proportion of their total health costs that are due to lifestyle factors (smoking, high blood pressure, cholesterol, etc.) and then allocate resources accordingly. This approach is often called health risk management[140] and utilizes the methodology of risk factor attributable risk,[141] that is, the percentage of a certain medical condition (heart disease) that is due to a specific risk factor (smoking). In the heart disease-smoking example, it is estimated that 18 percent of preventable heart disease is attributable to smoking. With these data, economic projections of potential benefits can be made and resource allocations can be justified.

Program Design and Management

Once approval is received to go ahead and plan a workplace health promotion program, it is essential to develop realistic and measurable program objectives. These objectives should reflect the motivation the company has for becoming involved in health promotion (employee health, health costs, morale, etc.) and should realistically reflect the outcomes that are possible from the resources that are available. All too often health promotion programs fail because they were unable to attain unrealistic objectives. The simple concept that there is a relationship between program input (resources) and outcomes (program impact) is often lost.[142]

Once realistic objectives are set, a quality and effective program can be designed. Unfortunately, neither quality nor effectiveness is easily defined or achieved. Health promotion is a newly evolving discipline and there is a general dearth of effective program guidelines and criteria. This problem is particularly pronounced in the workplace where the allure of financial gain has led to some less than effective programs. There have been some attempts to help to rectify this problem. A number of organizations,[143] including state health departments, business coalitions, and insurance companies, are developing guidelines to assist in the selection of health promotion vendors.

In an attempt to begin to define acceptable criteria for health promotion and education programs, the American Public Health Association in cooperation with the Centers for Disease Control has established draft criteria. At a minimum, it is recommended that workplace health promotion programs meet the following criteria:

1. Address one or more risk factors that are carefully defined, measurable, modifiable, and reasonably prevalent and that constitute a threat to health status and/or quality of life.
2. Consider the special characteristics, needs, and preferences of the target group.
3. Include interventions that are adequate to impact upon or reduce a targeted risk factor and appropriate for a particular setting.
4. Select and implement interventions that make effective use of available resources.
5. Be organized and planned from the outset in such a way that can be evaluated.

While these criteria relate to health promotion programs in general, some researchers have proposed specific guidelines for workplace programs.[144] Parkinson and Fielding[145] note that while workplace programs vary according to corporate culture, there are six key elements for success: (1) support of top management, (2) health risk assessment, (3) multiple opportunities for health improvement, (4) corporate culture efforts, (5) program evaluation, and (6) the organizational location and qualifications of program manager.

While there are key elements for success, there are also common pitfalls. Nay[146] identifies the following: (1) inadequate support for programs from the top down, (2) insufficient resources to implement the program, (3) fragmented implementation, (4) overlooking of unions and existing employee groups, (5) poor training of supervisory personnel, (6) insurance coverage limitations, and (7) inadequate evaluation.

In conclusion, quality workplace health promotion programs require effective managers who understand public health and prevention but are also adept at functioning successfully in a business environment. This includes skills such as program planning, budget justification, performance monitoring, and economic analysis—skills that are specific to the workplace but that would be beneficial in any health promotion setting.

Program Evaluation

As Nay has pointed out, program evaluation is often not a priority element of a workplace health promotion program.[147] It is erroneously felt that evaluation of workplace programs must be extremely costly, time consuming, or burdensome. While evaluation can be sophisticated and elaborate, this is not always necessary.[148] The important point to remember is that health promotion programs should be "evaluable," i.e., capable of being evaluated. This is consistent with the criteria of the American Public Health Association and makes good business sense.

There have been a number of attempts to evaluate specific elements of workplace health promotion programs and many of these have been reviewed in this chapter. There have also been attempts to evaluate the impact of comprehensive health promotion programs on employee health, behavior, costs, and job satisfaction.[149] These studies are more elaborate and require more time and resources. Despite this, a number of major companies and organizations are seriously committed to establishing the effectiveness of their health promotion efforts. The next few years should provide increasing data on the relative cost effectiveness of various workplace health promotion strategies.

Future Trends in Workplace Health Promotion

To better understand the relationship between employment and health, the National Institute of Occupational Safety and Health (NIOSH) and the Office of Disease Prevention and Health Promotion (ODPHP) of the Department of Health and Human Services commissioned a document entitled *The Future of Work and Health.*[150] This document will influence the direction and development of workplace health programs for the rest of the century and beyond. The document reveals a number of significant trends that have major implications for the development of corporate health promotion programs. One of the major trends recognizes employees as an important source of human capital. That is, each employee represents a significant corporate investment and is a "combination of innate talent, knowledge, skill and experience that makes each human a valuable contributor to economic production."[151]

To the extent that employees can be viewed as human capital, resources can be allocated for wellness program development and implementation. The document goes on to state:

> The key challenge is to fix the place of health promotion programs in the workplace within the emerging array of training, retraining, and human resource development programs which employers will increasingly turn to to enrich the work experience of employees and to enhance their productivity.[152]

The Future of Work and Health describes the characteristics of workplace health promotion in the year 2010. These characteristics are useful to consider in developing a corporate wellness strategy:

- Workplaces will be dramatically different, with smaller units, including the home. Work will emphasize information processing and sophisticated artificial intelligence.
- Employees will increasingly assert "expressive values," such as participation in management decisions and a concern for quality of products.
- Employee demographics will continue to be diverse, with more older workers, women, and workers with diverse racial and ethnic characteristics.
- Wellness will receive a new recognition of importance in the workplace. Wellness will be seen as central both to employee values and to management's recognition of the importance of enriching employees'

work experience and as an ethical and effective way of enhancing productivity.

- There will be dramatic advances in research and new technologies that will expand and enhance the impact of health promotion programs.
- The traditional providers of medical care—the hospital, clinic and laboratory—will gradually shrink in dominance. They will yield to the home, the community center, and the workplace.
- We will see the emergence of "total health care management" in the workplace concerned with all types of risks and hazards, the provision of medical care, and the advancement of health.

It is anticipated that these trends will shape the future of workplace health promotion—a future bright with potential if the current challenges are met.

For workplace health promotion to develop its potential, the challenge of program quality and effectiveness must be met. We must learn the relative effectiveness of different health interventions—what program works best with which employee under what conditions. We must learn to do a better job of integrating individual lifestyle interventions with organizational and environmental strategies that always support and are often more effective than the individual approach. We must learn to use and understand the new technologies—both the potential benefits and risks. And, most important, management, labor, and all other interested stakeholders must learn to work together to protect and promote the health and well-being of all employees to achieve the vast potential of workplace health promotion and to improve employee health.

NOTES

1. The Equitable Life Assurance Society of the United States, *The Equitable Health Care Survey: Options for Controlling Costs* (New York: Louis Harris and Associates, 1985).

2. Carter Center, *Closing the Gap: National Health Policy Consultation* (Atlanta: The Carter Center of Emory University, November 1984); and W.H. Foege, R.W. Amler, and C.C. White, "Closing the Gap: Report of the Carter Center Health Policy Consultation," *Journal of the American Medical Association* 254, no. 10 (1985): 1355–1358.

3. L. Goldman and E.F. Cook, "The Decline in Ischemic Heart Disease Mortality Rates: An Analysis of the Comparative Effects of Medical Interventions and Changes in Lifestyle," *Annals of Internal Medicine* 101 (1984): 826–838; and J. Stamler, "The Marked Decline in Coronary Heart Disease Mortality Rates in the United States, 1968–1981: Summary of Findings and Possible Explanations," *Cardiology* 72 (1985): 11–22.

4. U.S. Department of Health and Human Services, *National Survey of Worksite Health Promotion Activities*, Office of Disease Prevention and Health Promotion, Washington, DC, Monograph (in press, 1987).

5. J.E. Fielding and L. Breslow, "Health Promotion Programs Sponsored by California Employers," *American Journal of Public Health* 73 (1983): 538–542.

6. M.F. Davis et al., "Worksite Health Promotion in Colorado," *Public Health Reports* 99 (1984): 538–543.

7. Hewitt Associates, *Company Practices in Health Care Cost Management* (Hewitt Associates, 100 Half Day Road, Lincolnshire, IL 60015, 1984).

8. Business Roundtable Task Force on Health, *Corporate Health Care Cost Management and Private Sector Initiatives* (The Business Roundtable, Lilly Corporate Center, Indianapolis, IN 46285, 1984).

9. National Association of Employers on Health Care Alternatives, *1982 Survey of National Corporations on Health Care Cost Containment* (Minneapolis, 1983).

10. U.S. Department of Health and Human Services, 1986.

11. Towers, Perrin Forster & Crosby, *Health Care Cost Management: Attitudes of Management and Labor* (Towers, Perrin Forster and Crosby, 600 Third Avenue, New York, NY 10016, September 1984).

12. *The Equitable Health Care Survey: Options for Controlling Costs.*

13. *Corporate Health Care Cost Management and Private Sector Initiatives,* 1984.

14. Mercer-Meidinger, *Employer Attitudes Toward the Cost of Health* (Mercer-Meidinger, 1211 Avenue of the Americas, New York, NY 10036, October 1985).

15. M.A. Spilman et al., *Effects of a Corporate Health Promotion Program, Journal of Occupational Medicine* 28, no. 4 (1986): 285–289.

16. C.S. Wilbur, "The Johnson & Johnson Program," *Preventive Medicine* 12 (1983): 672–681.

17. M.P. Naditch, "The 'Staywell Program'," in *Behavioral Health: A Handbook of Health Enhancement and Disease Prevention,* ed. J.P. Matarazzo (New York: John Wiley, 1984).

18. U.S. Department of Health and Human Services, *National Survey,* 1987.

19. R.S. Parkinson and J.E. Fielding, "Health Promotion in the Workplace," in L.J. Cralley and L.V. Cralley (eds.), *Patty's Industrial Hygiene and Toxicology,* 2nd ed., vol. 3A, *The Work Environment* (New York: John Wiley, 1985).

20. R.W. Nay, "Worksite Health Promotion Programs," *Employee Benefits Journal,* June 1985, 17–27.

21. Ibid.

22. A.K. Kiefhaber and W.B. Goldbeck, "Worksite Wellness," in *Proceedings of the National Conference on Health Promotion Programs in Occupational Settings* (Washington, D.C.: Public Health Service, 1979).

23. American Cancer Society, *1986 Cancer Facts and Figures* (New York: American Cancer Society, Publication No. 5008-LE, 1986).

24. U.S. Department of Health and Human Services, *The Health Consequences of Smoking—Cardiovascular Disease: A Report of the Surgeon General* (Washington, D.C.: Public Health Service, DHHS Publication No. (PHS) 84-50204, 1983).

25. K.E. Warner, "The Effects of Publicity and Policy on Smoking and Health," *Business and Health* 2, no. 1 (1984): 7–14.

26. American Cancer Society, *1986 Cancer Facts and Figures.*

27. G.D. Friedman et al., "Mortality in Cigarette Smokers and Quitters: Effect of Baseline Differences," *New England Journal of Medicine* 304, no. 23 (1981): 1407–1410.

28. U.S. Department of Health, Education and Welfare, *Smoking and Health: A Report of the U.S. Surgeon General,* Public Health Service, DHEW Publication No. (PHS) 79-50066, 1979.

29. J.H. Lubin et al., "Modifying Risk of Developing Lung Cancer by Changing Habits of Cigarette Smoking," *British Medical Journal* 288 (1984): 1953–1956.

30. National Cancer Institute, *Cancer Control Objectives for the Nation: 1985–2000* (Bethesda, Md.: Division of Cancer Prevention and Control, U.S. Department of Health Services, Final Draft, February 1986).

31. J.E. Fielding, "Smoking: Health Effects and Controls (Part 1)," *New England Journal of Medicine* 313, no. 8 (1985): 491–497.

32. M.P. Eriksen, "Workplace Smoking Control: Rationale and Approaches," *Advances in Health Education and Promotion* 1(A) (1986): 65–103.

33. U.S. Department of Health and Human Services, *The Health Consequences of Smoking— Cancer: A Report of the Surgeon General,* Public Health Service, DHHS Publication No. (PHS) 82-50179, 1982.

34. Ibid., viii.

35. National Cancer Institute, *Cancer Control Objectives.*

36. Gallup Organization, *1983 Survey of Public Awareness and Use of Cancer Detection Tests* (Publication # GO 83261, The Gallup Organization, Inc., 53 Bank Street, Princeton, NJ 08542, 1984).

37. "Cancer News: Preliminary Findings on Smoking from ACS Cancer Prevention Study II," *Cancer News,* Winter 1986, 18.

38. National Cancer Institute, *Cancer Control Objectives.*

39. Ibid.

40. C.T. Orleans and R.H. Shipley, "Worksite Smoking Initiatives: Review and Recommendations," *Addictive Behaviors* 7 (1982): 1–16.

41. U.S. Department of Health and Human Services, *National Survey of Worksite Health Promotion Activities.*

42. Fielding and Breslow, *Health Promotion Programs,* 538–542.

43. R.H. Shipley and C.T. Orleans, "Evaluating Smoking Control Programs at the Worksite," *Corporate Commentary* 1, no. 4 (1985): 35–45.

44. L.C. Solomon, *Smoking Policies in Large Corporations* (Survey sponsored by the Tobacco Institute and conducted by Human Resources Policy Corporation, 1729 Casiano Road, Los Angeles, CA 90049, 1985).

45. M.P. Eriksen, "Smoking Policies at Pacific Bell," *Corporate Commentary* 1, no. 4 (1985): 24–34.

46. Office of Disease Prevention and Health Promotion and Office of Smoking and Health, *A Decision Maker's Guide to Reducing Smoking at the Worksite* (Washington, D.C.: U.S. Department of Health and Human Services/Washington Business Group on Health, 1985).

47. Eriksen, "Workplace Smoking Control," 65–103.

48. D.P. Rice et al., "The Economic Costs of Smoking: 1984," *Milbank Quarterly* (in press).

49. G. Oster, G.A. Colditz, and N.L. Kelly, *The Economic Costs of Smoking and Benefits of Quitting* (Lexington, Mass.: Lexington Books, 1984).

50. U.S. Department of Health and Human Sevices, *The Health Consequences of Smoking— Cancer and Chronic Lung Disease in the Workplace,* Public Health Service, DHHS Publication No. (PHS) 85-50207, 1985.

51. Office of Disease Prevention and Health Promotion, *A Decision Maker's Guide To Reduce Smoking.*

52. Ibid.

53. Personal communication with Len Beil, Director, Labor Relations, Pacific Northwest Bell, Seattle, Washington, May 1986.

54. American Dietetic Association, The Society for Nutrition Education, and Office of Disease Prevention and Health Promotion, *Worksite Nutrition: A Decision Maker's Guide* (Washington, D.C.: U.S. Department of Health and Human Services, 1986).

55. Carter Center, *Closing the Gap.*

56. U.S. Department of Health and Human Services, "Lowering Blood Cholesterol to Prevent Heart Disease," *National Institutes of Health Consensus Development Conference Statement* 5, no. 7 (1984).

57. Lipid Research Clinics Program, "The Lipid Research Clinics Coronary Primary Prevention Trial Results. II. The Relationship of Reduction in Incidence of Coronary Heart Disease to Cholesterol Lowering," *Journal of the American Medical Association* 251 (1984): 351–364.

58. G. Oster and A.M. Epstein, "Primary Prevention and Coronary Heart Disease: The Economic Costs of Lowering Serum Cholesterol," *American Journal of Public Health* 76 (1986): 647–656.

59. National Research Council, *Diet, Nutrition and Cancer* (Washington, D.C.: National Academy Press, 1982).

60. R. Doll and R. Peto, *The Causes of Cancer* (New York: Oxford Medical Publications, Oxford University Press, 1981).

61. *Cancer Control Objectives.*

62. S. Welch and R.M. Marston, "Review of Trends in Food Use in the United States: 1909–1980," *Journal of the American Dietetic Association* 81 (1982): 120–125.

63. *Cancer Control Objectives.*

64. U.S. Department of Health and Human Services, *National Survey, 1987.*

65. K. Glanz and T. Seewald-Klein: "Nutrition at the Worksite: An Overview," *Journal of Nutrition Education* 18, no. 1 (1986): S1–S12.

66. *Worksite Wellness Media Report: Nutrition Programs in the Workplace* (Washington, D.C.: Washington Business Group on Health/Office of Disease Prevention and Health Promotion, 1986).

67. Office of Disease Prevention and Health Promotion, *Worksite Nutrition.*

68. K. Glanz, ed., "Nutrition at the Worksite," *Journal of Nutrition Education* 18, no. 1 (Special Supplement, 1986).

69. Office of Disease Prevention and Health Promotion, *Worksite Nutrition.*

70. Ibid.

71. Ibid.

72. Ibid.

73. "Status of the 1990 Physical Fitness and Exercise Objectives," *Morbidity and Mortality Weekly Report,* Centers for Disease Control 34, no. 34 (1985): 521–531.

74. B. Marcotte and J.H. Price, "The Status of Health Promotion Programs at the Worksite—A Review," *Health Education,* July/August 1983, 4–8.

75. M.P. O'Donnell and T. Ainsworth, eds., *Health Promotion in the Workplace* (New York: John Wiley, 1984).

76. Parkinson and Fielding, "Health Promotion in the Workplace."

77. National Center for Health Statistics, "Provisional Data from the Health Promotion and

Disease Prevention Supplement to the National Health Interview Survey: United States, January–March 1985," *Advance Data* 113 (November 1985).

78. Parkinson and Fielding, "Health Promotion in the Workplace."

79. "Status of the 1990 Physical Fitness and Exercise Objectives," 521–531.

80. Ibid.

81. U.S. Department of Health and Human Services, *Promoting Health/Preventing Disease: Objectives for the Nation* (Washington, D.C.: ODPHP, Public Health Service, 1980).

82. U.S. Department of Health and Human Services, *National Survey,* 1987.

83. U.S. Department of Health and Human Services, *Promoting Health/Preventing Disease.*

84. L.D. Cady, P.C. Thomas, and R.J. Karwasky, "Program for Increasing Health and Physical Fitness of Fire Fighters," *Journal of Occupational Medicine* 27, no. 2 (1985): 110–114.

85. D.W. Bowne et al., "Reduced Disability and Health Care Costs in Industrial Fitness Program," *Journal of Occupational Medicine* 26 (1984): 809–816.

86. M.P. Naditch, "Workplace Preventive Medicine as an Employee Benefits Program, 1983," *Employee Benefit Symposium Proceedings,* 1983, 49–57.

87. M. Cox, R.J. Shephard, and P. Corey, "Influence of an Employee Fitness Programme upon Fitness, Productivity and Absenteeism," *Ergonomics* 24, no. 10 (1981): 795–806.

88. J.E. Fielding, "Effectiveness of Employee Health Promotion Programs," *Journal of Occupational Medicine* 24 (1982): 907–916; and J.J. Hoffman and C.J. Hobson, "Physical Fitness and Employee Effectiveness," *Personnel Administrator,* April 1984, 101–113.

89. S.N. Blair et al., "A Public Health Intervention Model for Work-Site Health Promotion: Impact on Exercise and Physical Fitness in a Health Promotion Plan after 24 Months," *Journal of the American Medical Association* 255, no. 7 (1986): 921–926.

90. National Institutes of Health Consensus Development Conference Statement, "Health Implications of Obesity," *Annals of Internal Medicine* 103 (1985): 1073–1077.

91. National Center for Health Statistics, *Plan and Operation of the National Health and Nutrition Examination Survey, 1976–1980* (Washington, D.C.: Public Health Service, DHHS Publication No. (PHS) 81-1317, 1981).

92. T.B. Van Itallie, "Health Implications of Overweight and Obesity in the United States," *Annals of Internal Medicine* 103 (1985): 983–988.

93. National Institutes of Health Consensus Development Conference Statement, 1985.

94. National Center for Health Statistics, *Plan and Operation,* 1981.

95. National Center for Health Statistics, "Provisional Data," 1985.

96. U.S. Department of Health and Human Services, *National Survey,* 1987.

97. K.D. Brownell, "Obesity: Understanding and Treating a Serious, Prevalent and Refractory Disorder," *Journal of Consulting and Clinical Psychology* 50, no. 6 (1982): 820–840.

98. K.D. Brownell et al., "Weight Loss Competitions at the Work Site: Impact on Weight, Morale and Cost-Effectiveness," *American Journal of Public Health* 74 (1984): 1283–1285; and L.S. Seidman, G.G. Sevelius, and P. Ewald, "A Cost-effective Weight Loss Program at the Worksite," *Journal of Occupational Medicine* 26, no. 10 (1984): 725–730.

99. J.L. Forster et al., "A Worksite Weight Control Program Using Financial Incentives Collected through Payroll Deduction," *Journal of Occupational Medicine* 27, no. 11 (1985): 804–808.

100. U.S. Department of Health and Human Services, *National Survey,* 1987.

101. Office of Disease Prevention and Health Promotion, *Worksite Nutrition.*

102. Parkinson and Fielding, "Health Promotion in the Workplace."

103. Office of Disease Prevention and Health Promotion, *Worksite Nutrition.*

104. Ibid.

105. Ibid.

106. Seidman, Sevelius, and Ewald, "A Cost-Effective Weight Loss Program," 725–730.

107. U.S. Department of Health and Human Services, "Worksite Health Promotion and Human Resources: A Hard Look at the Data," *Conference Proceedings,* Washington, D.C.: National Heart Lung and Blood Institute, October 1983.

108. Carter Center, *Closing the Gap.*

109. Ibid.

110. Ibid.

111. U.S. Department of Health and Human Services, "Worksite Health Promotion and Human Resources."

112. American Heart Association, *1986 Heart Facts* (Dallas: American Heart Association, Publication No. 55-005-J 11-85-150M, 1985).

113. Ibid.

114. Marcotte and Price, "The Status of Health Promotion Programs," 4–8.

115. American Heart Association, *1986 Heart Facts.*

116. Fielding, "Effectiveness," 907–916.

117. U.S. Department of Health and Human Services, "Worksite Health Promotion and Human Resources."

118. M.H. Alderman, "Hypertension Control Programs in Occupational Settings," *Public Health Reports* 95 (1980): 158–163.

119. U.S. Department of Health and Human Services, "Worksite Health Promotion"; Alderman, "Hypertension Control," 158–163; A. Foote and J.C. Erfurt, "Hypertension Control at the Worksite: Comparison of Screening and Referral Alone, Referral and Follow-Up, and On-Site Treatment," *New England Journal of Medicine* 308 (1983): 809–813; and J.C. Erfurt and A. Foote, "Cost-Effectiveness of Work-site Blood Pressure Control Programs," *Journal of Occupational Medicine* 26, no. 12 (1984): 892–900.

120. U.S. Department of Health and Human Services, *National Survey,* 1987.

121. J.E. Fielding, *Corporate Health Management* (Reading, Mass.: Addison-Wesley, 1985).

122. U.S. Department of Health and Human Services, "Worksite Health Promotion and Human Resources."

123. "Hypertension Control," 809–813.

124. B. Dorian and C.B. Taylor, "Stress Factors in the Development of Coronary Heart Disease," *Journal of Occupational Medicine* 26, no. 10 (1984): 747–756.

125. G.L. Stainbrook and L.W. Green, "Role of Psychosocial Stress in Cardiovascular Disease," *Houston Heart Bulletin* 3 (1983): 1–8.

126. National Center for Health Statistics, "Provisional Data."

127. R.E. Herzlinger and D. Calkins, "How Companies Tackle Health Care Costs, Part III," *Harvard Business Review,* January-February 1986, 70–80.

128. U.S. Department of Health and Human Services, *National Survey,* 1987.

129. "Health Promotion Programs," 538–542.

130. G.L. Stainbrook, L.W. Green, and C.T. Lovato, *An Overview of the Recent Introduc-*

tion of Health Promotion Concepts and Programs in U.S. Companies (Report prepared under contract for the National Institute of Occupational Safety and Health (NIOSH), 1986).

131. J. Manuso, "Management of Individual Stressors," in *Health Promotion in the Workplace,* ed. M. O'Donnell and T. Ainsworth (New York: John Wiley, 1985).

132. Parkinson and Fielding, "Health Promotion in the Workplace."

133. *Worksite Wellness Media Report: Stress Management in the Workplace* (Washington, D.C.: Washington Business Group on Health/Office of Disease Prevention and Health Promotion, 1986).

134. Ibid.

135. Ibid.

136. *Cancer Control Objectives.*

137. National Cancer Institute, *Cancer Control Objectives;* Gallup Organization, *1983 Survey of Public Awareness and Use of Cancer Detection Tests.*

138. Orleans and Shipley, "Worksite Smoking Initiatives," 1–16.

139. U.S. Department of Health and Human Services, *National Survey.*

140. J.E. Bernstein, "Using Risk Management To Predict and Control Health Costs," *Advanced Management Journal,* Spring 1983, 9–13; and J.E. Bernstein, "Handling Health Costs by Reducing Health Risk," *Personnel Journal,* November 1983, 882–887.

141. Carter Center, *Closing the Gap;* Rice et al., "The Economic Costs of Smoking."

142. Nay, "Worksite Health Promotion Programs"; and R.S. Parkinson et al., *Managing Health Promotion in the Workplace—Guidelines for Implementation and Evaluation* (Palo Alto, Calif.: Mayfield, 1982).

143. *Healthworks Northwest: Guidelines for Selecting Health Promotion Providers* (Seattle: Puget Sound Health Systems Agency, 1984); and Maine Department of Human Services, *Guidelines for Choosing Worksite Health Promotion Programs* (Augusta: State of Maine Department of Human Services, 1984).

144. Parkinson and Fielding, "Health Promotion in the Workplace"; O'Donnell and Ainsworth, eds., *Health Promotion in the Workplace;* and K.E. Kelly, "Building a Successful Health Promotion Program," *Business and Health,* March 1986, 44–45.

145. "Health Promotion in the Workplace."

146. "Worksite Health Promotion Programs," 17–27.

147. Ibid.

148. Parkinson et al., *Managing Health Promotion in the Workplace;* L.W. Green and F.M. Lewis, *Measurement and Evaluation in Health Education and Promotion* (Palo Alto, Calif.: Mayfield, 1986); R.A. Windsor et al., *Evaluation of Health Promotion and Education Programs* (Palo Alto, Calif.: Mayfield, 1984); and S.M. Shortell and W.C. Richardson, *Health Program Evaluation* (St. Louis: C.V. Mosby 1978).

149. Spilman et al., *Effects of a Corporate Health Promotion Program,* 285–289; and J.O. Gibbs et al., "Worksite Health Promotion: Five-year Trend in Employee Health Care Costs," *Journal of Occupational Medicine* 27, no. 11 (1985): 826–830.

150. C. Bezold, R. J. Carlson, and J. C. Peck, *The Future of Work and Health* (Dover, Mass.: Auburn House, 1986).

151. Ibid.

152. Ibid.

SUGGESTED READINGS

Atherosclerosis Study Group. "Optimal Resources for Primary Prevention of Atherosclerotic Diseases: Report of Intersociety Commission for Heart Disease Resources." *Circulation* 70 (1984): 157A–205A.

Bailar, J.C. and E.M. Smith. Progress Against Cancer? *The New England Journal of Medicine* 314 (1986): 1226–1232.

Berry, C.A. *Good Health for Employees and Reduced Health Care Costs for Industry.* Washington, D.C.: Health Insurance Association of America, 1981.

Brennan, A.J. Worksite Health Promotion Can Be Cost-effective. *Personnel Administrator,* April 1983, 39–42.

"Cancer News: Industry Cancer Control Programs Could Save Thousands of Lives, Billions of Dollars." *Cancer News,* Autumn 1982, 7–9.

Clement J., and D.A. Gibbs. "Employer Consideration of Health Promotion Programs: Financial Variables." *Journal of Public Health Policy,* March 1983, 45–55.

Collings, G.H. "Managing the Health of the Employee." *Journal of Occupational Medicine* 24, no. 1 (1982): 15–17.

Cunningham, R.M. *Wellness at Work: A Report on Health and Fitness Programs for Employees of Business and Industry.* Chicago: Blue Cross and Blue Shield Association of America, 1982.

Dickerson, O.B., and C. Mandelblit. "A New Model for Employer-Provided Health Education Programs." *Journal of Occupational Medicine* 25, no. 6 (1983): 471–474.

Feldman, R.H. "Strategies for Improving Compliance with Health Promotion Programs in Industry." *Health Education,* July/August 1983, 21–25.

Fielding, J.E. "Health Promotion and Disease Prevention at the Worksite." *Annual Review of Public Health* 5 (1984): 237–265.

Gelb, B.D. "Preventive Medicine and Employee Productivity." *Harvard Business Review,* March/April 1985, 12–13.

Health Insurance Association of America. *Your Guide to Wellness at the Worksite.* Washington, D.C.: HIAA, Public Relations Division, 1983.

Health Planning Council. *A Practical Guide for Employee Health Promotion Programs.* Madison, Wisc.: Health Planning Council, 1982.

Healthworks Northwest. *Employee Health Promotion: A Guide for Starting Programs at the Workplace.* Seattle: Puget Sound Health Systems Agency, 1983.

Healthworks Northwest. *Health Promotion Needs Assessment Manual.* Seattle: Puget Sound Health Systems Agency, 1984.

Healthy People Project. *How to Start a Health Promotion Program at the Worksite.* Baltimore: Maryland Department of Health and Mental Hygiene, 1982.

Ivancevich, J.M., M.T. Matteson, and E.P. Richards. "Who's Liable for Stress on the Job?" *Harvard Business Review,* March/April 1985, 60–72.

McLeroy, K.R., L.W. Green, K.D. Mullen, and V. Foshee. "Assessing the Effects of Health Promotion in Worksites: A Review of Stress Program Evaluations." *Health Education Quarterly* 11 (1984): 379–401.

Pelletier, K.R. *Healthy People in Unhealthy Places: Stress and Fitness at Work.* New York: Delacorte Press, 1984.

Russell, L.B. *Is Prevention Better Than Cure?* Washington, D.C.: The Brookings Institution, 1986.

Schwartz, R.M. and P.L. Rollins. "Cost Savings Through Participation in a Health Enhancement Program." *Journal of Occupational Medicine.*

Settergren, S.K., et al. "Comparison of Respondents and Nonrespondents to a Worksite Health Screen." *Journal of Occupational Medicine* 254, no. 6 (1983): 475–480.

Shepard, D.S., and L.A. Pearlman. "Healthy Habits That Pay Off." *Business and Health,* March 1985, 37–41.

U.S. Department of Agriculture. *Nutrition and Your Health, Dietary Guidelines for Americans.* Washington, D.C.: Office of Governmental and Public Affairs, USDA, 1985.

U.S. Department of Health, Education and Welfare. *Healthy People: The Surgeon General's Report on Health Promotion and Disease Prevention,* Public Health Service, DHEW (PHS) Publication No. 79-55071, Washington, D.C., 1979.

U.S. Department of Health, Education and Welfare. *Proceedings of the National Conference on Health Promotion Programs in Occupational Settings.* Washington, D.C.: Public Health Service, 1979.

U.S. Department of Health and Human Services. *Proceedings of Prospects for a Healthier America: Achieving the Nation's Health Promotion Objectives.* Washington, D.C.: Public Health Service, 1984.

Walsh, D.C. "Is There a Doctor In-house?" *Harvard Business Review,* July/August 1984, 84–94.

Warner, K.E., and H.A. Murt. "Economic Incentives for Health." *Annual Review of Public Health* 5 (1984): 107–113.

Wright, C.C. "Cost Containment Through Health Promotion Programs." *Journal of Occupational Medicine* 24, no. 12 (1982): 965–968.

Yenney, S.L. *Small Businesses and Health Promotion: The Prospects Look Good—A Guide for Providers of Health Promotion Programs.* Washington, D.C.: Office of Disease Prevention and Health Promotion, Department of Health and Human Services, March 1984.

Appendix 14-A

Corporations With
Health Promotion Programs

The following companies have effective and ongoing workplace health promotion programs. Although there are many other companies actively involved in workplace health promotion, these companies have distinguished themselves and are frequently cited in the health and business literature.

Adolf Coors Company
Apple Computer ·
AT&T
Bonne Bell
Burlington Industries
Campbell Soup
CIGNA Corporation
Control Data Corporation
DuPont
EXXON
Ford Motor Company
GTE
Honeywell
IBM
John Hancock
Johnson & Johnson
Kimberly Clark
Metropolitan Life Company
Mobil Oil
New York Telephone
Pacific Bell
Pepsico
Raytheon

Rolm
Scherer Brothers Lumber
Sentry Insurance Company
Southern California Edison
Southern New England Telephone Company
Speedball Corporation
Sperry Corporation
Tenneco
Union Carbide
Upjonn Corporation
Xerox

Index

A

Active listening, and patient cooperation, 174–175
Aerobics, 128, 139
Aerobics Master, 128, 139
Aging programs
  development of, 239–241
  evaluation of, 241
  example models
    AHOY/LIFE, 257
    Growing Younger/Growing Wiser, 255–256
    Health Promotion Programs (NCOA), 254
    Healthy Older People Campaign, 256
    Ken Dychtwal & Associates, 254–255
    Live Better Longer Project, 255
    Quality Aging Program, 258
    Staying Healthy After 50 Project, 258
    White Crane Senior Health Center, 259
    Wisdom Project, 257
  future and
    demographic trends and future, 244–245
    health care delivery system and, 245–246
    media, role of, 246–247
    peer models in, 243–244
    reimbursement and, 247
    role of family in, 242–243
  health fair approach, 240
  leadership in, 238
  major areas, 236
  networking approach, 241
  obstacles/problems in, 238–239
  present status of, 247–248
  qualities of successful program, 237
  settings for, 237
  See also Elderly.
AHOY/LIFE, 257
Analysis component, ethics, 102–103
Anatomy of an Illness (Cousins), 112

B

Bankers First, incentive system, 161
Basic versus incremental needs, 55
Be Your Own Coach, 128, 139
Belief systems, 13–15
  force field analysis, 15
Beneficience, ethics, 95–96
Bonne Bell, incentive system, 161–162
Bronx-Lebanon Hospital Center, The Hub, 265–266, 268–269, 273

C

Cancer screening, 304–305
Choice component, ethics, 104

Claims review procedure, 45
Community forum approach, data
    collection, 65
Community health advocacy, 261–277
    Community Health Participation
        Program (CHPP), 263–265, 268–
        269, 270–271
    facilitating factors, 266, 268–271
        funding, 269–270
        political climate, 270–271
        type of institution, 266, 268–269
    health professional's role, 271–276
        documentation, 271–272
        education/training, 272
        networking, 273
        political activities, 273–278
        research, 272–273
    organizations related to, 279–280
    process of, 261
    The Hub, 265–266, 268–269, 273
Community Health Participation
    Program (CHPP), 263–265, 268–
    269, 270–271
Community survey, data collection, 60–
    61
Competition, survey of, 81–82
Comprehensive/preventive-focused
    approach, workplace health
    promotion, 286
Comprehensive/risk-focused approach,
    workplace health promotion, 286
COMPUTE-A-LIFE (I and II), 126,
    138
Computers, 123–143
    computer terminology, 135–136
    hardware, 123–124
    software
        Aerobics, 128, 139
        Aerobics Master, 128, 139
        Be Your Own Coach, 128, 139
        COMPUTE-A-LIFE (I and II),
            126, 138
        Eating Machine, 128, 140
        Eliza, 130, 143
        Evrydiet, 128, 140
        FITCOMP, 129, 142

fitness and nutrition, 128–129,
    141–142
fitness software, 127–128, 139–
    140
guidelines in choice of software,
    124–125
for health, 125–127, 137–138
Health Risk Appraisal, 125–126,
    138
on health topics, 126–127
Healthpath, 128
Hospitalization Risk Assessment
    Program, 127, 137
Inshape, 128
integrated software, 130
interactive programs, 125–126,
    131–132
Janus F. Fixx Running Program,
    129, 142
Mind Prober, 130, 143
Nutri-Byte, 128
Nutri-Pack, 128, 140
NutriCalc, 128, 141
nutrition software, 128, 140–141
Nutritionist/The Nutritionist II,
    128, 142
Original Boston Computer Diet,
    128, 142
Personal Health II, 126
Personal Health Inventory, 126,
    137
Positive Lifestyling, 126
psychological software, 130, 143
Running Log, 128, 139
Running Program, 128, 139
SAS (Statistical Analysis System),
    130
STAYWELL Program, 132
STRESS ASSESS, 127
TESTWELL, 127
Total Health, 128
WHY SMOKE, 127
Consensus methods, data collection, 66
Cooperation, See Patient cooperation
Cost of health care, and elderly, 233–
    234

Cost-based reimbursement, 34
  and patient education, 39–42
    "incidental to care" programs, 40,
      41–42
    "separate" patient education, 40,
      44
    separate reimbursement, reasons
      for, 42
Cousins, Norman, 112
Critical incident technique, 66, 69

D

Dartmouth Self-Care Project, 235
Data collection, 60–65
  community forum approach, 65
  community survey, 60–61
  consensus methods, 66
    critical incident technique, 66, 69
    delphi technique, 66, 67
    Glaser's state-of-the art approach,
      66, 68
    NIH consensus development, 66,
      68
    nominal group technique, 66, 67
    Q-sort technique, 66, 69
  integrating information, 65–66
  key informant approach, 63–65
  secondary sources of population data,
    60–62
    National Case Reporting System,
      60
    National Morbidity and Mortality
      Reporting System, 61
    National Vital Registration System,
      60
    social statistics, 61–62
    state/local sources, 61
  service utilization records, 62
*Decision Maker's Guide to Reducing
  Smoking at the Worksite*, 290
Delphi technique, 66, 67
Deontological theories, ethics, 91
Desirability assessment, needs
  assessment, 58–60

Diagnosis Related Groups (DRGs), 35,
  37
  future and, 241–242
Documentation, community advocacy
  projects, professional's role, 271–272
Double standard, medical insurance, 45
DuPont, incentive system, 162–163
Dychtwal, Ken, 254–255

E

Eating Machine, 128, 140
Educational paradigms, 15–20
  applications, 19–20
  practical paradigm, 17
  strategic paradigm, 18
  technical paradigm, 15–17
  "technical rationality" and, 18–19
Elderly, 231–259
  chronic conditions related to, 235,
    244–245
  economic factors, 233–234
  health education programs, 236–241
  needs of, 232–234
  stereotypes, list of, 234
  view of health education, 235
  See also Aging programs.
Eliza, 130, 143
Employee-focused approach, workplace
  health promotion, 286
Ethics, 87–105
  decision making and, 92
  deontological theories, 91
  ethical analysis, 90
    macro level, 99–100
    meso level, 99
  ethical dilemmas, 100
  ethical obligations of educators, 89–
    90
  in expanding field, 88–89
  explanation of, 90–92
  morals, explanation of, 92
  normative ethics, 91
  organizations related to, 105
  principles of

beneficience, 95–96
justice, 97–98
nonmaleficience, 95–96
respect for person, 96–97
utility, 99
use in health education, 101–105
analysis component, 102–103
choice component, 104
goals in problem situations, 101–102
identification component, 102
justification component, 103–104
weighing component, 103
utilitarian theories, 91
values, explanation of, 92–94
Evrydiet, 128, 140

F

Family's role, aging program
development and, 242–243
Feasibility assessment, needs
assessment, 57–58
Financing, 31–46
insurance programs
Health Maintenance Organizations,
35
Medicaid, 33, 34–35
Medicare, 33, 34
private insurance, 34
patient education and, 37–46
cost-based reimbursement and, 39–42
current spending, 39
improvement of reimbursement
(case study), 42–44
key issues in, 46
problems in financing, 44–46
separate reimbursement, reasons
for, 42
prospective pricing system (PPS) and,
35–37
reimbursement
blank check, 34
"cost-based" policies, 34

UCR method, 33–34
use of term, 33
FITCOMP, 129, 142
Fitness programs, 295–298
appropriate physical activity, criteria
for, 296
health issues, 295
prevalence of, 295–296
workplace implications, 296–297
workplace programs, examples of,
297–298
Flexcon Company, incentive system,
163
Formal market research, 81
Freire, Paolo, 9
Freire's approach, program
development, 9–10, 12, 21, 27
Funding, community advocacy projects,
269–270
Future of Work and Health, The, 309

G

Glaser's state-of-the art approach, 66,
68
Griffin Hospital Self Care Program, 195
Growing Younger/Growing Wiser, 255–256

H

Healing Heart, The (Cousins), 112
Health educators, changing role of, 76–77
Health fair approach, aging programs,
240
Health Maintenance Organizations,
scope of, 35
"Health Partners" program, 247
Health problems, approach to study of,
55–57
Health promotion
components of, 27–28
See also Patient education programs.

Health Promotion and Disease
Prevention Supplement, 239
Health Promotion Programs (NCOA),
254
Health Risk Appraisal, 125–126, 138
Healthpath, 128
Healthy Older People Campaign, 256
High blood pressure
health issues, 300
prevalence of, 301
High blood pressure control, 300–302
workplace implications, 301
workplace programs, examples of,
302
Holistic health programs, 192
*Hospitalization Risk Assessment
Program*, 127, 137
The Hub, 265–266, 268–269, 273
Humor, 111–120
Cousin's case, 112
as health education tool, 115–116
communication tool, 116–117
gallows humor, 116
guidelines for patient care, 117
as health promotion tool, 117–119
guidelines for, 118–119
laughter, 112–114
Darwin's observations, 113
and exercise, 114
respiration, 113–114
types of laughing, 113
origins of, 114–115
resources related to, 119–120
types of, 115

I

Identification component, ethics, 102
Incentive systems
case examples, 161–166
Bankers First, 161
Bonne Bell, 161–162
DuPont, 162–163
Flexcon Company, 163
Intermatic, Inc., 163

L. L. Bean, 164
pay values used, 166
Scherer Brothers Lumber Co.,
164–165
Westlake Community Hospital,
165
Xerox, 165–166
Incentives, 145–158
advantages/disadvantages of, 147–
149
applications of, 145
definition of, 146
opportunities for use of, 153, 157
pay values, 149, 150–152, 166
formal pay values, 150, 151, 152
informal pay values, 150, 151, 152
reasons for use, 147
strength of, 153
maximization of behavior change,
153, 158
system design, 149, 153, 154–156
"Incidental to care" programs, 40, 41–
42
Informal market research, 80–81
Inshape, 128
Insurance programs
Health Maintenance Organizations,
35
history of, 33
Medicaid, 33, 34–35
Medicare, 33, 34
payment, determination of, 33
private insurance, 34
Integrating information, data collection,
65–66
Interactional model, program
development, 22–24, 25–27
Intermatic, Inc., incentive systems, 163
Interviewing skill, patient cooperation,
175–177

J

Janus F. Fixx Running Program, 129,
142

Justice, ethics, 97–98
Justification component, ethics, 103–104

K

Ken Dychtwal & Associates, 254–255
Key informant approach, data collection, 63–65
Knowles, Malcolm, 8–9
Knowles' andragogy, program development, 8–9, 20, 27

L

L. L. Bean, incentive system, 164
Laughter, 112–114
    Darwin's observations, 113
    and exercise, 114
    and respiration, 113–114
    types of laughing, 113
Linear approach, weaknesses of, program development, 24–25
Live Better Longer Project, 255
Lobbying
    community advocacy projects, professional's role, 274–276
    process of, 274–275

M

Macro level, ethical analysis, 99–100
Marketing, 75–86
    determining objectives, 77–78
    needs analysis/customer preferences, 79–81
        competition, survey of, 81–82
        imagination and, 79–80
        informal market research, 80–81
    reasons for, 75–77
    selecting target market, 78–79
    strategy for
        place, 83–84

price, 84–85
program, 82–83
publicity, 85–86
Medicaid, scope of, 34–35
Medical insurance, use of term, 32
Medicare
    cost-based reimbursement, 34
    prospective pricing system, 35–37
    scope of, 34
"Medicine on the Mall," 242
Meso level, ethical analysis, 99
Mind Prober, 130, 143
Montefiore Medical Center, Community Health Participation Program (CHPP), 263–265, 268–269, 270–271
Morals, explanation of, 92
Motivational versus functional needs, 53–54

N

National Case Reporting System, 60
National Health Interview Survey, 239
National Morbidity and Mortality Reporting System, 61
National Vital Registration System, 60
National Worksite Health Promotion Survey, 285
Needs assessment
    data collection, 60–65
        community forum approach, 65
        community survey, 60–61
        consensus methods, 66
        integrating information, 65–66
        key informant approach, 63–65
        secondary sources of population data, 60–62
        service utilization records, 62
    definitional ambiguity, 50–51
    desirability assessment, 58–60
    feasibility assessment, 57–58
    health problems, approach to study of, 55–57
    marketing and, 79–81

needs
  basic versus incremental needs, 55
  importance of, 55–57
  motivational versus functional
    needs, 53–54
  performance versus treatment
    needs, 54–55
  planning of, 66, 70
  purposes/functions of, 51
  self-care programs, 195–197
  values and, 52–53
Negotiation/decision making, patient
  cooperation, 178–182
Neighborhood Health Centers, 270
Networking
  aging programs, 241
  community advocacy projects,
    professional's role, 273
NIH consensus development, 66, 68
Nominal group technique, 66, 67
Nonmaleficience, ethics, 95–96
Normative ethics, 91
Nutrition education programs, 291–295
Nutrition software, 128, 140–141
  Nutri-Byte, 128
  Nutri-Pack, 128, 140
  NutriCalc, 128, 141
  Nutritionist/The Nutritionist II, 128,
    142
  Original Boston Computer Diet, 128,
    142
Nutritional problems, 291–295
  health issue, 291–292
  prevalence of, 292
  workplace implications, 293–294
  workplace programs, examples of,
    294–295

O

Obesity
  health issues, 298
  prevalence of, 298–299
Organizational delivery systems,
  strategic planning, 21–22, 27

Original Boston Computer Diet, 128,
  142

P

Participative learning, self-care, 199–
  200
Patient cooperation, 168–185
  active participation, necessity of,
    170–171
  establishment of, 172–178
    active listening, 174–175
    deterrents to, 177–178
    interviewing skill and, 175–177
    physical examination and, 176
    respect, communication of, 173–
      174
    setting in, 173
  factors in, 168–170
  negotiation/decision making and,
    178–182
  personal change components, 182–
    183
    explicit goals/protocols and, 183–
      184
    recall of medical information, 183
    reinforcement, 184–185
  and practitioners as educators, 172
  values of patient and, 172
Patient education, use of term, 32
Patient education programs
  aging programs, 231–259
  ethics in, 87–105
  financing of, 31–46
  as "incidental to care," 40, 41–42
  marketing, 75–86
  needs assessment, 49–70
  program development, 3–28
  program tools
    computers, 123–143
    humor, 111–120
  self-care education, 189–205
  as "separate activity," 40, 44
  workplace health promotion, 281–
    310

See also specific topics.
Pay values, 149, 150–152, 166
  formal pay values, 150, 151, 152
  incentive systems, 166
  informal pay values, 150, 151, 152
Peer teaching
  aging programs, 243–244
  self care, 201
Performance versus treatment needs,
  54–55
Personal Health II, 126
Personal Health Inventory, 126, 137
Physical examination, patient
  cooperation, 176
Place, marketing, 83–84
Planned Parenthood of New York City,
  The Hub, 265–266, 268–269, 273
Political factors, community advocacy
  projects, 270–271, 273–278
Positive Lifestyling, 126
Practical paradigm, 17
PRECEDE, program development, 8,
  10–11, 15, 19
Price, marketing, 84–85
Private insurance, scope of, 34
Problem-focused approach, workplace
  health promotion, 286
Program development
  approaches to, 4–12
    comparison of models, 10–12
    Freire's approach, 9–10, 12, 21,
      27
    interactional model, 22–24, 25–27
    Knowles' andragogy, 8–9, 20, 27
    linear approach, weaknesses of,
      24–25
    PRECEDE, 8, 10–11, 15, 19
  belief systems, 13–15
    force field analysis, 15
  definition of, 3
  educational paradigms, 15–20
    applications, 19–20
    practical paradigm, 17
    strategic paradigm, 18
    technical paradigm, 15–17
    "technical rationality" and, 18–19

empowerment of people and, 27–28
  guidelines for development, 12–13
  health promotion, components of,
    27–28
  obstacles to, 26–27
  organizational delivery systems,
    strategic planning, 21–22, 27
  program design as, 4
Program tools
  computers, 123–143
  humor, 111–120
Prospective pricing system (PPS), 35–
  37
  Diagnosis Related Groups (DRGs),
    35, 37
  patient education programs and, 37
  expansion of programs, 37–38
Publicity, marketing, 85–86

Q

Q-sort technique, 66, 69
Quality Aging Program, 258

R

Recall of medical information, personal
  change component, 183
Reimbursement
  blank check, 34
  "cost-based" policies, 34, 39–42
  UCR method, 33–34
  use of term, 33
Reinforcement
  personal change components, 184–
    185
  self-care, 198
Research
  community advocacy projects,
    professional's role, 272–273
  market research, 79–82
  See also Data collection.
Respect, communication of, and patient
  cooperation, 173–174

Respect for person, ethics, 96–97
Running Coach, 128, 139
Running Log, 128, 139
Running Program, 128, 139

S

SAS (Statistical Analysis System), 130
Scherer Brothers Lumber Co., incentive
  systems, 164–165
Secondary sources of population data,
  data collection, 60–62
Self-care, 189–205
  access to information and, 198–199
  client needs and program design,
    195–197
  critics of, 204
  definitions of self-care, 189–190
  evaluation of learning, 201–202
  future of, 204–205
  Griffin Hospital Self Care Program,
    195
  growth of, 190–191
    reasons for, 190–191
    women's movement in, 191
  holistic health programs, 192
  obstacles to, 203–204
  options, importance of, 199
  organizational integration and, 197
  organizations related to, 190
  outcomes, 192–193
  participants, 202–203
    avoiders, 202
    health hobbyists, 203
    seriously ill, 203
  participative learning, 199–200
    case studies, 200
    leadership training, 200–201
    peer teaching, 201
    role playing, 200
    simulations, 200
  reinforcing patient's knowledge, 198
  typical program, 191–192
  versus traditional health education,
    193–194

Yale University/Kellogg Foundation
  Self Care Project, 194–195, 198,
  200
"Separate" patient education, 40, 44
Service utilization records, data
  collection, 62
Smoking, 287–309
  control of, 287–291
  health issues, 287–288
  prevalence of, 288
  workplace implications, 289–290
  workplace programs, examples of,
    290–291
Social statistics, 61–62
Software, *See* Computers, software
Staying Healthy After 50 Project, 258
STAYWELL Program, 132
Strategic paradigm, 18
Strategic planning, and delivery
  systems, 21–22, 27
STRESS ASSESS, 127
Stress management, 302–304
  health issues, 302–303
  prevalence of adult stress, 303
  workplace implications, 303–304
  workplace programs, examples of,
    304

T

Technical paradigm, 15–17
Technical rationality, educational
  paradigms, 18–19
TESTWELL, 127
Total Health, 128
Training, community advocacy projects,
  professional's role, 272

U

UCR method, reimbursement, 33–34
Utilitarian theories, ethics, 91
Utility, ethics, 99

V

Values
    explanation of, 92–94
    and needs assessment, 52–53

W

Wallingford Wellness Project, 235
Weighing component, ethics, 103
Weight control, 298–300
    obesity
        health issues, 298
        prevalence of, 298–299
        workplace implications, 299
        workplace programs, examples of,
            299–300
Wellness programs, *See* Workplace
    health promotion
Westlake Community Hospital,
    incentive systems, 165
White Crane Senior Health Center, 259
WHY SMOKE, 127
Wisdom Project, 257
Women's movement, and self-care, 191
Workplace health promotion, 281–310
    cancer screening, 304–305
    corporations with health programs,
        319–320
    fitness programs, 295–298
    future trends, 309–310
    high blood pressure control, 300–302

implementation strategies, 285–287
    comprehensive/preventive-focused
        approach, 286
    comprehensive/risk-focused
        approach, 286
    employee-focused approach, 286
    problem-focused approach, 286
issues in, 306–308
    program design/management, 307–
        308
    program evaluation, 308
    program justification, 306–307
nutrition education programs, 291–
    295
reasons for establishment of, 282–
    283
smoking control, 287–291
status in U.S., 283–285
    growth of programs, 284
    types of worksites and, 284
stress management, 302–304
weight conrol, 298–300
See also individual programs.

X

Xerox, incentive systems, 165–166

Y

Yale University/Kellogg Foundation
    Self Care Project, 194–195, 198, 200